M. M. Eibl C. Huber H. H. Peter
U. Wahn (Eds.)

Symposium in Immunology I
Symposium in Immunology II

With 86 Figures and 29 Tables

Springer-Verlag
Berlin Heidelberg New York
London Paris Tokyo Hong Kong
Barcelona Budapest

Prof. Dr. Martha M. Eibl
Institut für Immunologie der Universität Wien
Borschkegasse 8 a
1090 Wien, Austria

Prof. Dr. Christoph Huber
Abteilung für Hämatologie
Johannes Gutenberg Universität
Langenbeckstr. 1
6500 Mainz, FRG

Prof. Dr. Hans H. Peter
Abteilung für Rheumatologie und
Klinische Immunologie
Medizinische Universitätsklinik
Hugstetter Str. 55
7800 Freiburg i.Br., FRG

Prof. Dr. Ulrich Wahn
Päd. Pneumologie und Immunologie
Univ.-Klinikum Rudolf Virchow
Standort Charlottenburg
Heubnerweg 6
1000 Berlin 19, FRG

ISBN-13: 978-3-540-56478-2 e-ISBN-13: 978-3-642-78087-5
DOI: 10.1007/978-3-642-78087-5

27/3145/5 4 3 2 1 0 - Printed on acid-free paper

Contents

Symposium in Immunology I – T-Cell Function and T-Cell Defects

T-Cell Function and T-Cell Defects

Clinical Aspects and Treatment

List of Contributors

L. Adorini
Preclinical Research 386-101, Sandoz Pharma Ltd., 4002 Basel, Switzerland

M. Armbruster
Pathologisches Institut der Universitätsklinik Freiburg, 7800 Freiburg, FRG

B. Arnold
Forschungsschwerpunkt Tumorimmunologie, Abteilung Somatische Genetik, Deutsches Krebsforschungszentrum, Im Neuenheimer Feld 280, 6900 Heidelberg, FRG

E. Baumert
Abteilung Rheumatologie und Klinische Immunologie, Medizinische Universitätsklinik, Hugstetter Str. 55, 7800 Freiburg, FRG

H. v. Boehmer
Basel Institute for Immunology, Grenzacherstr. 487, 4005 Basel, Switzerland

H. P. Buscher
Medizinische Klinik II, Gastroenterologie, Medizinische Universitätsklinik, 7800 Freiburg, FRG

E. Csernok
Medical University of Lübeck, Department of Clinical Rheumatology, Ratzeburger Allee 160, 2400 Lübeck, and Rheumaklinik Bad Bramstedt, 2357 Bad Bramstedt, FRG

R. Dräger
Abteilung Rheumatologie und Klinische Immunologie, Medizinische Universitätsklinik, Hugstetter Str. 55, 7800 Freiburg, FRG

M. M. Eibl
Institute of Immunology, University of Vienna, Borschkegasse 8a, 1090 Vienna, Austria

H. H. Euler
2nd Medical Clinic, Christian-Albrechts University, Chemnitzstr. 33, 2300 Kiel 1, FRG

B. K. Flesch
Medical University of Lübeck, Department of Clinical Rheumatology, Ratzeburger Allee 160, 2400 Lübeck, and Rheumaklinik Bad Bramstedt, 2357 Bad Bramstedt, FRG

W. Friedrich
Universitätskinderklinik Ulm, Prittwitzstr. 43, 7900 Ulm, FRG

E. Gleichmann
Division of Immunology, Medical Institute of Environmental Hygiene, Heinrich Heine University, Auf'm Hennekamp 50, 4000 Düsseldorf, FRG

C. Goebel
Division of Immunology, Medical Institute of Environmental Hygiene, Heinrich Heine University, Auf'm Hennekamp 50, 4000 Düsseldorf, FRG

P. Griem
Division of Immunology, Medical Institute of Environmental Hygiene, Heinrich Heine University, Auf'm Hennekamp 50, 4000 Düsseldorf, FRG

W. L. Gross
Medical University of Lübeck, Department of Clinical Rheumatology, Ratzeburger Allee 160, 2400 Lübeck, and Rheumaklinik Bad Bramstedt, 2357 Bad Bramstedt, FRG

G. J. Hämmerling
Forschungsschwerpunkt Tumorimmunologie, Abteilung Somatische Genetik, Deutsches Krebsforschungszentrum, Im Neuenheimer Feld 280, 6900 Heidelberg, FRG

W. Hartmann
Universitätskinderklinik Ulm, Prittwitzstr. 43, 7900 Ulm, FRG

K. Heeg
Institute of Medical Microbiology and Hygiene, Technische Universität München, Trogerstr. 9, 8000 München, FRG

E. W. Herbst
Pathologisches Institut der Universitätsklinik Freiburg, 7800 Freiburg, FRG

C. Huber
Department of Hematology, Johannes Gutenberg University, Langenbeckstr. 1, 6500 Mainz, FRG

V. Hurez
INSERM U 28 and Service d'Immunologie, Hôpital Broussais, 96 rue Didot, 75014 Paris, France

A. Jahreis
Abteilung Rheumatologie und Klinische Immunologie, Medizinische Universitätsklinik, Hugstetter Str. 55, 7800 Freiburg, FRG

S. H. E. Kaufmann
Department of Immunology, University of Ulm, Albert-Einstein-Allee 11, 7900 Ulm, FRG

M. D. Kazatchkine
INSERM U 28 and Service d'Immunologie, Hôpital Broussais, 96 rue Didot, 75014 Paris, France

A. Kliche
Abteilung Rheumatologie und Klinische Immunologie, Medizinische Universitätsklinik, Hugstetter Str. 55, 7800 Freiburg, FRG

C. Knobloch
Universitätskinderklinik Ulm, Prittwitzstr. 43, 7900 Ulm, FRG

H. Köhler
I. Medizinische Klinik und Poliklinik, Johannes Gutenberg Universität Mainz, Langenbeckstr. 1, 6500 Mainz, FRG

U. Krawinkel
Fakultät für Biologie, Universität Konstanz, Postfach 5560, 7750 Konstanz, FRG

M. Kubicka-Muranyi
Division of Immunology, Medical Institute of Environmental Hygiene, Heinrich Heine University, Auf'm Hennekamp 50, 4000 Düsseldorf, FRG

E.-M. Lemmel
Staatliches Rheumakrankenhaus, Rotenbachtalstr. 5, 7570 Baden-Baden, FRG

M. P. Manns
Department of Gastroenterology and Hepatology, Zentrum Innere Medizin, Medizinische Hochschule Hannover, Konstanty Gutschow Str. 8, 3000 Hannover 61, FRG

S. C. Meuer
Abteilung Angewandte Immunologie, Institut für Radiologie und Pathophysiologie, Deutsches Krebsforschungszentrum Heidelberg, Im Neuenheimer Feld 280, 6900 Heidelberg, FRG

L. Mucke
Department of Neuropharmacology, Division of Virology, The Scripps Research Institute, 10666 North Torrey Pines Road, La Jolla, CA 92037, USA

D. Niederwieser
Division of Internal Medicine, University of Innsbruck, 6020 Innsbruck, Austria

H. H. Peter
Abteilung Rheumatologie und Klinische Immunologie, Medizinische Universitätsklinik, Hugstetter Str. 55, 7800 Freiburg, FRG

G. Pluschke
Ciba-Geigy AG, 4002 Basel, Switzerland

L. Qiao
Abteilung Angewandte Immunologie, Institut für Radiologie und Pathophysiologie, Deutsches Krebsforschungszentrum Heidelberg, Im Neuenheimer Feld 280, 6900 Heidelberg, FRG

H.-G. Rammensee
Max-Planck-Institut für Biologie, Abteilung Immungenetik, Corrensstr. 42, 7400 Tübingen, FRG

C. Reiter
Institut für Immunologie, Universität München, Goethestr. 31, 8000 München 2, FRG

M. S. Reitz, Jr.
Laboratory of Tumor Cell Biology, National Cancer Institute, National Institutes of Health, Bethesda, MD 20892, USA

K. Resch
Institute of Molecular Pharmacology, Hannover Medical School, P.O.Box 610180, 3000 Hannover 61, FRG

E. P. Rieber
Institut für Immunologie, Universität München, Goethestr. 31, 8000 München 2, FRG

G. Riethmüller
Institut für Immunologie, Universität München, Goethestr. 31, 8000 München 2, FRG

J. A. Rump
Abteilung Rheumatologie und Klinische Immunologie, Medizinische Universitätsklinik, Hugstetter Str. 55, 7800 Freiburg, FRG

Y. Samstag
Abteilung Angewandte Immunologie, Institut für Radiologie und Pathophysiologie, Deutsches Krebsforschungszentrum Heidelberg, Im Neuenheimer Feld 280, 6900 Heidelberg, FRG

A. Schirren
Abteilung Angewandte Immunologie, Institut für Radiologie und Pathophysiologie, Deutsches Krebsforschungszentrum Heidelberg, Im Neuenheimer Feld 280, 6900 Heidelberg, FRG

M. Schlesier
Abteilung Rheumatologie und Klinische Immunologie, Medizinische Universitätsklinik, Hugstetter Str. 55, 7800 Freiburg, FRG

G. Schönrich
Forschungsschwerpunkt Tumorimmunologie, Abteilung Somatische Genetik, Deutsches Krebsforschungszentrum, Im Neuenheimer Feld 280, 6900 Heidelberg, FRG

B. Schraven
Abteilung Angewandte Immunologie, Institut für Radiologie und Pathophysiologie, Deutsches Krebsforschungszentrum Heidelberg, Im Neuenheimer Feld 280, 6900 Heidelberg, FRG

H.-C. Schuppe
Dermatological Clinic, Heinrich Heine Universität, 4000 Düsseldorf, FRG

M. Szamel
Institute of Molecular Pharmacology, Hannover Medical School, P.O.Box 610180, 3000 Hannover 61, FRG

E. Tschachler
Department of Dermatology I, Division of Cutaneous Immunobiology, University of Vienna Medical School, Alser Str. 4, 1090 Wien, Austria

J. Uetrecht
Faculties of Pharmacy and Medicine, University of Toronto and Sunnybrook Medical Centre, Toronto, Canada

P. Vaith
Abteilung Rheumatologie und Klinische Immunologie, Medizinische Universitätsklinik, Hugstetter Str. 55, 7800 Freiburg, FRG

H. Völpel
Abteilung Angewandte Immunologie, Institut für Radiologie und Pathophysiologie, Deutsches Krebsforschungszentrum Heidelberg, Im Neuenheimer Feld 280, 6900 Heidelberg, FRG

H. Wagner
Institute of Medical Microbiology and Hygiene, Technische Universität München, Trogerstr. 9, 8000 München, FRG

U. Wahn
Päd. Pneumologie und Immunologie, Univ.-Klinikum Rudolf Virchow, Standort Charlottenburg, Heubnerweg 6, 1000 Berlin 19, FRG

M. E. Weinblatt
Brigham and Women's Hospital, 75 Francis Street, Boston, MA 02115, USA

H. Wekerle
Max-Planck-Institut für Psychiatrie, Am Klopferspitz 18 A, 8033 Martinsried, FRG

H. M. Wolf
Institute of Immunology, University of Vienna, Borschkegasse 8 a, 1090 Vienna, Austria

G. Wolff-Vorbeck
Abteilung Rheumatologie und Klinische Immunologie, Medizinische Universitätsklinik, Hugstetter Str. 55, 7800 Freiburg, FRG

Symposium in Immunology I
T-Cell Function and T-Cell Defects

T-Cell Function and T-Cell Defects

Self-Nonself Discrimination by Developing and Mature T Cells

H. von Boehmer

Introduction

The question of self-nonself discrimination by the immune system is still awaiting a complete solution. The problem was recognized long ago, and Owen's observation (1945) [1] in dizygotic cattle twins which were chimeric with regard to their blood cells indicated that self tolerance was acquired rather than inherited. Ideas by Burnet and Fenner (1949) [2] which were reinforced by Ledenberg (1963) [3] offered a simple-possibly too simple-solution to the problem of self tolerance: it was argued that clones of lymphocytes, each bearing a distinct antigen receptor, go through an early phase in development in which contact with antigen is lethal rather than inducing effector function. Thus, tolerance to self was thought to be due to the elimination of self reactive clones early during their development. This concept had two weaknesses in explaining all self tolerance. First, it was difficult to imagine that all self antigens could reach developing lymphocytes in primary lymphoid organs. Second, considering the enormous diversity of antigen receptors themselves, it was difficult to see how deletion of lymphocytes induced by diverse receptors on other lymphocytes would leave anything substantial behind fit to deal with foreign antigens [4]. Possible solutions to these considerations were, first, that clonal deletion was not the only mechanism of tolerance, and, second, that tolerance induction required a certain threshold amount of antigen, which is probably not reached by most idiotypic antigen-receptor sequences. The main question was clearly not whether clonal deletion was the only way to achieve tolerance, but whether clonal deletion exists at all as central tolerance mechanism possibly aided by some additional mechanisms responsible for silencing already matured lymphocytes which had escaped clonal deletion simply because they did not encounter their self antigen early in development.

For decades this question was extremely difficult to address because of the lack of clonotypic receptor markers. This was especially so for T lymphocytes, where antigen binding by surface receptors could not be visualized. This left an ambiguity to the interpretation of results obtained with most tolerance models. Tolerance models by Billingham et al. (1953) [5] and Hasek (1953) [6] confirmed that tolerance can be acquired. Neonatal tolerance could not be established in all mouse strain combinations, and it was not clear whether the relative ease by which tolerance can be induced in some neonatal mice reflects the immaturity of lymphocytes or simply their relatively small numbers. Conceptually more clearcut were models in which hemopoietic stem cells develop in the presence of foreign antigen in hemopoietic chimeras prepared by injecting stem cells into lethally X-irradiated histoincompatible hosts. In this model mature T lymphocytes were deliberately removed from the donor cells, and it turned out that this tolerance model worked in all strain combinations. These experiments showed that there is something special about developing lymphocytes with regard to tolerance, as they can be adapted to tolerate a large variety of strong histocompatibility antigens [7]. However, the experiments could not establish that clonal deletion was the mechanism. The read-out in all the models depended on activation of lymphocytes in vivo or in vitro and therefore did not establish whether tolerance is due to silence or to absence of lymphocytes bearing specific receptors for the tolerogen. More conclusive studies became feasible only in the mid-1980s when it was possible to raise antibodies specific for clonotypic receptors on T lymphocytes [8–10]. Even this technological advance was not sufficient to yield conclusive results because the frequency of cells bearing one particular T cell receptor (TCR) was extremely low, such that one clone could not be visualized during lymphocyte development. This was different with cells specific for so-called superantigens which are recognized by particular V_β protein sequences shared by heterogenous TCRs. Here a relatively large fraction of heterogenous T cells appeared specific for one superantigen [11]. Studies employing superantigens provided some clues to repertoire selection during T cell development [12], but the essential points became clear only when the selection of a single TCR specific for "conventional" antigens, i.e., peptides bound by major histocompatibility complex (MHC) encoded molecules, was studies in TCR transgenic mice [13]. The latter studies clearly established two rules of self-nonself discrimination by the immune system: they showed that tolerance can result from clonal deletion of immature T lymphocytes being confronted with the specific peptide as well as the MHC molecule early in T cell maturation [14, 15]. In addition, they showed that T cell maturation required the recognition of the MHC molecule in the absence of the specific peptide early in T cell development [15–17]. As these studies have been published elsewhere, only a brief summary is provided below to introduce the experimental system which was used to study further details of intrathymic and postthymic selection on the T cell repertoire.

Negative and Positive Selection of a Transgenic Receptor Specific for the Male-Specific Peptide Presented by Class I H-2D^b MHC Molecules

The α- and βTCR genes from the CD4$^-$8$^+$ cytolytic B6.2.16 clone specific for the male-specific peptide presented by H-2D^b MHC molecules were cloned, and cosmids containing flanking sequences which harbored T cell specific

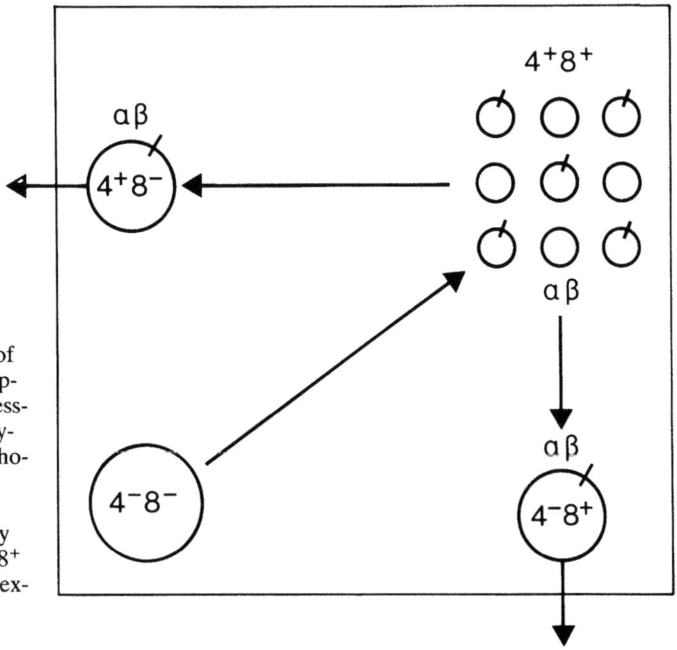

Fig. 1. A scheme of intrathymic development of cells expressing the αβTCR. Cycling $CD4^-8^-$ lymphoblasts differentiate into noncycling $CD4^+8^+$ and finally $CD4^+8^-$ and $CD4^-8^+$ thymocytes which express the αβTCR (symbolized by -)

regulatory elements (enhancers) were injected into fertilized eggs [18–20]. Transgenic mice which expressed both genes were crossed onto the SCID background to produce mice expressing essentially only one TCR [21]. Negative selection (deletion) was studied by comparing male and female αβTCR transgenic SCID mice expressing H-$2D^b$ MHC molecules. Positive selection was studied by comparing female αβTCR transgenic SCID mice expressing or lacking H-$2D^b$ MHC molecules. The studies involved the analysis of thymocyte subpopulations in the various mice. In an oversimplified way, one can picture the development of thymocytes as going from $CD4^-8^-$ thymocytes, which begin to express TCRs, through receptor-positive but functionally incompetent $CD4^+8^+$ intermediates into $CD4^+8^-$ or $CD4^-8^+$ TCR-positive, functionally competent T cells (Fig. 1).

Figure 2 shows the analysis of the thymus of the experimental mice compared to a normal thymus by staining thymocytes with CD4 and CD8 antibodies. As is evident from Fig. 2, the thymus of male αβTCR transgenic SCID mice as compared to female littermates is largely devoid of $CD4^+8^-$ and $CD4^-8^+$ as well as $CD4^+8^+$ thymocytes but contains comparable numbers of $CD4^-8^-$ thymocytes as female littermates. Because single-positive and double-positive thymocytes comprise approximately 90 % of all thymocytes, the total number of thymocytes in male animals is only one-tenth of that in females. The interpretation of this result is that clonal deletion eliminates even the earliest $CD4^+8^+$ immature thymocytes which express the transgenic receptor.

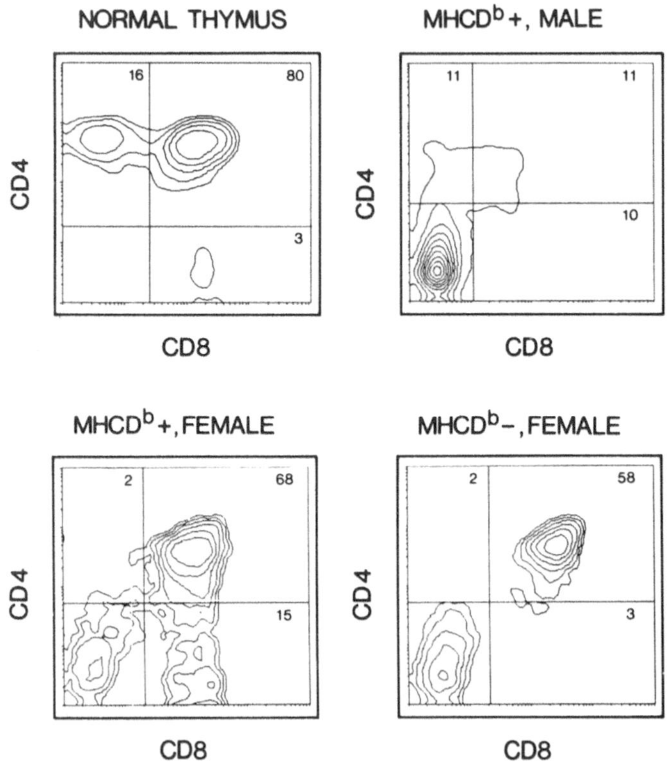

Fig. 2. The subset composition of the thymus from normal mice and four experimental mice by lymphocytes expressing CD4 and CD8 coreceptors. *Numbers in quadrants,* percentage of cells in these quadrants

When one compares female αβTCR transgenic SCID mice which either lack or express H-2D^b MHC molecules, one finds that thymuses from both types of animals contain CD4$^-$8$^-$ as well as CD4$^+$8$^+$ thymocytes, but that only those from the latter have CD4$^-$8$^+$ but not CD4$^+$8$^-$ mature thymocytes (Fig. 2). Here the interpretation is that the generation of mature thymocytes requires binding of the αβTCR to H-2D^b MHC molecules in the absence of the male-specific peptide. Furthermore, binding of the TCR to H-2D^b MHC molecules induces maturation of CD4$^-$8$^+$ thymocytes only, while binding to class II MHC molecules generates mature CD4$^+$8$^-$ thymocytes only [22, 23]. The latter conclusion is well supported by more recent independent experiments employing β_2-microglobulin deficient – and therefore class I MHC molecule deficient – mice which have CD4$^-$8$^-$, CD4$^+$8$^+$, and CD4$^+$8$^-$ but lack CD4$^-$8$^+$ thymocytes [24].

Lack of Allelic Exclusion of the αTCR Chain in αβTCR Transgenic Mice

The picture of thymocyte subsets in αβTCR transgenic mice which were not crossed with SCID mice was slightly more complicated due to the fact that endogenous α-but not βTCR genes could rearrange in these mice. In spite of the fact that the αβTCR was expressed early on the surface of $CD4^-8^-$ thymocytes, endogenous αTCR genes were expressed at later stages at the RNA and protein level such that many cells contained transcripts from both endogenous and from the transgenic αTCR gene. While in some cases this led to the expression of roughly equimolar amounts of endogenous and transgenic αTCR chains paired with the transgenic βTCR chain, most T cells expressed either high levels of the transgenic or high levels of endogenous αTCR chain on the cell surface, presumably due to preferential pairing with the transgenic βTCR chain. In the absence of productive rearrangements of endogenous αTCR gene segments, of course, only the transgenic αTCR chain is expressed. These αβTCR transgenic mice contain significant numbers of $CD4^+8^-$ T cells both in the thymus (Fig. 3) and in the periphery which all expressed high levels of endogenous αTCR chains at the cell surface. In contrast, most $CD4^-8^+$ thymocytes expressed high levels of the transgenic αTCR chain and a variable proportion of peripheral $CD4^-8^+$ T cells expressed high levels of endogenous αTCR chains. Thus, the early expression of the transgenic αTCR chain did not prevent endogenous αTCR rearrangement. In contrast, the early expression of the βTCR transgene prevented rearrangement of V_β gene segments. Some of the receptors containing endogenous αTCR chains were selectable by thymic class I or class II MHC molecules, and mature T cells bearing these receptors could, therefore, be detected in the thymus as well as peripheral lymph organs [13], and this must be taken into

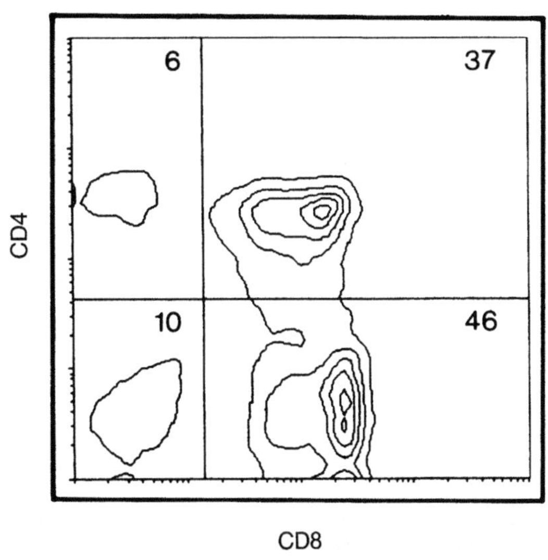

Fig. 3. H-2^b αβ transgenic female: the subset composition of the thymus from αβTCR transgenic mice not crossed onto the SCID background. *Numbers in quadrants,* percentage of cells in these quadrants

consideration in the following experiments, which were conducted with αβTCR transgenic mice which were not backcrossed onto the SCID background.

Mutations in the Peptide-Binding Groove of MHC Molecules Affect Antigenicity and Negative as well as Positive Selection

Two naturally occurring mutants of the D^b MHC molecule have been isolated, namely in the bm13 and the bm14 mutant strains. The latter contains a single mutation of the inward-pointing residue 70 (Glu → Asp) of the α_1 domain while the bm13 contains three changed residues 114 (Leu → Glu), 116 (Phe → Tyr), and 119 (Glu → Asp) at the bottom of the groove (Fig. 4) [25]. According to the Bjorkman-Wiley model [26], these residues would appear to be inaccessible for the TCR and are considered to be involved in peptide binding. In contrast to cells from male B6 mice, cells from male bm13 and bm14 mice fail to stimulate the B6.2.16 clone from which the genes for the male-specific receptor were isolated. This agrees with earlier studies in these mice which showed that cells from female mutant mice cannot be stimulated by cells from male littermates to produce male-specific cytolytic T lymphocytes [27]. It was therefore expected that cells with the transgenic αβTCR in mice backcrossed onto the bm13 or bm14 background would show no deletion in animals homozygous for the bm13 or bm14 mutation. This was indeed the case, as shown for the bm13 homozygous male mice in Fig. 5, which contain a high proportion of $CD4^+8^+$ thymocytes expressing intermediate levels of the transgenic receptor on the cell surface. In contrast, in male D^b/bm13 heterozygous mice this population is entirely deleted [25].

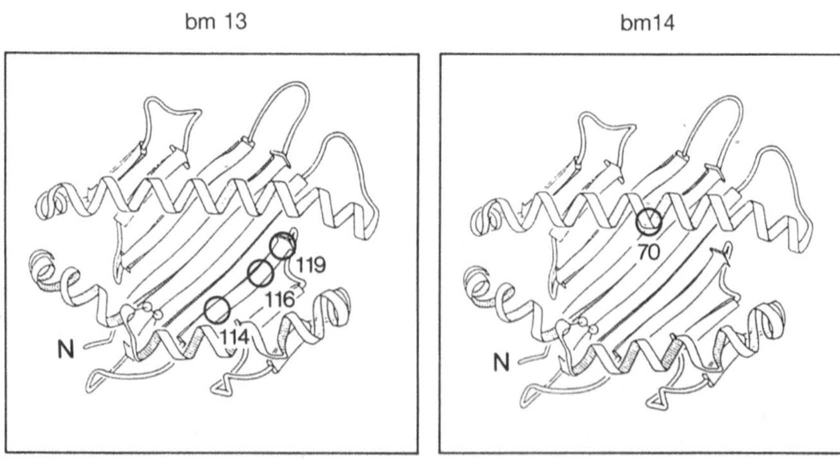

Fig. 4. Position of residues in the mutant bm13 and bm14 MHC molecules which differ from the wildtype D^b MHC molecule

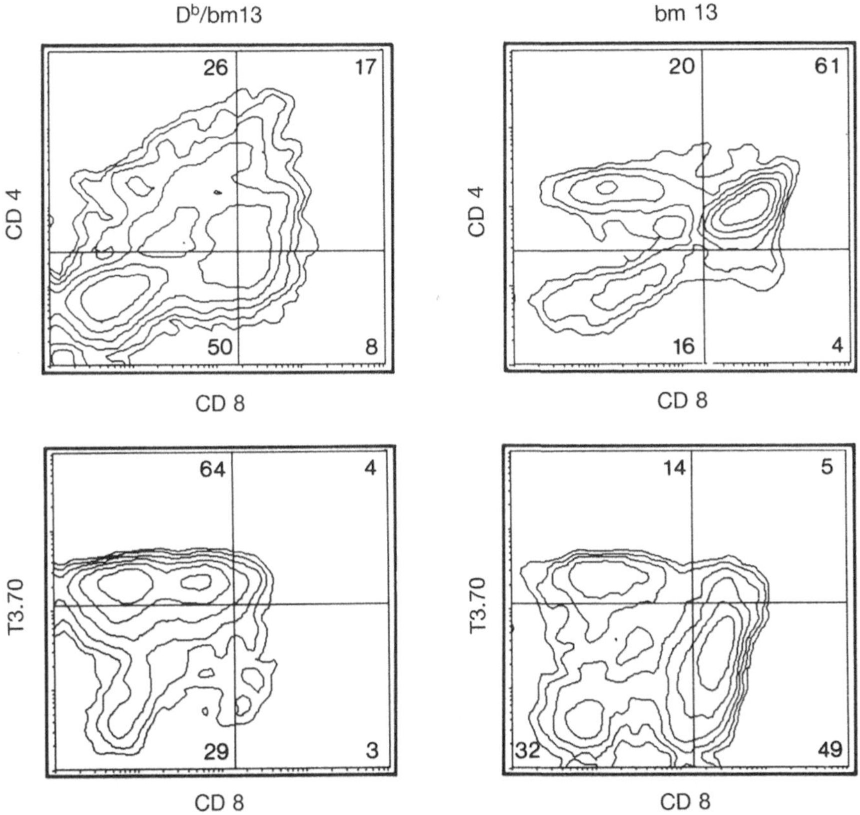

Fig. 5. Male αβ transgenic thymus: the absence of negative selection of male-specific thymocytes in the bm13 mutant strain. Note the absence of $CD4^+8^+$ T cells expressing low levels of the transgenic αTCR chain in the D^b/bm13 heterozygous, but not bm13 homozygous mice

As positive selection proceeds in the absence of the specific peptide, one may or may not have anticipated that MHC mutations restricted to the peptide-binding groove would not affect positive selection. The fact that MHC molecules seldom exist on the surface of cells without a bound peptide [28] creates difficulties with the view that positive selection would simply be achieved by the binding of TCR to upward-pointing residues of MHC molecules without the positive or negative interference of the MHC-bound peptides. It may therefore not be surprizing that indeed, as a rule, mutations which affect antigenicity also affect positive selection [25, 29, 30]. This is shown in Fig. 6 for the bm14 mutation: in hemopoietic chimeras produced by injecting T cell depleted bone marrow cells from H–2^b αβTCR transgenic female mice into lethally X-irradiated H-$2D^b$(B6) homozygous or bm14 homozygous recipient mice, it is evident that positive selection of $CD4^-8^+$,

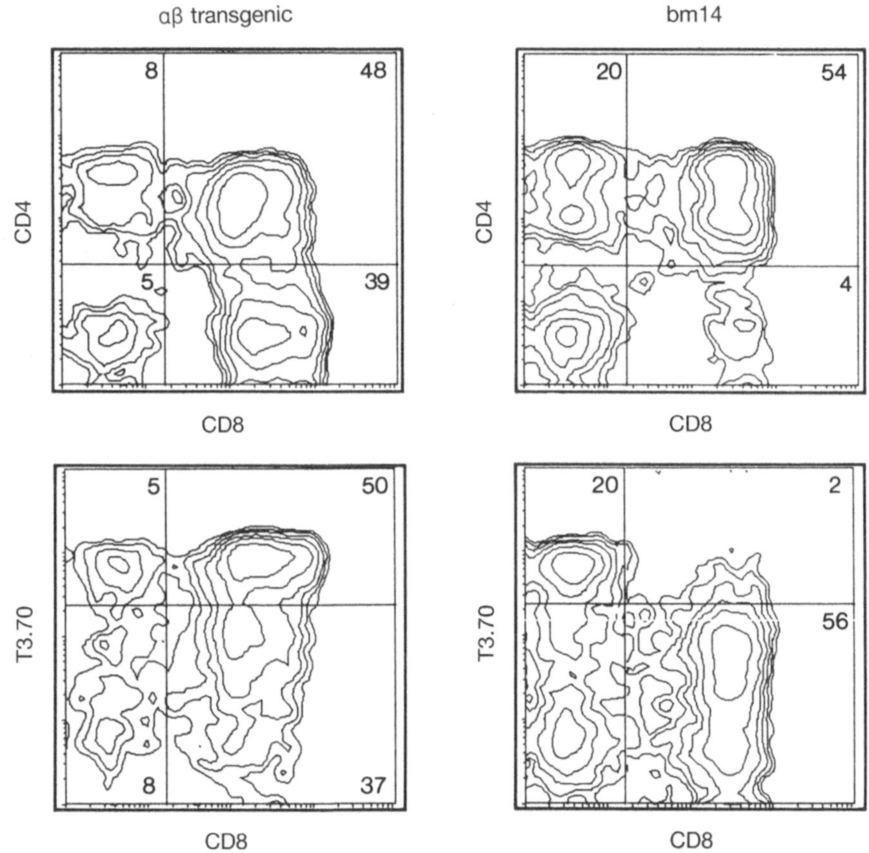

Fig. 6. Thymus: Lack of positive selection in bm14 homozygous mice. Note the absence of $CD8^+$, T3.70 high cells in the thymus of bm14 homozygous mice compared to αβ transgenic $H\text{-}2^b$ mice

T3.70 cells occurs in the former but not the latter recipients. Unfortunately, these experiments do not tell us whether the role of the peptide in positive selection is facilitating or interfering with positive selection by MHC molecules; they simply tell us that peptides are not ignored during positive selection.

Positive Selection: Expansion of Mature Thymocytes or Maturation of Immature Thymocytes?

We have addressed the question of whether positive selection is reflected in expansion of mature T cells rather than maturation of immature resting cells by labeling experiments employing bromodeoxyuridine (BrdU), which

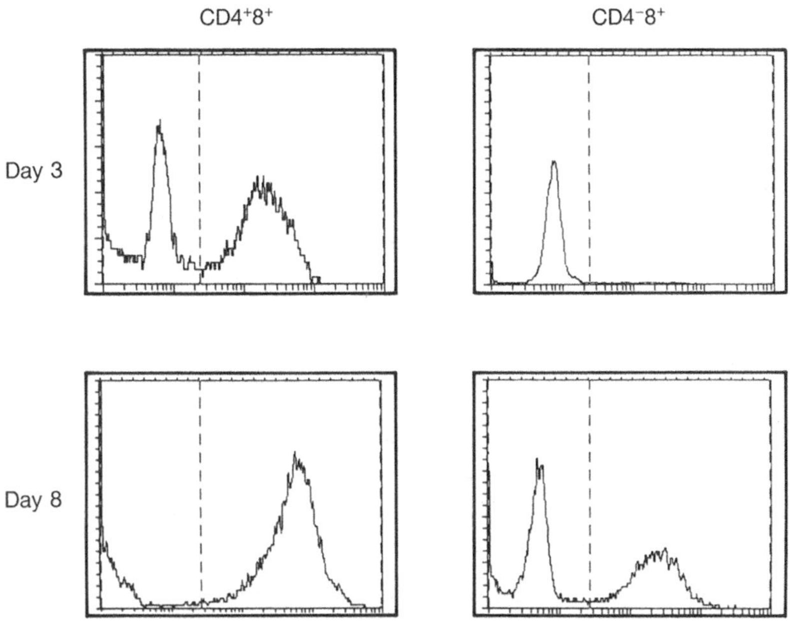

Fig. 7. The proportion of BrdU-labeled $CD4^+8^+$ and $CD4^-8^+$ cells after 3 and 8 days of continuous labeling

incorporates into newly synthesized DNA and can be visualized by a monoclonal antibody specific for BrdU [31]. Continuous labeling experiments (BrdU injected intraperitoneally every day early in the morning and late in the evening) show that in female H-2^b αβTCR transgenic mice, most $CD4^+8^+$, but none of the $CD4^-8^+$ thymocytes are labeled after 4 days of continuous labeling. This indicates that $CD4^-8^+$ thymocytes do not divide in these mice (Fig. 7). Whereas the label accumulates linearly in the $CD4^+8^+$ compartment during the first 5 days, it accumulates nonlinearly in the $CD4^-8^+$ compartment from day 5 onwards (Fig. 8): at day 5 there is a steep increase in the proportion of labeled $CD4^-8^+$ cells. Thereafter, the label accumulates more slowly. The nonlinear slope in the $CD4^-8^+$ compartment may be due to the fact that the time of migration from this compartment into the periphery is not related to the time of entry into it, i.e., the first cells which have entered are not necessarily the first ones to leave. This means that the accumulation of labeled cells in this compartment has kinetics that do not parallel the new generation of $CD4^-8^+$ thymocytes. If one extrapolates the line with the same slope as observed from day 4 to day 5, one can obtain two parallel lines indicative of the new production of cells with the $CD4^+8^+$ and the $CD4^+8^-$ phenotype. Because approximately 40% of thymocytes are $CD4^-8^+$ cells in these mice, this could mean that almost all $CD4^+8^+$ precursors turn into $CD4^-8^+$ progeny. In any case, if one compares the absolute numbers of labeled $CD4^+8^+$ and $CD4^-8^+$ cells in αβ transgenic and

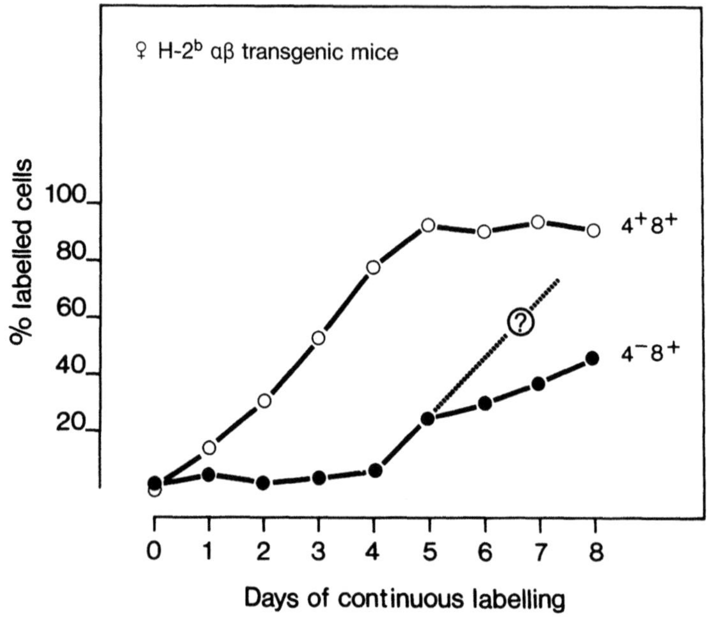

Fig. 8. The increase in percentage of labeled CD4$^+$8$^+$ and CD4$^-$8$^+$ cells during continous labeling of female αβTCR transgenic H-2^b mice. The linear extrapolation of the line of labeld CD4$^-$8$^+$ cells may represent the real accumulation of labeled cells

normal B6 mice, it is clear that in the former the transition of CD4$^+$8$^+$ precursors into CD4$^-$8$^+$ progeny is much more efficient than in the latter (Fig. 9).

Postthymic Expansion of Mature T Cells

Once mature T cells are formed, they can leave the thymus and undergo considerable expansion in peripheral lymph organs. The expansion potential of T cells has been shown in a variety of experiments, probably most directly by transferring small numbers of peripheral T cells into T cell deficient, thymusless nu/nu mice in which both CD4$^+$8$^-$ and CD4$^-$8$^+$ expand considerably [32]. It is not clear whether this peripheral expansion randomly amplifies patterns of TCR specificities as they were selected in the thymus, or whether it is not random and modifies patterns which were initially selected in the thymus. To study these questions, mature T cells from female αβTCR transgenic mice were transferred into female and male nu/nu recipients. The remarkable observation in these experiments was that the entire increase in T cells in the T cell deficient recipients could be attributed to CD4$^+$8$^-$ and CD4$^-$8$^+$ T cells expressing endogenous αTCR chains even though approxi-

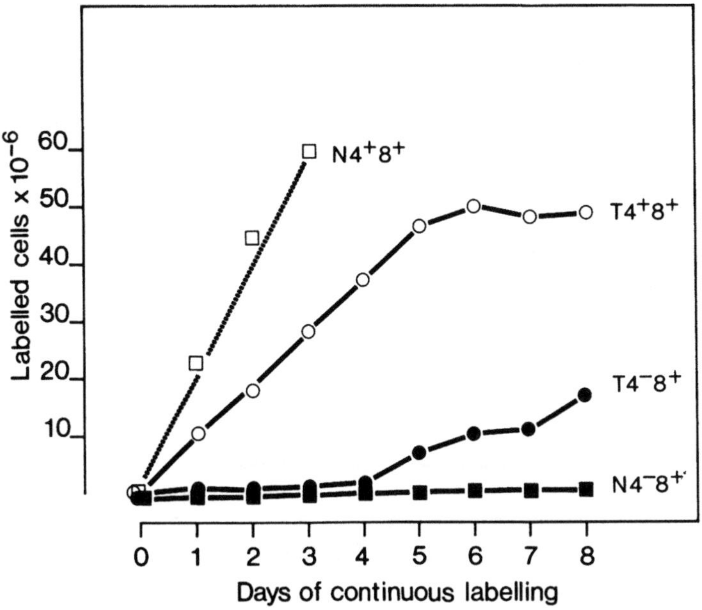

Fig. 9. The absolute numbers of labeled $CD4^{+}8^{+}$ and $CD4^{-}8^{+}$ thymocytes in normal (*N*) and αβTCR transgenic (*T*) mice during continous labeling with BrdU

mately half of the inoculated $CD4^{-}8^{+}$ T cells expressed the male-specific transgenic αβTCR. In fact, these male-specific cells did not expand at all, and the total number of cells with this phenotype was the same at day 5 and at day 60 after transfer (Fig. 10a). This indicates that postthymic repertoire selection is totally different from thymic selection with regard to both specificity and mechanism; the former selects specificities of nontransgenic TCRs and involves expansion of cells, the latter selects predominantly the specificity of the transgenic TCR and involves maturation rather than expansion.

Postthymic Tolerance

We have begun to address the induction of unresponsiveness in mature T cells by transferring T cells from female αβTCR transgenic B6 mice into male nu/nu B6 mice and by following the fate of male-specific T cells in these animals. As shown in Fig. 10b, these cells proliferate initially vigorously such that by day 5 after transfer the number of peripheral T cells is four times higher than that observed in female recipients injected with the same numbers of cells. After this, the number of male-specific $CD4^{-}8^{+}$ T cells declines steadily, but significant numbers can still be detected even 8 weeks after transfer. When these cells are analyzed more carefully, one finds that

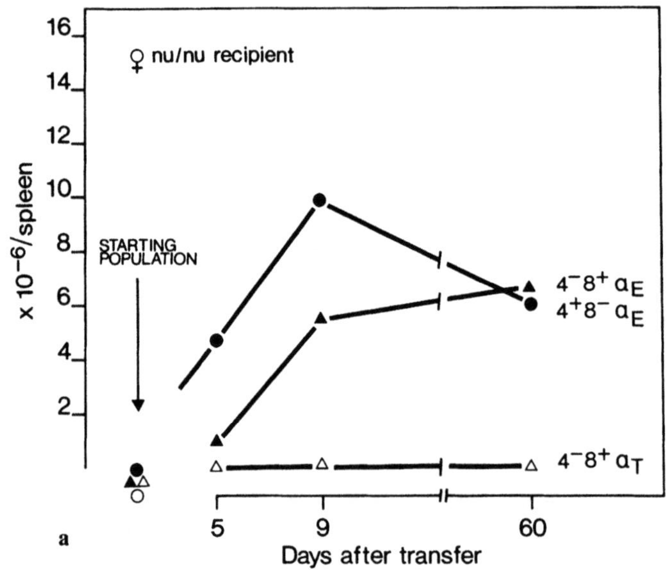

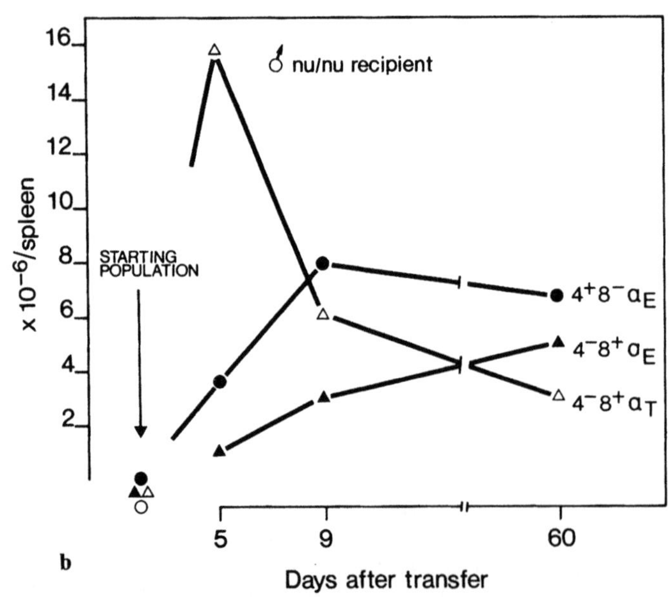

Fig. 10 a, b. a The total number of T cells in spleen and lymph nodes from female nu/nu mice injected with T cells from female αβTCR transgenic H-2^b mice. α_E, endogenous αTCR chains; α_T transgenic αTCR chains. **b** The total number of T cells in spleen and lymph nodes from male nu/nu mice injected with T cells from female αβTCR transgenic H-2^b mice

Table 1. Proliferative response of T cells from nu/nu mice injected with T cells from transgenic mice

Cells	+ IL-2		nu/nu ♂	nu/nu ♀
	nu/nu ♂	nu/nu ♀		
♀ αβ CD8	150000	4800	37400	600
♀ αβ CD8 from nu/nu ♂ d5	74500	35200	17500	5000
♀ αβ CD8 from nu/nu ♂ d9	42300	46000	1000	1700
♀ αβ CD8 from nu/nu ♂ d20	7400	5800	600	700

Responder cells (5×10^4; B cell and CD4 cell depleted lymph node cells) from various mice were cultured with 5×10^5 X-irradiated (3000 R) spleen cells from male or female nude mice in the presence or absence of exogenous interleukin 2 (IL-2). Values represent the mean cpm of [^{3}H] thymidine of triplicate cultures. Standard errors $\leq$10%.

their size is equal to that of cells with the transgenic receptor in female mice, but that the levels of CD8 coreceptors as well as that of the transgenic receptor is lower in the male compared to the female recipients. In fact, the cells from the male recipients no longer proliferate in response to antigenic stimulation by male cells in vitro, even in the presence of interleukin 2, while proliferation of such male-specific cells is easily detected with cells from female recipients (Table 1). Thus, as postthymic "positive selection" differs from thymic "positive selection", so does thymic "negative selection" differ from postthymic "negative selection." Postthymic "negative selection" involves initial expansion and subsequent elimination of cells and/or down-regulation of antigen receptors as well as coreceptors; thymic "negative selection" involves deletion of cells at an immature stage without prior expansion.

Discussion

Monoclonal antibodies specific for clonotypic TCRs and TCR transgenic mice have made it possible to study thymic [13–23] and postthymic T cell repertoire selection in previously unknown detail. The conclusions are that T cell maturation depends on "assertion" of self, namely the binding of the αβTCR to thymic MHC molecules in the absence of the specific peptide recognized by the receptor when expressed on mature T cells. This event is called "positive selection", rescues $CD4^+8^+$ thymocytes from programmed cell death [33, 34], and induces maturation into mature single-positive thymocytes in the absence of cell division. An important feature of this selective step is that binding of the αβTCR to class I or class II MHC molecules determines that the mature T cells are of the $CD4^-8^+$ and $CD4^+8^-$ phenotype, respectively [16, 17, 22, 23].

In the presence of the specific peptide, one observes the opposite: $CD4^+8^+$ thymocytes are not even allowed to persist throughout their programmed lifespan but are deleted as soon as they start to express the CD4/CD8 coreceptors [14, 15]. This event is called "negative selection" and prevents the entry of autoaggressive T cells into the peripheral lymphocyte pool.

Once the cells have passed through positive selection and avoided negative selection, they can expand considerably in peripheral lymph organs [32, 35]. This expansion depends, again, on the specificity of the αβTCR but in a different way than in intrathymic positive selection; here the receptor must bind to both the peptide and the presenting MHC molecule. The consequence of "positive selection" in peripheral lymph organs is also different from that in the thymus: in the former it is expansion and maturation into effector cells, while in the latter the consequence is differentiation into mature lymphocytes.

As predicted by Burnet and Fenner [2] and by Lederberg [3], "negative selection" of mature T cells in peripheral or secondary lymph organs differs from that in primary lymph organs. In the thymus cells can be deleted without prior stimulation to expand, while in secondary lymph organs cells expand considerably but then disappear and/or down-regulate antigen receptors and coreceptors such that the cells become refractory to antigenic stimulation even in the presence of exogenous interleukin 2. This mode of peripheral tolerance which we observe in male nu/nu mice injected with male-specific cells from αβTCR transgenic mice differs from that seen in transgenic animals in which certain antigens are expressed exclusively by "nonprofessional antigen" presenting cells; in these experiments the antigens induce a state of anergy in antigen-specific T cells which can be overcome by the addition of exogenous interleukin 2 [36]. Thus, in addition to one central tolerance mechanism, there appear to be at least two and possibly more peripheral tolerance mechanisms, hopefully including some which are mediated by so-called suppressor cells.

While the biological sense of negative selection of potentially autoaggressive cells is obvious, the biological meaning of positive selection has confused immunologists to some extent [37]: the high frequency of alloreactive T cells, many of which probably recognize some peptides presented by foreign MHC antigens, in a repertoire selected by self MHC antigens appears to make positive selection superfluous. It has been demonstrated in the past by experiments employing hemopoietic chimeras that this is not true: experiments in X-irradiated, MHC homozygous animals reconstituted with cells from donors expressing either completely allogeneic or semiallogeneic MHC molecules have shown that positive selection has a considerable impact on the "immunological fitness:" immune responses in allogeneic chimeras (as long as one does not study responses to a multitude of allogeneic major or minor histocompatibility antigens [38]) are very much reduced even after in vivo priming (which, as we have shown in the transfer experiments reported here, can lead to enormous expansion of peripheral T cells); likewise, responses "restricted" by MHC molecules not encountered in the thymus are very much lower, or even absent, in semiallogeneic chimeras [39]. Thus, after negative selection, responses restricted by MHC molecules not encountered in the thymus are as a rule orders of magnitude lower than those restricted by MHC molecules which were encountered in the thymus.

But does positive selection increase the frequency of self MHC restricted cells compared to the unselected repertoire? This question is difficult to address experimentally but the following consideration may indicate that this is so. From the data on positive selection of several transgenic αβTCRs which have been studied so far, it is apparent that different MHC molecules rarely select the same αβTCR, and thus in a first approximation one can look at the unselected repertoire of immature T cells as a collection of 50 or so repertoires which can be selected by 50 different MHC molecules. Considering this assumption and the data in allogeneic or semiallogeneic chimeras, one comes to the conclusion that in the unselected repertoire, the frequency of self MHC restricted T cells will always be lower than in the selected repertoire. Thus, positive selection serves to increase the "immunological fitness" of the mature T cell pool in spite of some confusion raised by earlier experimental data. In summary, one may conclude that the experimental demonstration of allorestricted T cells has not been a good argument against the beneficial effect of positive selection, but that the low frequency of T cells restricted by MHC antigens not present on the thymus in allogeneic or semiallogeneic chimeras has documented the usefulness of positive selection.

References

1. Owen RD (1945) Science 102: 400
2. Burnet FM, Fenner F (1949) In: The production of antibodies Macmillan, Melbourne
3. Lederberg J (1959) Science 129: 1649–1653
4. Jerne NK (1974) Ann Immunol 125: 373
5. Billingham RE, Brent L, Medowar PB (1953) Nature 172: 603
6. Hasek M (1953) Czech Biol 2: 265
7. von Boehmer H, Sprent J, Nabholz M (1975) J Exp Med 141: 322
8. Allison JP, McIntyre BW, Bloch D (1982) J Immunol 129: 2293
9. Meuer SC, Fitzgerald KA, Hussey RE, Hodgdon JC, Schlossman SF, Reinherz EL (1983) J Exp Med 157: 705
10. Haskins K, Kubo R, White J, Pigeon M, Kappler JW, Marrack PC (1983) J Exp Med 157: 1149
11. Marrack P, Kappler J (1990) Science 248: 705
12. Kappler JW, Roehm N, Marrack PC (1987) Cell 49: 273–280
13. von Boehmer H (1990) Annu Rev Immunol 8: 531
14. Kisielow P, Teh HS, Blüthmann H, von Boehmer H (1988) Nature 335: 730
15. Sha WC, Nelson CA, Newberry RD, Kranz DM, Russell JH, Loh DY (1988) Nature 335: 271
16. Teh HS, Kisielow P, Scott B, Kishi H, Uematsu Y, Blüthmann H, von Boehmer H (1988) Nature 335: 229

17. Kisielow P, Blüthmann H, Staerz UD, Steinmetz M, von Boehmer H (1988) Nature 335: 229
18. Uematsu Y, Ryser S, Dembic Z, Borgulya P, Krimpenfort P, Berns A, von Boehmer H, Steinmetz M (1988) Cell 52: 831
19. Krimpenfort P, de Jong R, Uematsu Y, Dembic Z, Ryser S, von Boehmer H, Steinmetz M, Berns A (1988) EMBO J 7: 745
20. Blüthmann H, Kisielow P, Uematsu Y, Malissen M, Krimpenfort P, Berns A, von Boehmer H, Steinmetz M (1988) Nature 334: 156
21. Scott B, Blüthmann H, Teh HS, von Boehmer H (1989) Nature 338: 591–593
22. Berg LJ, Pullem AM, Fazekas de St Groth B, Mathis D, Benoist C, Davis MM (1989) Cell 58: 1035–1046
23. Kaye J, Hsu ML, Sauron ME, Jameson JC, Gascoigne RJ, Hedrick SM (1989) Nature 341: 746–749
24. Zijlstra M, Bix M, Simister NE, Loring JM, Raulet DH, Jaenisch R (1990) Nature 344: 742
25. Jacobs H, von Boehmer H, Melof CJM, Berns A, Eur J Immunol, (in press)
26. Bjorkman P, Saper M, Samraouri B, Bennet W, Strominger J, Wiley D (1987) Nature 329: 512–518
27. de Waal LP, Melvold RM, Melof CJM (1983) J Exp Med 158: 1537
28. Ljunggren H, Stam NJ, Oehlen C, Neefjes JJ, Höglund P, Heemels M, Bastin J, Schumacher TNM, Townsend A, Kärre K, Ploegh HL (1990) Nature 346: 476
29. Nikolic-Zugic J, Bevan MJ (1990) Nature 344: 65–67
30. Sha C, Nelson CA, Newberry RP, Pullen JK, Pease LR, Russell JH, Loh DY (1990) Proc. Natl Acad Sci USA (in press)
31. Dolbeere F, Gretner H, Pallovicini MG, Gray JV (1983) Proc Natl Acad Sci USA 80: 5573
32. Rocha B, Dautigny N, Pereira P (1989) Eur J Immunol 19: 905–911
33. von Boehmer H (1986) Immunol Today 7: 333
34. von Boehmer H (1988) Annu Rev Immunol 6: 309–326
35. Miller R, Stutman OJ (1984) Immunol 133: 2925–2932
36. Lo D, Burkly L, Flavell R, Palmiter R, Brinster RJ (1989) J Exp Med 169: 779
37. Matzinger P (1981) Nature 292: 497
38. Matzinger P, Mirkwood, G (1978) J Exp Med 184: 84
39. von Boehmer H, Teh HS, Bennink JR, Haas W (1985) In: Watson, J D, Mabrook, J (eds) Recognition and regulation in cell mediated immunity. Dekker, New York

Vaccination in Immunodeficiency

S. C. Meuer, L. Qiao, A. Schirren, H. Völpel, and *H. Köhler*

Introduction

Immunodeficient individuals frequently suffer from persistent and severe infections with microbial pathogens and carry an enhanced risk of developing malignant disease. Because of reduced immune responsiveness, these same individuals are, however, less likely to benefit from vaccination in conventional form. Obviously, correction of immunodeficiencies by means of clinical immune intervention represents the only realistic approach to induce protection in immunocompromised hosts. Therefore, elucidation of the molecular events that underlie immunodeficiencies in man seems crucial for the development of successful strategies for disease prevention.

The vast majority of immunodeficiencies observed in adults are of secondary origin. A number of infectious diseases caused by viruses – including Epstein-Barr virus, cytomegalovirus, measles virus, and human immunodeficiency virus – lead to suppressed immune functions. Moreover, immunodeficiency can result from drug treatment (immunosuppressive therapy, chemotherapy), irradiation, malnutrition, and perhaps stress. Finally, metabolic disorders secondary to organ failure as observed, for example, in diseases of the kidney and the liver have severe negative influences on the immune system.

The present report summarizes some of the new approaches to studying immunodeficiencies at the cellular level in vitro. Experimental procedures are delineated which, by means of monoclonal antibodies, allow the analyis of functional capacities of individual ligand receptor systems that govern the cellular immune response. Moreover, preliminary results are presented where such information was used to develop a successful clinical strategy to induce vaccine responses in a particular group of immunodeficient patients.

Cell Interaction Molecules Involved in T Cell Activation

One of the central processes underlying specific immune responses is the generation of activated regulatory and effector T lymphocytes. T cell activation consists of a complex series of sequential and parallel ligand/receptor interactions which, in concert, lead to the generation of activated T cells. These then contribute to B lymphocyte activation for antibody production, macrophage activation, and, in addition, execute themselves effector functions such as cell-mediated lysis. At present, T cell activation represents the main target for clinical immune intervention in autoimmune disease, transplantation, cancer, and immunodeficiencies.

Recently, a number of important cell/cell interaction molecules that are required for efficient T cell activation in the immune response have been discovered and characterized at the molecular level. As shown in Figure 1, these structures include the CD3-Ti antigen receptor [8] recognizing antigenic peptides in MHC association. Moreover, the CD4 and CD8 glycoproteins interact with monomorphic regions of the MHC class II and MHC class I determinants on antigen-presenting and -effector cells, respectively [7]. It has been well recognized that additional ligand receptor systems facilitate adhesion of lymphocytes to a large number of other cell types of hematopoietic and nonhematopoietic origin [20]. These structures mediate initial contact, for example, between T cells and antigen-presenting cells which is believed to represent a crucial prerequisite for the subsequent processes of specific recognition by the T cell receptor and the following activation processes. In particular, lymphocyte recirculation seems to be dependent on expression of adhesion molecules such as intercellular adhesion molecule 1 (ICAM-1; CD54) [6] and lymphocyte function associated antigen (LFA-3; CD58) [22]. Besides mediating cell-to-cell contact, the interaction between CD2 and LFA-3 appears to be intimately involved in amplifying lymphocyte activation [2, 4, 11].

Immunodeficiencies can exist at the level of each individual molecular interaction system [14]. Thus, blockade of only one of these mechanisms results in profound reduction in antigen-directed immune responses both in vitro and in vivo. Due to the availability of monoclonal antibodies that are capable of mimicking the physiologic activity of a given natural ligand [9] and the existence of recombinant sources of human cytokines, it has recently

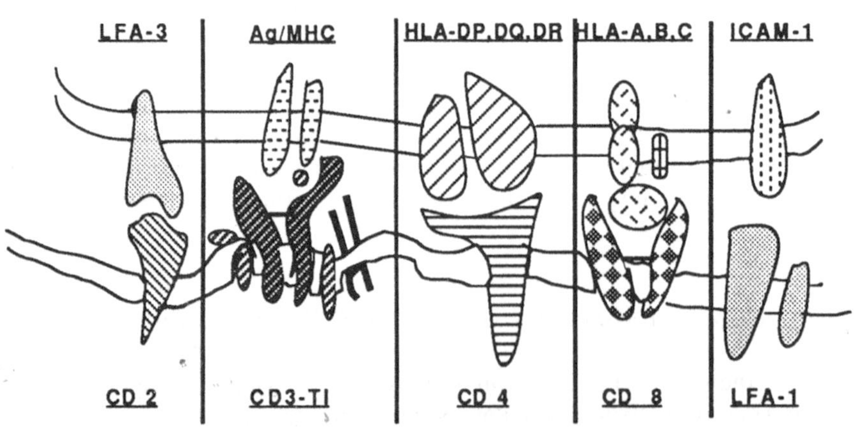

Fig. 1. Cell surface structures involved in effector target/antigen presenting cell interactions (*bottom*, T cell side; *top*, effector/antigen presenting cell side)

become possible to establish diagnostic in vitro systems that help to analyze the functions of individual receptor/ligand systems in T cell activation [13].

A Model of Human T Cell Activation

To explain and localize the molecular basis of immunodeficiencies at the level of T cell activation, it is first necessary to summarize the current knowledge regarding these processes in a contemporary, yet simplified, operational model of T cell activation. As shown in Figure 2, purified resting T lymphocytes receive the initial triggering signal for differentiation through the T cell antigen receptor complex with recognizes antigenic peptides in appropriate MHC association. An analogous signal can be mediated experimentally by surface-linked monoclonal antibodies directed at either constant or variable determinants of the T cell antigen receptor complex [8–10] which consists of the Ti-heterodimer and the associated CD3 subunits. Antigen recognition results in rapid acquisition of responsiveness to the lymphokine interleukin-2 (IL-2), however, does not lead to T cell proliferation (stage T_{A1}) [12].

T_{A1} lymphocytes interact with cells of the monocyte lineage which appear to be specialized to provide additional signals that eventually mediate their clonal expansion and differentation into activated regulatory and effector cells. T cell/monocyte interaction appears to represent a bidirectional process in which the T lineage restricted glycoprotein CD2 and the LFA-3 molecule seem to play a central role [3]. We and others have, most recently, recognized that engagement of the LFA-3 molecule expressed on monocytes induces their production of monokines, including interleukin-1 (IL-1) and interleukin-6 (IL6) [5, 24]. On the other hand, binding of LFA-3 to CD2 represents one mechanism which enables T lymphocytes to respond to IL-1 and IL-6 (stage T_{A2}) [3]. The function of IL-1 appears to be related to the induction of the secretion of IL-2 by T cells which acts in an autocrine fashion on its own cell surface receptor (stage T_{A3}). This is concluded from the finding that IL-1

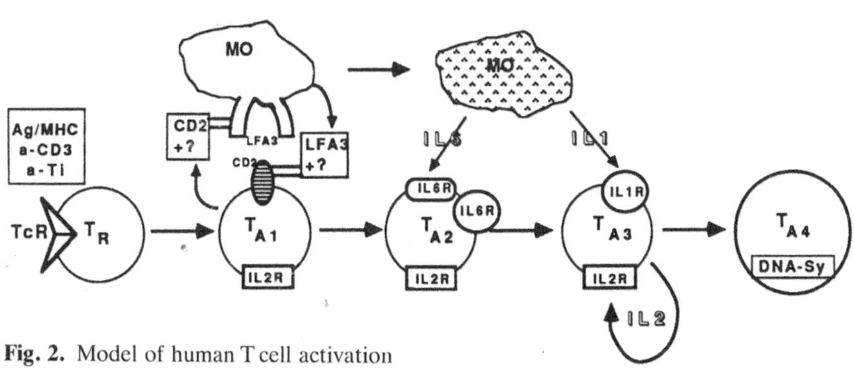

Fig. 2. Model of human T cell activation

mediated amplification of signals delivered through CD2 can be inhibited by monoclonal antibodies directed at the IL-2 receptor (anti-CD25). This indicates that IL-1 promotes T cell proliferation through the IL-2/IL-2 receptor system. In contrast, anti-CD25 antibodies do not inhibit proliferation induced through CD2 plus IL-6, suggesting that IL-6 itself represents a growth factor for T cells or, alternatively, mediates its activity through an as yet unknown additional cytokine (stage T_{A3}). Under the influence of IL-6 and IL-2, T cells are induced to synthesize DNA and to upregulate genes encoding four crucial effector molecules [3].

Note that all signals which regulate the CD2/LFA-3 system (i.e., alternative pathway of T cell activation) are not completely known at present. Experimentally, these activation processes can be initiated employing monoclonal antibodies that bind to individual epitopes of the CD2 [11] and LFA-3 molecules [5, 24]. The respective unknown natural activities could be executed by short-lived mediators. This view is, however, a current hypothesis which will require substantiation by experimental data.

Some Recent Facts Concerning T Cell Unresponsiveness

Physiologic unresponsiveness of the immune system could be considered as "relative immunodeficiency." For example, host immune responses would be harmful in locations which are constantly exposed to foreign antigens, for example, the gastrointestinal and respiratory tracts. In the gastrointestinal tract a considerable proportion of the host immune system, particularly T lymphocytes, homes to the mucosal areas. Apparently these cells fulfill a protective function yet do not generate detectable systemic immune responses toward the multitude of antigens to which these cells are permanently exposed. On the other hand, intestinal T cells must represent a major source of helper activity which enable B lymphocytes to produce, for example, antibody of the IgA subclass.

Recent investigations on T lymphocytes that were freshly recovered from mucosal areas of the human intestine have demonstrated that these cells, despite normal expression of a T cell receptor complex, do not or only weakly respond to signals mediated through CD3-Ti with clonal expansion and mediator production [17, 18]. On the other hand, these same cells can be easily induced to secrete cytokines through the CD2/LFA-3 interaction system and the CD28 cell surface receptor (Fig. 3). Unresponsiveness to triggering of the T cell antigen receptor complex appears to be induced through local environmental conditions which exist in the mucosal environment and lead to downregulation of early second messenger responses such as calcium mobilization and IP3 generation [18]. This physiologic state of low responsiveness to antigens may be one reason to explain the failure of attempts to achieve protective immune responses through oral vaccination with inactivated antigenic material. As a consequence, attempts to elicit immune responses upon oral introduction of antigenic material by immuno-

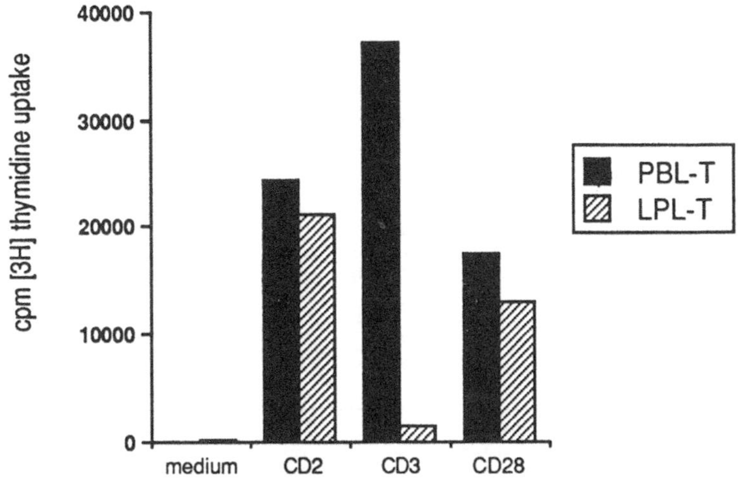

Fig. 3. Proliferative responses of peripheral blood (*PBL-T*) versus lamina propria T (*LPL-T*) lymphocytes to stimulation with monoclonal antibodies directed at CD2, CD3, and CD28

modulation may result in severe side effects, including inflammatory responses of the bowel, since one would have to interfere considerably with the local mucosal milieu.

Escape Mechanisms Employed by Malignant Cells

To escape immune surveillance, tumors not unfrequently develop strategies which interfere with cell/cell interaction molecules. Downregulation or even loss of expression of MHC determinants required for recognition by the T cell antigen receptor has been well documented [16]. We have recently found that an inverse relationship exists between tumor spread and the surface density of adhesion molecules ICAM-1 (CD54) and/or LFA-3 (CD58) [21]. Thus, high peripheral white blood cell counts in some T and B cell leukemias correlate significantly with low expression of CD54 and CD58 (Fig. 4). This is in sharp contrast to nontransformed lymphocytes which usually express higher densities of CD54 and CD58 with enhanced proliferation (not shown).

Autologous cytotoxic T effector cells that were generated from tumor samples in vitro employing IL-2 are not capable of killing the respective tumor cell blasts. Importantly, under the influence of cytokines such as tumor necrosis factor expression of CD54 and CD58 can be reinduced on tumor cells in vitro. Once this is achieved, malignant blast cells become susceptible to lysis through autologous T and natural killer effector cells (Fig. 5). The fact that this cytolytic effector function can be inhibited by monoclonal antibodies directed at CD58 stresses the role of adhesion molecules for immunologic effector functions toward malignant cells and, in addition, provides impor-

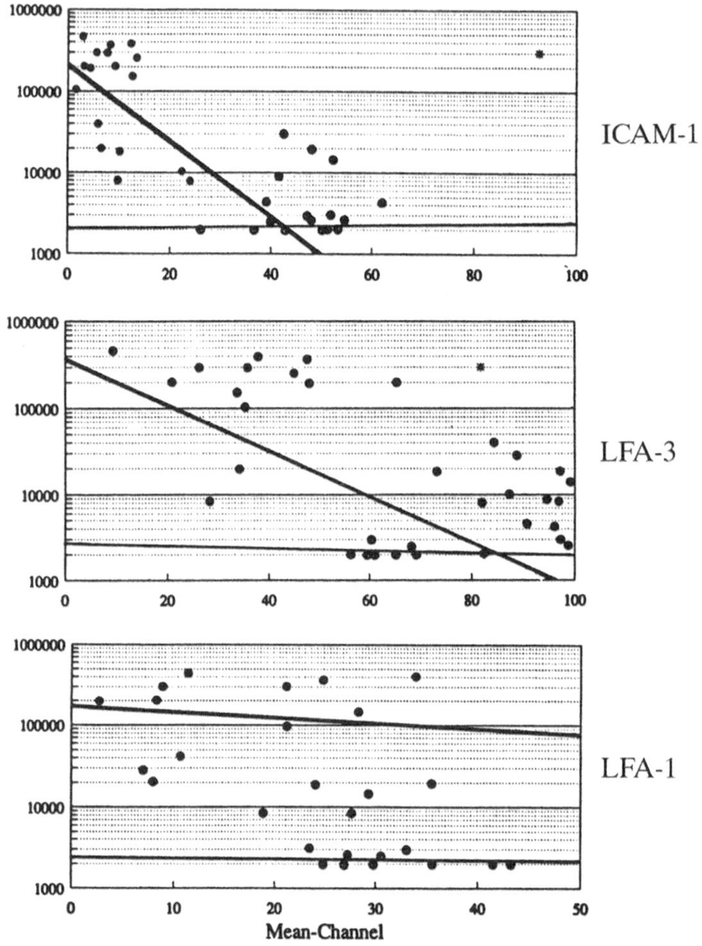

Fig. 4. Downregulation of adhesion molecules on human T cell leukemias correlates with accelerated leukemia spread in vivo (*each point*, one individual freshly recovered tumor cell sample)

tant perspectives for immune therapy of such tumors. It seems obvious that attempts to achieve immunity against tumor cells by vaccination with tumor material will have to take into consideration these recent findings and therefore need to be accompanied by rational cytokine applications in vivo.

Secondary Immunodeficiencies

A large group of secondary immunodeficiencies exist at the level of the immune processes underlying T cell activation. Such situations pose serious

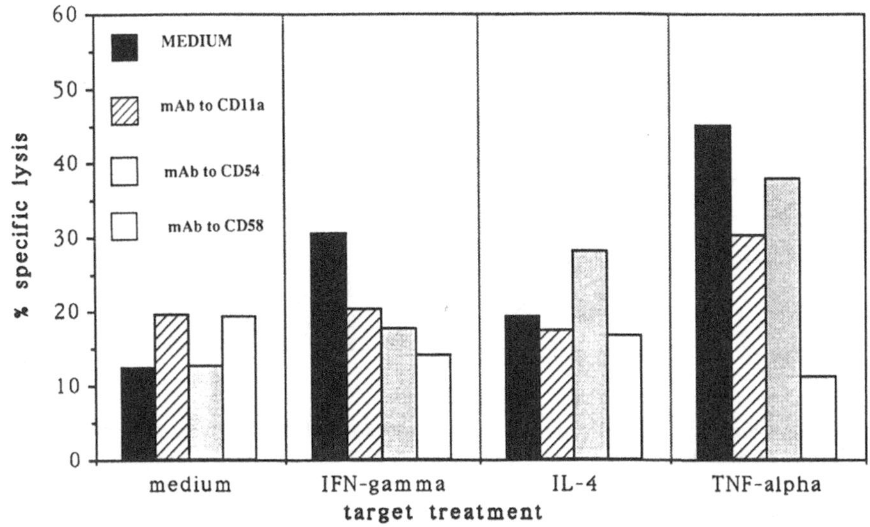

Fig. 5. Lysis of T leukemic blast by autologous cytotoxic effector cells. Tumor necrosis factor (*TNF*) alpha induces expression of LFA-3 and ICAM-1 on leukemic blasts and renders malignant cells susceptible to lysis. Monoclonal antibodies, particularly those directed at CD58, have strong blocking effects on this reaction. *IFN*, interferon

constraints on our attempts to achieve host protection in immunocompromised individuals. Particularly these individuals, however, carry an enhanced risk to encounter chronic infections with viruses, for example, that cause organ damage or are even associated with the development of cancer.

We have intensively investigated cellular immune responses of patients with chronic renal failure who are known to be highly susceptible to chronic infection with hepatitis B virus [13]. In vitro investigations helped to identify a severe dysfunction of the monocyte population with regard to its capacity to support the process of T cell activation in primary immune responses to antigens (Fig. 6; compare Fig. 2). That monocytes are deficient in patients with renal failure has recently been confirmed by others [19, 23]. Thus, when T cells of such patients are exposed to stimuli that mediate signals through the T cell antigen receptor (such as surface-linked anti-CD3 monoclonal antibody), clonal T cell expansion and cytokine production are markedly reduced because monocytes are required by T lymphocytes to proceed from stage T_{A1} to stage T_{A2}. The fact that expression of receptors for IL-2, however, occurs in such individuals following antigen encounter, is in accordance with the model proposed in Fig. 2.

Indeed, antigen receptor triggering resulted in even higher expression of IL-2 responsiveness in immunodeficient individuals as compared to normal healthy control persons [13]. In addition, responses through the CD2-dependent alternative pathway could be experimentally triggered in vitro, which indicated a normal function of the T cell population (Fig. 7). In a similar

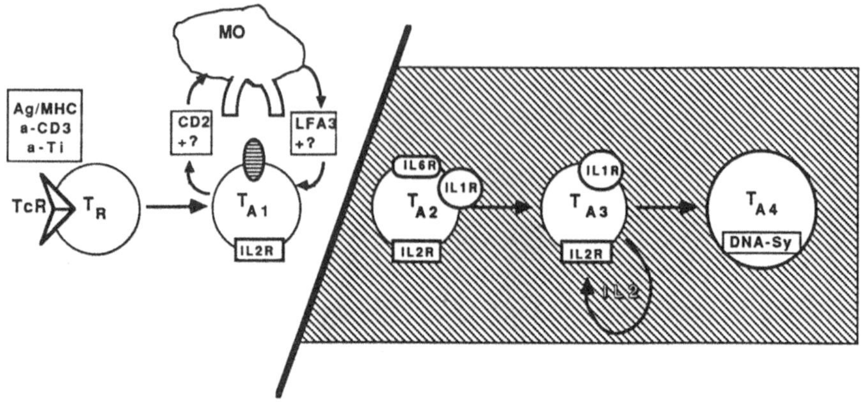

Fig. 6. A monocyte defect leads to a selective blockade of T cell activation in patients with chronic renal failure

fashion, in patients with acquired immunodeficiency syndrome (AIDS) T cell receptor triggering also does not result in clonal T cell expansion (Table 1). There, however, the defect appears to be unrelated to monocyte function with regard to providing help for T cell activation. Rather, there exists a deficiency in the T cell population to interact with monocytes and to induce monokines. While monocytes from AIDS patients can provide help to T cells from healthy individuals, monocytes from patients with chronic renal failure are inefficient.

An important difference between these groups of immunocompromised individuals exists in that the T cell system in patients with chronic renal failure appears to be normal whereas, as shown in numerous reports, there is a

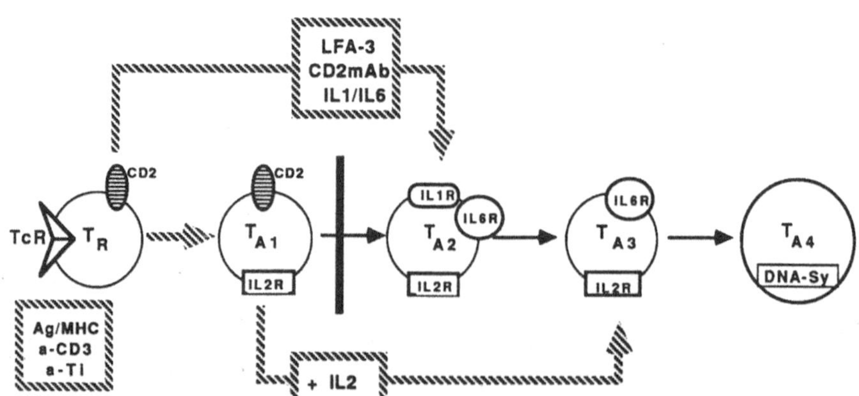

Fig. 7. Strategies for circumvention of immune deficiency in patients with chronic renal failure (compare Fig. 6)

Table 1. T Cell activation in immunodeficiency

Responder cells	Stimulus	Disease and origin of T lymphocytes		
		Healthy donor	AIDS patient	Dialysis patient
T	Medium	64a	54	246
T	Anti-CD3 Sepharose	700	956	332
T + Mo (healthy)	Anti-CD3 Sepharose	18301	2035	20961
T + Mo (AIDS)	Anti-CD3 Sepharose	19185	1798	NT
T + Mo (dialysis patient)	Anti-CD3 Sepharose	6055	NT	1569
T + IL-2	Anti-CD3 Sepharose	26523	30558	36089
T	Anti-$T11_2$ + anti-$T11_3$	11597	12310	14870

Separated T cells and monocytes from representative donors as indicated were exposed to stimulation via the Ti-T3 complex (anti-CD3 Sepharose) or the alternative pathway (anti-$T11_2$ plus anti-$T11_3$). Mo, monocytes
[a] [^{3}H] Thymidine incorporation cpm

severe lack of the $CD4^+$ inducer population in AIDS [1]. It seems rather unlikely that this phenotypic abnormality is in itself sufficient to explain our in vitro results since isolated $CD8^+$ plus T lymphocytes from normal individuals can well interact with monocytes in the experimental in vitro system. Since this does not seem to be possible in AIDS patients, a severe functional deficiency within the T cell population must exist. Whether this failure involves expression of cell/cell interaction molecules required for T cell – monocyte cooperation or loss of a particular T cell subset has not been investigated so far.

A Strategy for Immune Intervention

The finding that in a group of immunocompromised patients with chronic renal failure, deficient monocyte function results in reduced IL-2 production while triggering of the T cell antigen receptor leads to enhanced IL-2 receptor expression (Fig. 5) prompted us to develop a clinical protocol aimed at correcting the deficient immune response to hepatitis B vaccine by providing exogenous IL-2 along with the antigen preparation (Fig. 6). Based on our previous investigations on cellular immune responses of these individuals in vitro, we subjected a selected group of individuals to such a treatment. These individuals had been unresponsive to multiple previous attempts to induce antibodies against hepatitis B surface antigen by standard vaccination.

Upon combined vaccination with IL-2 plus hepatitis B vaccine [15], however, a major proportion (eight out of ten individuals) responded with antibody production following three vaccinations and have maintained antibody titers similar to those of healthy individuals (Fig. 8). Importantly,

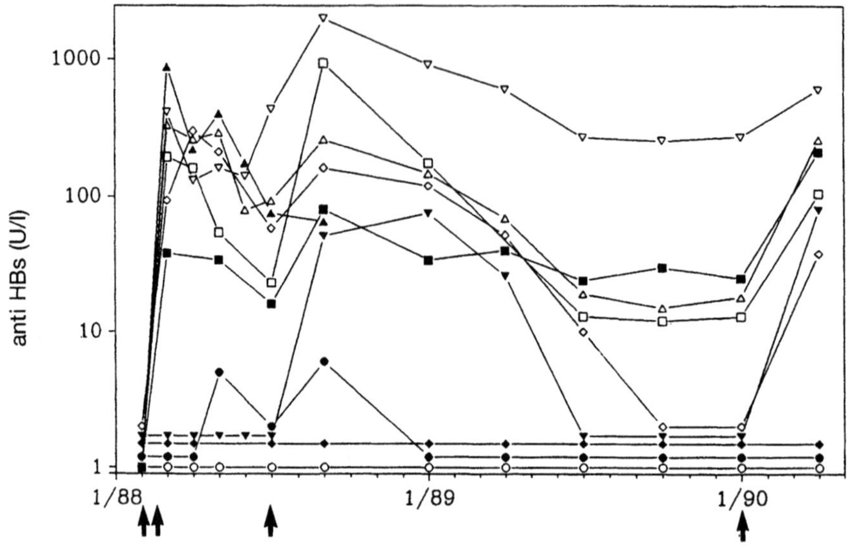

Fig. 8. Low-dose IL-2 therapy induces systemic immune responses against hepatitis B surface antigen in previous non responders to hepatitis B vaccination. *Arrows*, time points of combined vaccination with hepatitis B vaccine and local IL-2 injection

since secondary (memory) immune responses appear to be less dependent on monocyte help, it has been possible to booster anti-hepatitis B surface, antibody titers by administering the vaccine alone.

Conclusions

Recent developments in the field of T cell activation have opened up a new area for investigations on human immunodeficiencies. It has become possible to create in vitro systems which allow analysis of the functions of individual cellular receptor systems at the molecular level. Despite the fact that a considerable number of as yet unknown variables exist within the multitude of functional processes that are required for efficient generation of regulatory and effector T lymphocytes, the example of immune reconstitution in patients suffering from chronic renal failure has clearly demonstrated the potency of this approach.

Recombinant sources of human cytokines appear particularly suited to reconstituting immune responses in immunodeficient individuals. Strategies based on live viral vectors containing immunogen and lymphokine genes may not be applicable there, since these individuals cannot sufficiently control replication of recombinant viral organisms.

The present investigations stress the point that one of the most relevant variables that can be influenced to favor responses to vaccines exists at the level of the host immune system. Therefore, besides efforts to optimize vaccine antigens, information on immune functions in immunocompromised hosts will likely provide important clues for attempts to design successful vaccination strategies in the future.

References

1. Cohn ZA, Steinman RM (1988) The immunological and infectious sequelae of the acquired immune deficiency syndrome. J Exp Med 168: 2415–2323
2. Dustin ML, Sanders ME, Shaw S, Springer TA (1987) Purified lymphocyte function-associated antigen 3 binds to CD2 and mediates T lymphocyte adhesion. J Exp Med 165: 677–692
3. Endler-Jobst B, Schraven B, Hutmacher B, Meuer SC (1991) Human T cell responses to IL-1 and IL-6 are dependent on signals mediated through CD2. J Immunol 146: 1736–1742
4. Hünig T, Tiefenthaler G, Meyer zum Büschenfelde KH, Meuer SC (1987) Alternative pathway activation of T cells by binding of CD2 to its cell-surface ligand. Nature 326: 298–301
5. Le PT, Vollger LW, Haynes BF, Singer KH (1990) Ligand binding to the LFA-3 cell adhesin molecule induces IL-1 production by human thymic epithelial cells. J Immunol 144: 4541–4547
6. Makgoba MW, Sander, ME, Luce GEG, Gugel EA, Dustin ML, Springer TA, Shaw S (1988) Eur J Immunol 18: 637–640
7. Meuer SC, Schlossman SF, Reinherz EL (1982) Clonal analysis of human cytotoxic T lymphocytes: $T4^+$ and $T8^+$ effector T cells recognize products of different major histocompatibility complex regions. Proc Natl Acad Sci USA 79: 4395–4399
8. Meuer SC, Fitzgerald KA, Hussey RE, Hodgdon JC, Schlossman SF, Reinherz EL (1983 a) Clonotypic structures involved in antigen-specific human T cell function. J Exp Med 157: 705–719
9. Meuer SC, Hodgdon JC, Hussey RE, Protentis JP, Schlossman SF, Reinherz EL (1983 b) Antigen-like effects of monoclonal antibodies directed at receptors on human T cell clones. J Exp Med 158: 988–993
10. Meuer SC, Hussey RE, Cantrell DA, Hodgdon JC, Schlossman SF, Smith KA, Reinherz EL (1984 a) Triggering of the T3-Ti antigen-receptor complex results in clonal T cell proliferation through an interleukin-2-dependent autocringe pathway. Proc Natl Acad Sci USA 81: 1509–1513
11. Meuer SC, Hussey RE, Fabbi M, Fox D, Acuto O, Fitzgerald KA, Hodgdon JC, Protentis JP, Schlossman SF, Reinherz EL (1984) An alternative pathway of T cell activation: a functional role for the 50 kd T11 sheep erythrocyte receptor protein. Cell 36: 897–906
12. Meuer SC, Meyer zum Büschenfelde KH (1986) T cell receptor triggering induces responsiveness to interleukin-1 and interleukin-2 but does not lead to T cell proliferation. J Immunol 136: 4106–4112
13. Meuer SC, Hauer M, Kurz P, Meyer zum Büschenfelde KH, Köhler H (1987) Selective blockade of the antigen-receptor-mediated pathway of T cell activation in Patients with impaired primary immune responses. J Clin Invest 80: 743–749
14. Meuer SC, Roux MM, Schraven B (1989) The alternative pathway of T cell activation: biology, pathophysiology, and perspectives for immunopharmacology. Clin Immunol Immunopathol 50: 133–139
15. Meuer SC, Dumann H, Meyer zum Büschenfelde KH, Köhler H (1989) Low-dose interleukin-2 induces systemic immune responses against HBsAg in immunodeficient nonresponders to Hepatitis-B vaccination. Lancet I: 15–18

16. Momburg F, Ziegler A, Harprecht J, Möller P, Moldenhauer G, Hämmerling GJ (1989) Selective loos of HLA-A or HLA-B antigen expression in colon carcinoma. J Immunol 142: 352–358
17. Pirzer UC, Schürmann G, Post S, Betzler M, Meuer SC (1990) Differential responsiveness ot CD3-Ti versus CD2-dependent activation of human intestinal T lymphocytes. Eur J Immunol 20: 2339–2342
18. Qiao L, Schürmann G, Betzler M, Meuer SC (1991) Activation and signalling status of human lamina propria T lymphocytes. Gastroenterology 101: 1529–1536
19. Ruiz P, Gomez F, Schreiber D (1990) Impaired function of macrophage Fc gamma receptors in end-stage renal disease. N Engl J Med 322: 717–722
20. Sanchez-Madrid F, Krensky AM, Ware CF, Robbins E, Strominger JL, Burakoff SJ, Springer TA (1982) Three distinct antigens associated with human T lymphocyte mediated cytolysis: LFA-1, LFA-2, and LFA-3, Proc Natl Acad Sci USA 79: 7489–7493
21. Schirren CA, Völpel H, Meuer SC (1992) Adhesion molecules on freshly recovered T leukemias promote tumor directed lympholysis 79: 138–143
22. Springer TA (1990) Adhesion receptors of the immune system. Nature 346: 425–434
23. Tolkoff-Rubin NE, Rubin RH (1990) Uremia and host defenses. N Engl J Med 322: 770–772
24. Webb, SA, Shimizu Y, Seventer GA, Shaw S, Gerrard TL (1990) LFA-3, CD44, and CD45: physiologic Triggers of human monocyte TNF and IL-1 release. Science 249: 1295–1297

Induction of Peripheral Tolerance to Class I MHC Alloantigenic Cells in Adult Mice

H. Wagner and *K. Heeg*

A major goal in transplantation immunology is to define gentle methods able to convert immune reactivity to MHC-encoded transplantation antigens into a state of immune unresponsiveness (tolerance). It is known that this conversion can be achieved in neonates: introduction of foreign antigens into a developing immune system prevents the system from responding further to these antigens (Nossal 1983). Recent evidence indicates that both in natural tolerance and in experimentally induced neonatal unresponsiveness maturing antigen-reactive thymocytes become either clonally deleted (White et al. 1989; MacDonald et al. 1988) or at least clonally silenced (Stockinger 1984). Induction of tolerance in the mature peripheral T cell pool poses problems since receptor occupancy by antigens primarily causes sensitization rather than tolerization (Lafferty et al. 1980; Mueller et al. 1989). On the other hand, there is evidence that gentle methods, for example, the use of noninvasive methods, may have effects on the immune reactivity of the peripheral T cell pool in adults. These include "pretransplant transfusion" effects (Van der Kwast et al. 1981; Sano et al. 1987) and the veto cell concept (Miller 1980; Fink et al. 1988). Since intraveneous transfusion represents a gentle method, we analyzed the efficacy of intraveneous allogenic cell transfusion to induce unresponsiveness in adult mice. The main findings have been:

- Injected mice develop a long-lasting chimerism that is paralleled by a state of tolerance to skin allografts.
- Injected mice display a state of split tolerance, i.e., peripheral but not intrathymic cytotoxic T cell precursors (CTL-p) bearing high-affinity tolerogen-reactive T cell receptors (TCRs) are clonally silenced.
- $L3T4^+$ recipient T cells are necessary for induction of tolerance.
- Donor-derived lymphocytes isolated from chimeric mice display effective veto activity in vitro.

Since details of this work have been published elsewhere (Heeg and Wagner 1990), we proceed immediately to the findings. It should be stressed that we are discussing induction of tolerance only to class I MHC incompatible allogenic cells. Addition of MHC class II disparities means a change in the rules presented here.

When adult B6 recipient mice are intraveneously transfused with about 5×10^7 allogeneic bm1 splenocytes, the in vivo and in vitro reactivity of the recipients changes dramatically. First, and not anticipated, the recipients show no signs of graft-versus-host reactivity, even though high numbers of recipient reactive T cells are transferred. Second, the frequency of anti-bm1 reactive CTL-p and IL-2 producing T lymphocyte precursors in the recipient spleen drops within 24 h upon transfusion from about 1/500 (control) to less than 1/10000. Third, the majority of B6 recipient mice tolerate bm1 skin grafts but not third-party skin grafts. Essentially similar results were obtained using recombinant mice differing at the H-2D locus. Further, when splenocyte subsets were titrated for their efficacy to induce tolerance to class I MHC antigens expressed by the donor cells, $CD8^+$ T cells were found to be most effective. We conclude that upon intravenous injection of class I MHC incompatible $CD8^+$ T cells a profound and immediate state of tolerance toward the disparate class I MHC antigens occurs in the mature T cells of the recipient mouse.

This selective loss of reactivity affected only the peripheral T cell pool. Thus the frequencies of CTL-p within thymocytes of the recipient mice remained normal, while that of the peripheral T cells decreased rapidly upon donor cell injection (split tolerance). Furthermore, the loss of frequencies in the peripheral T cell pool affected primarily peripheral CTL-p bearing high-affinity TCRs, i.e., CTL-p which were resistant to blockade with anti-CD8 monoclonal antibodies (mAb).

Surprisingly, recipient mice depleted for CD4 T cells (by pretreatment with high doses of anti-CD4 mAb) were resistant to tolerance induction by the protocol used. This aspect is not understood, and helpful comments on this would be appreciated. On the other hand, B6 recipients treated with cyclosporin A remained susceptible for tolerance induction. In other words, in vivo tolerance induction as studied here appeared to be resistant to cyclosporin A.

Using fluorescein isothiocyanate labeled anti-H-$2D^d$ mAb, we analyzed the state of chimerism in the B10.A → B10.BR mouse combination. While in bone marrow or thymus no donor cells were found, significant numbers (3%–9%) of D^d positive B10.A donor cells were detected for up to 20 days in the spleen of recipient B10.BR mice. We conclude that the state of tolerance is paralleled by a state of chimerism in the recipient's peripheral lymphocyte pool.

Using cell sorter technology, we next analyzed whether upon in vitro depletion of donor splenocytes from chimeric splenocytes (4 days after intravenous transfusion), recipient T cells express CTL responsiveness to donor's MHC antigens. Since unresponsiveness remained, we conclude that it was not due to active suppression mediated via donor cells. Thus the profound reduction in CTL-p frequencies in (tolerant) recipient $CD8^+$ splenocytes must be explained by other mechanisms.

One observation might represent a clue in understanding the mechanism(s) of tolerance studied here. We noted that inasmuch as donor $CD8^+$ T lymphocytes (from chimeric splenocytes) were tolerant, i.e., clonally depleted for anti-recipient (anti-D^K) reactive CTL-p, the very same cells efficiently suppressed the primary activation of naive CTL-p to donor class I MHC antigens. Specifically, responsiveness of naive B10.BR T cells to B10.A stimulator cells (anti-D^d) was suppressed by addition of B10.A T cells purified via cell sorter technology from chimeric splenocytes. This suppression was antigen specific, since the reactivity to third-party MHC antigens was not affected. It must be noted that B10.A T cells from control mice did not exhibit suppressive activity. In other words the "suppressor cells" displayed the hallmarks of veto cells. We thus conclude that by "parking" class I MHC incompatible donor $CD8^+$ T cells via the intravenous route in adult recipients, these cells become "activated" to a state defined by the ability to "veto" the recipients' $CD8^+$ T cells to respond to donor cell MHC antigens.

Why do donor and recipent T cells not reject each other, or at least cause symptoms resembling those of graft-versus-host or host-versus-graft disease? We have shown that peripheral tolerance is not due to active suppression but rather to clonal anergy of antigen-reactive $CD8^+$ CTL-p and interleukin 2 producing $CD8^+$ T cells. Since donor lymphocytes exhibit clonal anergy to recipient class I MHC antigens, yet express at the same time remarkably efficient veto activity, we believe that the reciprocal peripheral tolerance in adult chimeric mice is caused, and maintained, by veto activity induced both in the donor and in the recipient $CD8^+$ T cells.

Short-term mixed lymphocyte cultures of murine $CD8^+$ T cells reactive to MHC alloantigens have shown that CTLs can inactivate ("veto") CTL-p that recognized them (Miller 1980). This process does not involve the receptor of CTL being recognized and can occur in the presence of efficient APCs and factors such as interleukin-2, known to support activation (Fink et al. 1988). Recent evidence indicates that it is the CD8 molecule expressed by veto cells which is essential for the veto cell function (Hamber et al. 1990). Further, CD8 structures expressed by $CD8^+$ veto cells recognize the α-3 domain of class I MHC (Connolly et al. 1990) and by doing so appear to signal "programmed cell death" (apoptosis) to the CTL-p recognizing allogenic class I MHC antigen expressed by the veto cell (Suryaprakash and Miller 1991). If the latter data are confirmed, the veto phenomenon detailed could represent a mechanism of deleting antigen-reactive CTL-p, provided that potentially immunogenic peptides are recognized in association with MHC on cells expressing CD8 molecules. Accordingly, CD8 expressing APCs and CD8 not expressing APCs could initiate two functionally opposite pathways in CTL-p recognizing their antigenic peptide, the former inducing apoptosis and the latter activation. Thus, vetoing APCs might represent a peripheral mechanism to induce via apoptosis clonal deletion of CTL-p.

Lately we stumbled upon the phenomenon of apoptosis in resting peripheral T cells while titrating the optimal concentrations of immobilized anti-α/β TCR mAb to cause activation. We noticed that ligation of TCRs of resting $CD8^+$ T cells with submitogenic concentrations of immobilized anti-TCR mAb is not biologically inert but represents a powerful signal to propel $CD8^+$ T cells within 24 h into apoptosis (Welwert-Kossik et al. 1991).

Rescue from apoptosis was brought about by ligation of CD8 molecules, in addition. The mechanisms of "rescue from apoptosis" were genestein sensitive, suggesting that ligation of CD8 molecules caused activation of $p56^{lck}$, known to be associated with the transcytoplasmatic tail of CD8 and CD4 structures. These findings led us to conclude that limited TCR ligation of antigen-reactive CTL-p "sensitizes" the reactive cell for two functional opposite options, i.e., activation versus apoptosis. The decision for this option is brought about by signal pathways controlled by so-called "coreceptors." CD8 coreceptors appear to be prime candidates to initiate activation, while the coreceptors for inducing "programmed cell death," i.e., clonal deletion via apoptosis, are yet unknown. A candidate is ligation of class I MHC structures, or members of the nerve growth factor – tumor necrosis factor receptor family (Itoh et al. 1991). If, as we hope, this successful meeting will be repeated by the organizers, it may well be that the physiological ligand responsible for inducing apoptosis in $CD8^+$ T cells upon limited cross-linking of their TCR structures will be defined.

Acknowledgements. This work was supported by the Bundesministerium für Forschung und Technologie and by the Deutsche Forschungsgemeinschaft (Sonderforschungsbereich 322).

References

Conolly JM, Hanson TH, Ingold L, Potter TA (1990) Recognition by CD8 on cytotoxic T lymphocytes is ablated by several substitutious in the class I α-3 domain: CD8 and the T cell receptor recognize the same class I molecule. Proc Natl Acad Sci USA 87: 2137

Fink PJ, Shimonkevitz RP, Bevan MJ (1988) Veto cells. Annu Rev Immunol 6: 115

Hamber JE, Kaplan DR, Tycocinski ML (1990) CD8 functions as an inhibitory ligand in mediating the immunoregulatory activity of $CD8^+$ cells. J Immunol 145: 1646

Heeg K, Wagner H (1990) Induction of peripheral tolerance to class I MHC alloantigens in adult mice: transfused class I MHC incompatible splenocytes veto clonal responses of antigen-reactive Lyt 2^+ T cells. J Exp Med 172: 719

Itoh N, Yonehara S, Ishii A, Yonehara M, Miushima SI, Sameshima M, Hase A, Seto Y, Nagata S (1991) The polypeptide encoded by the c-DNA for human cell surface antigens fas can mediate apoptosis. Cell 66: 233

Lafferty KJ, Andrus L, Prowse SJ (1980) Role of lymphokine and antigen in the control of specific T cell responses Immunol Rev 51: 279

MacDonald HR, Schneider R, Lees K, Howe RC, Acha-Orbea H, Festenstein RM, Zinkennagel R, Hengartner H (1988) T cell receptor Vβ use predicts reactivity and tolerance to MLs^a-encoded antigens. Nature 332: 40

Miller RG (1980) An immunological suppressor cell inactivating cytotoxic T lymphocyte precursor cells recognizing it. Nature 287: 544

Mueller DL, Jenkins MK, Schwartz RH (1989) Clonal expansion versus functional clonal inactivation: a costimulatory signalling pathway determines the outcome of T cell receptor occupancy Annu Rev Immunol 7: 445

Nossal GJV (1983) Cellular mechanisms of immunologic tolerance. Annu Rev Immunol 1: 33

Sano S, Suda T, Quiau JH, Sato S, Ikegami R, Hamaoka T, Fujiwara H (1987) Abrogation of the capacity of delayed-type hypersensitivity responses to alloantigens by intraveneous injection of neuramimidase-treated allogenic cells J Immunol 139: 3625

Stockinger B (1984) Cytotoxic T cell precursor revealed in neonatally tolerant mice Proc Natl Acad Sci USA 81: 220
Suryaprakash RS, Miller RD (1991) Programmed cell death of T cells signalled by the T cell receptor and the α-3 domain of class I MHC. Science 252: 1424
Van der Kwast TH, Binanchi AJJ, Bril H, Benner R (1981) Suppression of antigraft immunity by preimmunisation. Transplantation 31: 79
White J, Herman A, Pullen AM, Kubo R, Kappler JW, Marrak P (1989) The Vβ-specific superantigen staphylococcal enterotoxin B: stimulation of mature T cells and clonal deletion in neonatal mice. Cell 56: 27
Welwet-Kossik A, Wagner H, Heeg K (1991) Limited T cell receptor ligation induces programmed cell death in resting peripheral CD8 T lymphocytes: rescue via ligation of CD8 coreceptors (to be published)

Analysis of Human Immunodeficiency Virus 1 Envelope Proteins: Contribution of Cysteine Residues to Envelope Function

E. Tschachler and *M. S. Reitz, Jr.*

Introduction

Human immunodeficiency virus type 1 (HIV-1) is the etiologic agent which causes the acquired immunodeficiency syndrome. Various HIV-1 isolates show a high level of genetic diversity. The envelope gene is the most variable (Alizon et al. 1986; Gurgo et al. 1988; Hahn et al. 1985; Srinivasan et al. 1987; Starcich et al. 1986; Willey et al. 1986); the amino acid sequence of the envelope proteins of different strains differ from each other by as much as 30 % of their residues. In spite of this variation there are 21 cysteine residues in the HIV-1 envelope which are perfectly conserved in all reported isolates (Gurgo et al. 1988). Even more surprising is the conservation of the same cysteine residues within the envelope proteins of simian immunodeficiency virus (Franchini et al. 1987; Hirsch et al. 1987; Chakrabarti et al. 1987) and HIV-2 (Guyader et al. 1987), which have only 30 %–40 % amino acid identity with the envelope of HIV-1. This conservation of cysteine residues suggests that they are highly important to HIV-1 envelope function, most likely through the contribution of disulfide bridges to the tertiary structure of the envelope proteins.

The envelope proteins of HIV-1, like those of other retroviruses, are synthesized as a precursor polypeptide (Allan et al. 1985; diMarzo-Veronese et al. 1985) glycosylated in the Golgi complex, modified by glycosyl trimming enzymes, and transported to the cell surface. The glycosylated envelope precursor protein (gp 160) is subsequently cleaved proteolytically into the mature gp120 outer membrane protein and the gp41 transmembrane protein. The gp120 binds to the CD4 molecule on the surface of the target cell (Dalgleish et al. 1984; Klatzmann et al. 1984; McDougal et al. 1986 a). After binding to CD4, the virion is internalized by fusion, either at the cell membrane (Stein et al. 1987) or within endocytosed vacuoles (Maddon et al. 1986). After the uncoating of the virion, reverse transcription of viral DNA is started.

To investigate the relationship of each of these steps to the viral life cycle and to analyze the contribution of cysteine residues in maintaining the necessary envelope protein structure, we constructed a series of HIV-1 envelope mutants in which cysteine residues were replaced by other amino acids and characterized them with respect to their biological activity (Tschachler et al. 1990).

M. M. Eibl, C. Huber, H. H. Decker, U. Wahn (Eds.)
Symposium in Immunology I
Symposium in Immunology II

Results and Discussion

Construction of HIV-1 Envelope Mutants

HIV-1 mutants in which cysteine residues in the envelope protein gp120 were replaced by other amino acids were constructed by subcloning either a 2.7-kb (*Sal*1 to *Bam*H1) or a 0.6 kb (*Bgl*II) restriction endonuclease fragment from the biologically active molecular clone pHXB2D (Fisher et al. 1986) into M13, performing site-directed mutagenesis using the method of Zoller and Smith (1984) and then inserting the mutagenized fragment back into pHXB2D. Clones were identified by differential hybridization with the appropriate mutagenic oligomers. The final constructs were all verified by direct DNA sequence analysis using plasmid DNA. The positions of the substituted cysteine residues and the amino acids substituted in their stead are listed in Fig. 1.

```
  1  M R V K E K Y Q H L W R W G W R W G T M L L G M L M I C S A
 31   T E K L W V T V Y Y G V P V W K E A T T T L F C A S D A K A
 61  Y D T E V H N V W A T H A C V P T D P N P Q E V V L V N V T
 91  E N F N M W K N D M V E Q M H E D I I S L W D Q S L K P C V
                         G  (cys-131)
121  K L T P L C V S L K C T D L K N D T N T N S S S G R M I M E
151  K G E I K N C S F N I S T S I R G K V Q K E Y A F F Y K L D
                                  V  (cys-196)
181  I I P I D N D T T S Y T L T S C N T S V I T Q A C P K V S F
211  E P I P I H Y C A R A G F A I L K C N N K T F N G T G P C T
241  N V S T V Q C T H G I R P V V S T Q L L L N G S L A E E E V
                                                    V (cys-296
271  V I R S A N F T D N A K T I I V Q L N Q S V E I N C T R P N
301  N N T R K S I R I Q R G P G R A F V T I G K I G N M R Q A H
     V  (cys-296)
331  C N I S R A K W N N T L K Q I D S K L R E Q F G N N K T I I
                                                  V  (cys-385)
361  F K Q S S G G D P E I V T H S F N C G G E F F Y C N S T Q L
                                          (cys-418)  S
391  F N S T W F N S T W S T K G S N N T E G S D T I T L P C R I
                                                  G  (cys-445)
421  K Q I I N M W Q E V G K A M Y A P P I S G Q I R C S S N I T
451  G L L L T R D G G N S N N E S E I F R P G G G D M R D N W R
481  S E L Y K Y K V V K I E P L G V A P T K A K R R V V Q R E K
511  R || A V

   gp120 -- gp41
```

Fig. 1. Amino acid sequence of gp120 of HTLV-IIIB as deduced from BH10 (Ratner et al. 1985). *Rectangles*, cysteine residues which have been mutated; *above*, the new amino acids. *Underlining*, unaltered cysteines

Biological Activity of Cysteine Substitution Mutants

Plasmids containing the respective cysteine substitution mutants were transfected into cos-1 cells. At 48 h after transfection, reverse transcriptase activity was assayed in the supernatant of transfected cos-1 cells. All mutant proviruses were able to release comparable amounts of reverse transcriptase into the media. Analyses by transmission electron microscopy of the transfected cos-1 cells revealed the presence of mature and immature viral particles in the cell medium or budding from the cell membrane (data not shown).

To measure virus transmission, transfected cos-1 cells were cocultivated with cell lines susceptible to HIV-1 infection for 24 h. With the exception of the Cys-385 mutant, none of the mutant viruses was demonstrably transmissable to any of the target cells (Fig. 2). The Cys-385 mutant could be transmitted to the T cell lines MT-2, H9, and CEM. Unlike the wild-type virus, however, the Cys-385 mutant was not transmissable to the monocytoid cell line U937. The rate of spread to the T cell lines, moreover, was considerably slower with the Cys-385 mutant than with the parental virus (Fig. 2).

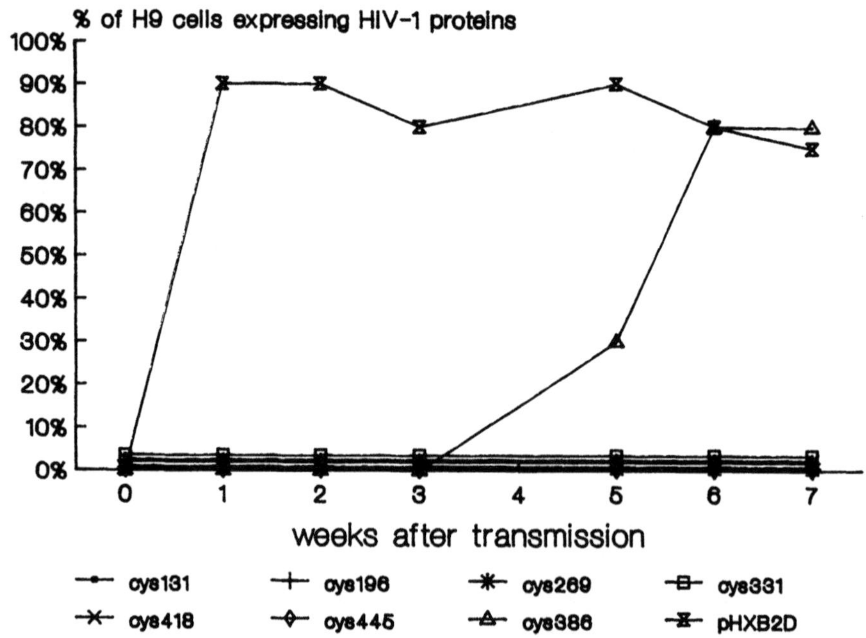

Fig. 2. Transmission of wild type and mutant viruses from transfected cos-1 cells to MT-2 cells. Either wild-type pHXB2D or the respective Cys mutant plasmids were transfected into cos-1 cells by electroporation. After 48 h cos-1 cells were cocultivated for 24 h with 2×10^6 H9 cells. Transmission of virus was monitored weekly by indirect immunofluorescence using defined sera of HIV-1 seropositive patients as first step reagents. *y-Axis*, percentage of HIV-1 positive cells within the different individual cultures

Biochemical Analysis of Envelope Expression by the Cysteine Substitution Mutants

After transfection into cos-1 cells the cysteine substitution mutants were analyzed for protein expression by radioimmuno-precipitation assays. As depicted in Fig. 3A, the HIV-1 gag protein p24 was detectable at comparable levels in lysates of cos-1 cells transfected with the different cysteine substitution mutants. The processing of the envelope precursor gp160, however, was impaired in Cys-296, Cys331, and Cys-418. Practically no gp120 was detectable in the cell lysates of these mutants, while the envelope precursor protein corresponded in size to the gp160 of wild-type virus. The quantify of cell-associated gp120 was reduced compared to wild-type with the Cys-445 mutation, whereas the amount of both gp160 and gp120 was reduced in cells transfected with the Cys-385 mutation. Immunoprecipitation of HIV-1 proteins from the supernatant of transfected cos-1 cells (Fig. 3B) confirmed the data obtained from the cell lysates; media gp120 was readily detectable with the three mutants for which cell-associated gp120 was

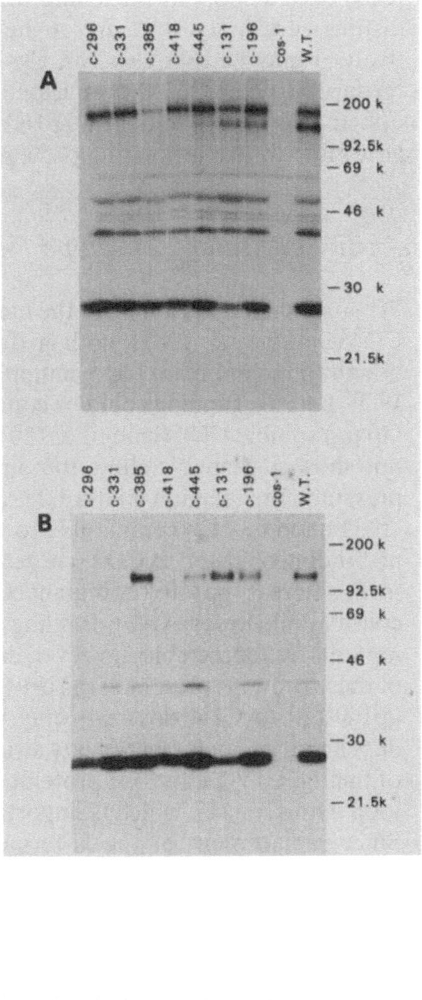

Fig. 3 A, B. Immunoprecipitation of viral proteins produced by cos-1 cells after transfection of wild-type (pHXB2D) or mutant HIV-1 genomes. pHXB2D or the different Cys-mutant plasmids were transfected into cos-1 cells by electroporation. After 24 h cells were cultured in cysteine/methionine-free medium substituted with [^{35}S] cysteine/methionine for 12 h. Cells were lysed in a NP40-containing lysis buffer as described (Tschachler et al. 1990). Immunoprecipitation was carried out by incubating the cell lysate with 10 µl mixture of sera from three HIV-1 seropositive patients followed by protein A-Sepharose beads. Immunoprecipitates were analyzed on a 10% polyacrylamide/sodium dodecyl sulfate (*A*) under reducing conditions. For detection of the viral proteins in the supernatant of transfected, readiolabeled cos-1 cells, the supernatant was cleared of residual cells by centrifugation and concentrated lysis buffer (4×) was added at a 1:4 ratio. Radioimmunoprecipitation was performed as described above (*B*)

demonstrated. Surprisingly, cells transfected with the Cys-385 mutant, which contained only low amounts of cell-associated gp120 and gp160, expressed levels of media gp120 comparable to those seen in pHXB2D. We were not able to detect gp160 in the media of cells transfected with either the wild-type virus or any of the mutants, which is in agreement with other reports (McCune et al. 1988; Guo et al. 1990) that suggest cleavage of the envelope precursor protein to be an obligatory step preceding its incorporation into virions.

The abrogation of the cleavage of gp160 of these mutants was not due to retention of envelope proteins in intracellular compartments since they were readily detectable by immunostaining on the surface of transfected viable cells (data not shown). We and others (McCune et al. 1988; Guo et al. 1990) have previously shown that alteration of the primary sequence at the envelope protein cleavage site abrogates cleavage. With the Cys-296, -331, -418, and -445 mutants, however, a modification of the primary sequence recognized by the cellular protease can presumably be excluded since the mutagenized cysteine residues are located 100–200 amino acids upstream of the cleavage site (residues 511, 512; di Marzo-Veronese et al. 1985). Our data suggest that the protease responsible for HIV-1 envelope cleavage not only recognizes a short linear amino acid sequence but is also dependent on a distinctive tertiary structure of the envelope precursor molecule. Alternatively, it may be that Cys-296, Cys-331, and Cys-418 are important for the tertiary structure of the envelope protein so that elimination of either cysteine residue results in a gp160 in which the cleavage site is no longer accessible to the processing protease.

Ability of Mutant Envelope Proteins to Bind to CD4

When we tested the ability of the mutant envelope proteins to bind to soluble CD4 (Smith et al. 1987), both gp160 and gp120 from wild-type virus readily bound to recombinant CD4 immobilized on CNBr-Sepharose beads (Fig. 4; W.T., lane a). Binding could be completely blocked by the addition of excess (10 μg) soluble CD4 (lane b) or (10 μg) OKT-4A monoclonal antibody (data not shown). Lanes c show the amount of radiolabeled envelope protein present in the reaction mixture. The gp160 and gp120 of mutants Cys-131 and -196 bound to CD4 comparable to wild-type envelope proteins. In contrast, no binding of gp160 to CD4 was detectable in mutants Cys-296, -331, -385 or -418 whereas gp160 of mutant Cys-445 bound to CD4 although to a considerable lower extent. Binding of gp120 proteins of the Cys-385 and -445 mutants was detectable, however, difficult to evaluate due to the low quantity of these proteins present in the cell lysates. These data suggest that binding of gp160/120 to CD4 does not only involve a linear epitope but is crucially dependent on an intact tertiary structure involving a relatively large portion of the the HIV-1 envelope protein. It has been inferred that Cys-418 forms a loop with Cys-445, which is important for CD4 binding (Lasky et al. 1987). Since replacement of the N-terminal cysteine of this loop (Cys-418), as

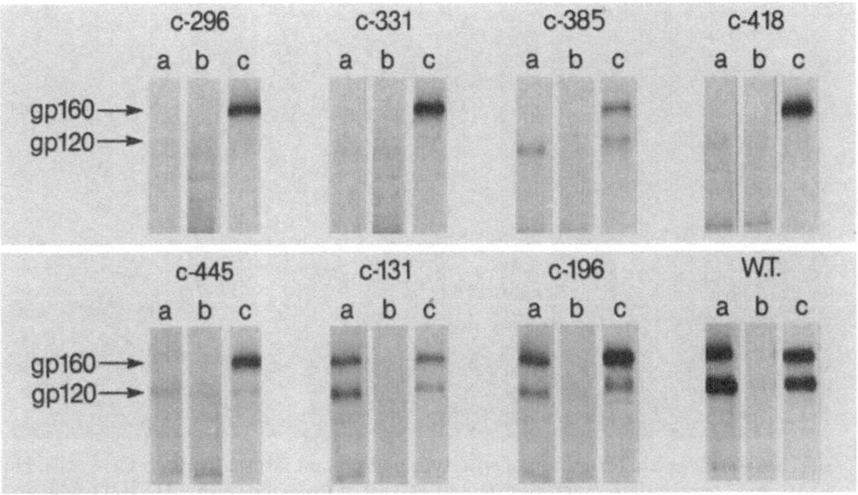

Fig. 4. Binding of wild-type and Cys-mutant envelope proteins to CD4. Cell lysates of radiolabeled cos-1 cells transfected with pHXB2D or the respective cysteine mutants were prepared as described in Fig. 3. Soluble CD4 immobilized on CNBr-Sepharose beads was added to equal amounts of cell lysates in the absence of free soluble CD4 (*lanes a*) or after preincubation of the lysates with 10 μg soluble CD4 (*lanes b*) and incubated for 16 h. After extensive washes in lysis buffer, samples were denatured by boiling in Laemmli buffer for 3 min and analyzed on a 8 % polyacrylamide sodium dodecyl sulfate gel. *Lanes c* show the immunoprecipitation of envelope proteins remaining in the lysate after the reaction for lane b has been performed

mentioned above, abrogates both envelope cleavage and CD4 binding, whereas replacement of the C-terminal cysteine (Cys-445) results in a gp160 which is processed to gp120 and retains some ability to bind to CD4, our data suggest that these two cysteine residues are not partners in a disulfide bond. Additional support for the importance of disulfide bonds in maintaining the proper tertiary structure of the HIV-1 envelope for envelope-CD4 interaction comes from data by McDougal et al. (1986 b), who found that reduction and alkylation of gp120 abrogate its capacity to bind to CD4.

Ability of Mutant HIV-1 Envelope Proteins to Form Syncytia

To test the ability of the mutant viruses to form syncytia, the cysteine mutant plasmids were transfected into HeLa CD4 cells (Maddon et al. 1986). Syncytium formation was evaluated 12–24 and 48 h posttransfection as described elsewhere (Tschachler et al. 1990). As shown in Fig. 5, wild-type pHXB2D induced the formation of large syncytia; however, the ability of all seven of the cysteine mutant viruses to form syncytia was vastly reduced with respect to both size and number, even in the case of the Cys-385 mutant (Fig. 5), which retains some infectivity.

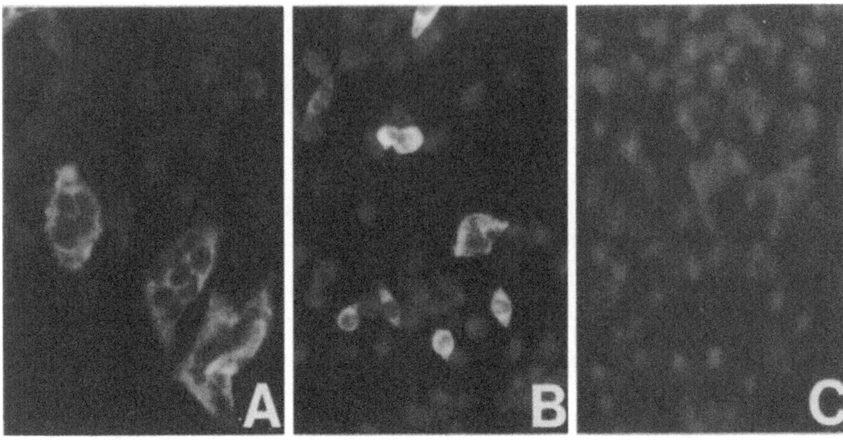

Fig. 5 A–C. Syncytia formation of wild-type and mutant viruses in HeLa CD4 cells. HeLa CD4 cells were either mock-transfected (*C*) or transfected with pHXB2D (*A*) or the Cys-385 mutant (*B*). Transfected cells were cultured in chamber slides for 12–24 h and subsequently fixed in methanol/acetone. Expression of HIV-1 proteins was detected by indirect immunofluorescence using a defined serum of a HIV-1 seroposive individual and a fluoresceinated goat anti-human Ig antiserum

The inability of the Cys-296, -331, and -418 mutants to form syncytia was not surprising since they are defective in both envelope cleavage and CD4 binding, both of which are indispensable for this function. In the case of Cys-385, the low amount of cell-associated envelope proteins could explain this functional impairment. Surprisingly, however, the replacement of the cysteines in the N-terminal part of gp120 (Cys-131 and -196) also abrogated the ability to form syncytia, even though neither envelope processing nor CD4 binding of these mutants was impaired. The lack of syncytia formation by these mutants argue for a function of gp120 subsequent to receptor binding, which is dependent at least in part on the structure of the N-terminal part of the gp120, and which is essential for cell fusion.

It was not clear whether the primary defect was in syncytium formation, resulting in an inability to infect target cells, or whether some other post-CD4 binding step, such as uncoating of the viral core, was adversely affected, and this lack of signicant syncytia formation was simply due to a lack of virus spread.

Summary

We report here the construction and characterization of mutants of a biologically active molecular clone of HIV-1, $\text{HTLV-III}_{\text{HXB2D}}$, in which individual cysteine residues within the large envelope protein gp120 were replaced by other amino acids. The strong conservation of cysteine residues in

HIV-1 envelope proteins had suggested that they were important in envelope function, probably at least in part by establishing and maintaining the protein tertiary structure through the formation of disulfide bridges during protein folding. The critical nature of cysteine residues in normal envelope function was confirmed by our data, which show that six of the seven cysteine substitution mutants tested lacked the ability reproducibly to infect any of the target cells used in these studies. The remaining mutant, in which Cys-385 was replaced by valine, was able to infect various T-cell lines but spread much more slowly than the wild-type virus. Substitutions in the N-terminal part of HIV-1 gp120 do not impair envelope cleavage, excretion, or CD4 binding but no abrogate detectable syncytium formation and infectivity. Substitutions in the carboxy half of the gp120 impair envelope cleavage, excretion, and CD4 binding (positions 296, 331 and 418) as well as syncytia formation and infectivity (postions 296, 331, 418, and 445). The results suggest that most or all of the cysteine residues of the HIV-1 large envelope protein are required for its functional integrity, and that an intact tertiary structure of the carboxy half of the gp120 is important for envelope cleavage and receptor binding and fusion, while that of the amino half is important in fusion or other post-CD4 binding events.

References

Alizon M, Wain-Hobson S, Montagnier L, Sonigo P (1986) Genetic variability of the AIDS virus: nucleotide sequence analysis of two isolates from African patients. Cell 46: 63–74

Allan JS, Coligan JE, Barin F, McLane MF, Sodroski JG, Rosen CA, Haseltine WA, Lee TH, Essex M (1985) Major glycoprotein antigens that induce antibodies in AIDS patients are encoded by HTLV-III. Science 228: 1091–1094

Chakrabarti L, Guyader M, Alizon M, Daniel MD, Desrosiers RC, Tiollais P, Sonigo P (1987) Sequence of simian immunodeficiency virus from macaque and its relationship to other human and simian retroviruses. Nature 328: 543–547

Dalgleish AG, Beverly PC, Clapham PR, Crawford DH, Greaves MF, Weiss RA (1984) The CD4 (T4) antigen is an essential component of the receptor for the AIDS retrovirus. Nature 312: 763–767

diMarzo Veronese FD, DeVico AL, Copeland TD, Oroszlan S, Gallo RC, Sarngadharan MG (1985) Characterization of gp41 as the transmembrane protein coded by the HTLV-III/LAV envelope gene. Science 229: 1402–1405

Fisher AG, Feinberg MB, Josephs SF, Harper ME, Marselle LM, Reyes G, Gonda MS, Aldovini A, Debouk C, Gallo RC et al. (1986) The trans-activator gene of HTLV-III is essential for virus replication. Nature 320: 367–371

Franchini G, Gurgo C, Guo HG, Gallo RC, Collalti E, Fargnoli KA, Hall LF, Wong-Staal F, Reitz MS Jr (1987) Sequence of simian immunodeficiency virus and its relationship to the human imunodeficiency viruses. Nature 328: 539–543

Guo H-G, diMarzo Veronese F, Tschachler E, Pal R, Kalynaraman VS, Gallo RC, Reitz MS Jr (1990) Characterization of a point mutation blocked in envelope glycoprotein cleavage. Virology 174: 217–224

Gurgo C, Guo H-G, Franchini G, Aldovini A, Collalti E, Farrell K, Wong-Staal F, Gallo RC, Reitz MS Jr (1988) Envelope sequences of two new United States HIV-1 isolates. Virology 164: 531–536

Guyader M, Emerman M, Sonigo P, Clavel F, Montagnier L, Alizon M (1987) Genome organization and transactivation of the human immunodeficiency virus type 2. Nature 326: 662–669

Hahn BH, Gonda MA, Shaw GM, Popovic M, Hoxie JA, Gallo RC, Wong-Staal F (1985) Genomic diversity of the acquired immune deficiency szndrome virus HTLV-III: different viruses exhibit greatest divergence in their envelope genes. Proc Natl Acad Sci USA 82: 4813–4817

Hirsch V, Riedel N, Mullins JI (1987) The genome organization of STLV-3 is similar to that of the AIDS virus except for a truncated transmembrane protein. Cell 49: 307–319

Klatzman D, Champagne E, Chamaret S, Gruest J, Guetard D, Hercend T, Gluckman JC, Montagnier L (1984) T-lymphocyte T4 molecule behaves as the receptor for human retrovirus LAV. Nature 312: 767–768

Lasky LA, Nakamura G, Smith DH, Fennie C, Shimasaki C, Patzer E, Berman P, Gregory T, Capon DJ (1987) Delineation of a region of the human immunodeficiency virus type 1 gp120 glycoprotein critical for interaction with the CD4 receptor. Cell 50: 975–985

Lifson JD, Feinberg MB, Reyes GR, Rabin L, Banapour B, Chakrabarti S, Moss B, Wong-Staal F, Steimer KS, Engleman EG (1986) Induction of CD4-dependent cell fusion by the HTLV-III/LAV envelope glycoprotein. Nature 323: 725–728

Maddon PJ, Dalgleish AG, McDougal JS, Clapham PR, Weiss RA, Axel R (1986) The T4 gene encodes the AIDS virus receptor and is expressed in the immune system and the brain. Cell 47: 333–348

McCune JM, Rabin LB, Feinberg MB, Lieberman M, Kosek JC, Reyes GR, Weissman IL (1988) Endoproteolytic cleavage of gp160 is required for the activation of human immunodeficiency virus. Cell 53: 55–67

McDougal JS, Kennedy MS, Sligh JM, Cort SP, Mawle A, Nicholson JK (1986 a) Binding of HTLV-III/LAV to T4+ Tcells by a complex of the 110K viral protein and the T4 molecule. Science 231: 382–385

McDougal JS, Nicholson JK, Cross GD, Cort SP, Kennedy MS, Mawle AC (1986 b) Binding of the human retrovirus HTLV-III/LAV/ARV/HIV to the CD4 (T4) molecule: conformation dependence, epitope mapping, antibody inhibition, and potential for idiotypic mimicry. J Immunol 137: 2937–2944

Ratner L, Haseltine W, Patarca R, Livak KJ, Starcich B, Josephs SF, Doran ER, Rafalski JA, Whitehorn EA, Baumeister K et al. (1985) Complete nucleotide sequence of the AIDS virus, HTLV-III. Nature 313: 277–284

Smith DH, Byrn RA, Marsters SA, Gregory T, Groopman JE, Capon DJ (1987) Blocking of HIV-1 infectivity by a soluble, secreted form of the CD4 antigen. Science 238: 1704–1707

Srinivasan A, Anand R, York D, Ranganathan P, Feorino P, Schochetman G, Curran J, Kalyanaraman VS, Luciw PA, Sanchez-Pescador R (1987) Molecular characterization of human immunodeficiency virus from Zaire: nucleotide sequence analysis identifies conserved and variable domains in the envelope gene. Gene 52: 71–82

Starcich BR, Hahn BH, Shaw GM, McNeely PD, Modrow S, Wolf H, Parks ES, Parks WP, Josephs SF, Gallo RC, Wong-Staal F (1986) Identification and characterization of conserved and variable regions in the envelope gene of HTLV-III/LAV, the retrovirus of AIDS. Cell 45: 637–648

Stein BS, Gwoda SD, Lifson JD, Penhallow RC, Bensch KG, Engleman EG (1987) pH-independent HIV entry into CD4-positive T cells via virus envelope fusion to the plasma membrane. Cell 49: 659–668

Tschachler E, Buchow H, Gallo RC, Reitz MS Jr (1990) Functionol contribution of cysteine residues to the human immunodeficiency virus type 1 envelope. J Virol 64: 2250–2259

Willey RL, Rutledge RA, Dias S, Folks T, Theodore T, Buckler CE, Martin MA (1986 Jul) Identification of conserved and divergent domains within the envelope gene of the acquired immunodeficiency syndrome retrovirus. Proc Natl Acad Sci USA 83(14): 5038–42

Zoller MJ, Smith M (1984) Oligonucleotide-directed mutagenesis: a simple method using two oligonucleotide primers and a single-stranded DNA template. DNA 3: 479–488

Clinical Aspects and Treatment

Immunodeficiency and Graft-versus-Host Disease: Opposing Features of Allogenic Bone Marrow Transplantation

C. Huber and *D. Niederwieser*

Introduction

Intensive chemo- and radiotherapy followed by allogenic bone marrow transplantation still represents the most successful modality for treatment of acute myelogenous leukemia [1]. The most prominent transplant-related complications are graft-versus-host disease (GvHD) and cytomegalovirus disease (CMVD). Whereas GvHD is caused by expansion of alloimmune T cells, CMVD is related to the severe immunodeficiency state following transplantation [1]. Interestingly, GvHD and CMVD are expressed simultaneously in many patients [2]. The negative effects of alloimmune hyperreactivity and immunodeficiency are counterbalanced by protection against recurrency of leukemia [3]. Although the graft-versus-leukemia (GvL) effect of allogenic bone marrow transplantation is clinically well established, the cellular mechanisms involved and their relationship to GvHD and CMVD are poorly understood. We summarize here recent experiments aimed at elucidating some of these questions.

In Vitro Characterization of Cellular Effector Mechanisms Directed Against Target Tissues of GvHD

To unravel cellular effector mechanisms responsible for GvHD a panel of cytotoxic T cell lines (CTL lines) were established from posttransplant T cells of allogenic bone marrow transplant recipients by stimulation with irradiated mononuclear blood cells harvested from the recipients prior to transplantation [4]. In the presence of interleukin-2 (IL-2) CTL lines and clones were established which exclusively lysed pretransplant hemopoietic cells but failed to kill donor targets. Such GvHD lines were established exclusively from patients suffering from clinical manifestation of GvHD. They expressed the CD8 phenotype and lysed targets carrying the appropriate minor histocompatibility antigen (mHA) in a class I MHC restricted fashion [4]. The latter was established by blocking experiments using monoclonal antibodies with specificity for class I MHC antigens and by formal segregation analyses in family studies.

GvHD lines which readily lysed hemopoietic cells such as mononuclear blood or bone marrow cells or PHA blasts carrying the appropriate mHA antigens were also tested for their capacity to destroy epidermal cells, which represent the natural targets of GvHD. Quite unexpectedly, both fresh epidermal cells and keratinocytes of recipients in vitro grown were found to resist lysis by GvHD CTL lines. This failure to lyse mHA^+ epidermal targets was bypassed by pretreatment with natural or recombinant interferon-gamma (IFN-γ). Pretreatment with interferon-alpha (IFN-α), tumor necrosis factor-alpha (TNF-α), or combinations of these cytokines failed to render the targets susceptible to CTL lysis.

Our interpretation of these findings is that GvHD-derived CTL lines recognize mHA antigens in context with class I MHC antigens. Whereas hemopoietic cells carry an abundent expression of the restricting class I MHC elements, epidermal cells reveal a low constitutive expression which is inadequate appropriately to present immunogenic peptides to CTLs. Inappropriate expression of the class I MHC restricting elements can be enhanced by IFN-γ [4, 5].

Characterization of Prerequisites for Clinical Manifestation of GvHD

We further examined whether prerequisites for in vitro lysis of keratinocytes were also required for the clinical manifestation of GvHD. The prediction from our in vitro experiments was that three factors are essential to cause tissue destruction by mHA-reactive CTLs. These are the presence of high frequencies of mHA-reactive CTL precursor cells (CTL-p) in context with in vivo expression of IFN-γ and enhanced class I MHC antigen biosynthesis. CTL-p frequencies were assessed by means of limiting dilution analyses [6] and endogenous IFN-γ levels by radioimmuno-assay measurements [7]. Assessments of seric levels of β_2 microglobulin (β_2m) and the polymorphic chain of HLA-A, B represented the means to estimate the overall endogenous MHC class I biosynthesis [5, 7, 8]. Measurements were performed prospectively in a large group of allogenic bone marrow transplant recipients during the first months following grafting. Results indicated that clinical disease expression was invariably preceded by and associated with detectable frequencies of mHA-reactive CTL-p in context with expression of endogenous IFN-γ levels and increased class I MHC antigen production [6, 7]. In contrast, patients who failed to demonstrate extensive GvHD also lacked detectable frequencies of mHA-reactive CTL-p and revealed low serum levels of IFN-γ and components of HLA-A, B [6]. These data suggest that IFN-γ mediated enhancement of HLA-A, B biosynthesis also represents an in vivo prerequisite for the clinical manifestation of GvHD.

CMVD Is Associated with Enhanced Endogenous Expression of IFN-γ and HLA-A, B Biosynthesis

As discussed previously, CMVD frequently precipitates GvHD. We therefore asked whether CMVD leads to enhanced expression of endogenous IFN-γ, thereby increasing susceptibility of GvHD target tissues to lysis by mHA-reactive T cells. Again, a large group of allogenic bone marrow transplant recipients were followed prospectively for reactivation of primary infection with CMV. In parallel IFN-γ levels and serum levels of HLA-A, B components were investigated [7]. Results demonstrated that patients with active CMV also exhibit high levels of endogenous IFN-γ and HLA-A, B components. We may conclude therefore that CMV infection, by its capacity to induce endogenous IFN-γ production, renders epidermal cells more susceptible to lysis by mHA-reacitve CTLs.

Characterization of Cellular Effector Mechanisms of GvL

In an attempt to characterize cellular effector mechanisms of GvL we established mHA-reactive clones from GvHD CTL lines. Clones were tested in parallel against mHA^+ normal targets and autologous leukemic cells (9). First clones derived from two patients with chronic myelogenous leukemia were able to lyse both autologous hemopoietic and epidermal targets as well as leukemic cells harvested prior to transplantation. These clones also inhibited clonal growth of leukemic cells in soft agar cultures. Destruction of leukemic cells and inhibition of their clonal growth both occurred without pretreatment with IFN-γ. Our present preliminary data suggest that the same cellular mechanisms mediating GvHD reactivity, at least in certain patients, are also responsible for GvL effects. These data, however, require further support by testing a larger group of leukemia patients.

References

1. Thomas ED, Appelbaum FR, Buckner CD et al. (1983) Marrow transplantation for acute nonlymphocytic leukemia. In: Gale RP (ed) Recent advances in bone marrow transplantation. Proceedings of the UCLA symposia, Vol. 61, Liss, New York
2. Tilg H, Vogel W, Herold M, Aulilzky WE, Huber C (1991) Cachexia and tumor necrosis factor alpha in CMN infection. J Clin Pathol 44: 519–520
3. Weiden P, Sullivan KM, Flurnoy N, Storb R, Thomas ED (1981) Antileukemic effect of chronic graft-versus-host disease. Contribution to improve survival after allogeneic marrow transplantation N Engl J Med 304: 15219
4. Niederwieser D, Huber C (1990) Cytokines in the regulation of MHC restricted T-cell functions: a human graft versus host disease model. In: Pichler WJ, Stadler BM, Dahinden CA et al. (eds) Progress in allergy and clinical immunology. Hogrefe and Huber, Toronto, 506
5. Niederwieser D, Auböck J, Troppmaier J, Herold M, Schuler G, Boeck G, Lotz J, Fritsch P, Huber C (1988) IFN-mediated induction of MHC antigen expression on human

keratinocytes and its influence on in vitro alloimmune responses. J Immunol 140: 2556–2561
6. Irschick E, Hladik F, Niederwieder D, Nußbaumer W, Holler E, Kolb HJ, Kminski E, Huber C (1992) Studies on the mechanism of tolerance of graft-versus-host disease (GvH-D) in allogeneic bone marrow recipients at the level of CTL-precursor frequencies. Blood 79: 1622–1628
7. Niederwieser D, Herold M, Woloszcuk W, Aulitzky W, Meister B, Tilg H, Gastl G, Bowden R, Huber C (1990) Endogenous IFN-gamma during human bone marrow transplantation: analysis of serum levels of interferon and interferon-dependent secondary messages. Transplantation 49: 1074–1080
8. Aulitzky WE, Grosse-Wilde H, Westhoff U, Tilg H, Aulitzky W, Gastl G, Herold M, Huber C (1991) Enhanced serum levels of soluble HLA class I molecules are induced by treatment with recombinant interferon gamma. Clin Exp Immunol 86: 236–239
9. Niederwieser D, Grasegger A, Auböck T, Herold M, Nachbaur D, Rosenmayr A, Gächter A, Nussbaumer W, Geissler D, Ritter M, Huber CH: Correlation of minor histocompatibility antigen (Mi-HA)-specific cytotoxic T-lymphocyte (CTL) with GvH-D status and analyses of tissue distribution. Blood (in press)

Clinical and Immunological Approach to the Diagnosis of Immunodeficiencies

H.H. Peter, M. Armbruster, E. Baumert, H.P. Buscher, R. Dräger, E.W. Herbst, A. Jahreis, A. Kliche, J.A. Rump, P. Vaith, G. Wolff-Vorbeck, and *M. Schlesier*

Introduction

The rational diagnosis of immunodeficiencies is increasingly gaining importance in clinical practice. The availibility of highly complex and expensive immunologic and molecular methods to identify subtle defects in the immune apparatus often contrasts with the limited immunological knowledge of the physicians in charge of immunocompromised patients. In this situation a practical guide for the diagnosis of immunodeficiencies may be helpful. Any evaluation should start with simple, informative, and inexpensive measures before proceeding to more complex, specialized, and expensive diagnostic procedures. Prime emphasis is placed on defects of the specific immune system, which account for 80%–90% of clinically relevant immunodeficiencies. The ultimate aim of each immunodiagnostic measure is the establishment of a validated diagnosis, the identification of etiological factors, and the proposal of a causal therapy. Our current knowledge on the ever-increasing number of primary and secondary immunodeficiencies and their classification is regularly updated in reports of an expert committee of the World Health Organization [1]:

Combined specific immunodeficiencies
- Severe combined immunodeficiency (SCID)
  - X-linked
  - Autosomal recessive
- Adenosine desaminase deficiency
- Purin nucleoside phosphorylase deficiency
- MHC class II deficiency
- Reticular dysgenesis

Predominant antibody deficiencies
- X-linked agammaglobulinemia
- X-linked agammaglobulinemia with growth hormone deficiency
- Ig deficiency with high IgM (hyper-IgM syndrome)
- Ig heavy-chain deficiency
- Kappa-chain deficiency
- IgA deficiency
- Selective IgG subclass deficiencies
- Common variable immunodeficiency (CVID)
- Transient hypogammaglobulinemia of infants
- Hypogammaglobulinemia associated with thymoma

M. M. Eibl, C. Huber, H. H. Decker, U. Wahn (Eds.)
Symposium in Immunology I
Symposium in Immunology II

Immunodeficiencies associated with other defects
- Wiskott-Aldrichsyndrome
- Ataxia teleangiectasia
- DiGeorge's syndrome

Complement deficiencies

Defects of phagocyte function
- Chronic granulomatous disease
  - X-linked
  - Autosomal recessive
- Leukocyte adhesion deficiency
- Chediak-Higashisyndrome
- Glucose-6-phosphate dehydrogenase deficiency
- Myeloperoxidase deficiency
- Deficiency of secondary granula

Basically, the immune defense is brought about by four modalities. A *physicochemical barrier protection* is conferred by the body surfaces of skin, respiratory system, gastrointestinal (GI) tract, and urogenitial (UG) tract. Penetration of these natural barriers by pathogenic agents immediately mobilizes *nonspecific cellular defenders* such as granulocytes, mononuclear phagocytes, and natural killer (NK) cells. Their activity is supported by *nonspecific humoral defense mechanisms* such as the bactericidal properdin and complement system, acute-phase proteins, and natural antibodies. Only if these immediately available natural defense principles fail to control invading pathogens does the highly specific and clonally organized *T and B cell system* localized in the lymphatic tissues move into action [2, 3]. The specificity of T and B cells resides in their receptors for antigen which are encoded for by variable gene segments; their rearrangement and selection during differentiation ensure an enormous combinatorial diversity. Activitation of T and B cells via specific antigen leads to amplification of the relevant cells and specific antibodies which ultimately outnumber and neutralize the invading pathogens.

The Clinical Approach

Of great clinical importance is a relevant definition of the "immunocompromised host." One consequence of such a definition is that it entails a series of diagnostic procedures to specify the defect. From our clinical experience we would consider someone as immunologically compromised if he presents with at least three infectious episodes of more than 4 weeks per year. Under these circumstances the clinician has a good chance to unravel some pathological abnormalities either by clinical or laboratory examinations.

Below we list 11 essential points in the clinical approach to diagnosis of immunodeficiency.

1. *Medical history:* family history, vaccinations, allergies, tumors, frequency and type of infections (upper and lower respiratory tract, skin, GI tract, UG tract), blood transfusions, drugs, sexual behavior, travel in tropical countries, nutrition.
2. *Clinical examinations:* exclusion of lymphoreticular diseases, malignancies, chronic bacterial, viral or parasitic infections, metabolic and autoimmune diseases, intoxications.
3. *Laboratory examinations:* blood formula, urinalysis, routine liver and kidney function tests, electrophroresis, clotting tests, zinc, iron, vitamins.
4. *Microbiology:* titers of lymphotropic viruses – human immunodeficiency virus (HIV), cytomegalovirus (CMV), Epstein-Barr virus (EBV), hepatitis B virus (HBV), herpes simplex virus (HSV) – isoagglutinins, tetanus and diphtheriaantitoxins, AST.
5. *Immunology:* quantitative immunoglobulins (IgM, A, G, E), possibly IgG and IgA subclasses, ANA, rheumatoid factors, etc.
6. *Exclusion of paraproteinemia:* immunoelectrophoresis, immunofixation.
7. *Complement diagnosis:* CH50, C3, C4, C3d.
8. *Delayed-type skin reactions (Multitest Merieux)*
9. *Cellular immune status in vitro:* this battery of tests is indicated if the above points make primary immunodeficiency seem likely, or if secondary immunodeficiencies are to be quantitated.
10. *Purin metabolism enzymes adenosine desaminase, purin nucleoside phosphorylase, and 5'-ectonucleotidase:* indicated only if SCID is suspected.
11. *Granulocyte function tests:* chemotaxis, phagocytosis, bactericidal activity, O_2^-, adhesion markers (indicated only if defective phagocyte function is suspected).

Information regarding points 1–8 is readily available in every outpatient clinic and private practice. Only for points 9–11 are specialized services and laboratories required. There is no rationale to proceed to points 9–11 unless points 1–8 clearly indicate a necessity.

A careful *medical history* is absolutely mandatory. We ask for type and frequency of infections, body surfaces involved (e.g., skin, upper or lower respiratory tract, GI tract, UG tract), allergies, tumors, and wound-healing problems. The inquiry also includes questions as to the family history (early child deaths, frequent infections, dwarfism, hormonal disturbances, consanguinity), vaccination history, sexual behavior, working conditions, drug, alcohol, and nicotin abuse, excessive sun exposure, infusion of blood products, and excessive exposure to toxic substances or radiation. A thorough *clinical examination* including chest X-ray and abdomen sonography helps to exclude lymphoma, nonlymphoid malignancies, severe chronic infections, autoimmunopathies, and chronic liver or kidney failure. *Routine laboratory tests* such as blood formula, electrolytes (including iron and zinc), serum proteins, and liver and kidney function tests complement the clinical findings. By means of *immunological screening tests* specific questions can be asked with regard to the defects in B and T cells, phagocytes, and complement system. These examinations include *for the B cell compartment:* quantitative determinations of serum IgG, A, M, and E, detection of paraproteins (immunofixation), measurement of specific antibodies to blood group antigens (isoagglutinins), vaccination recall antigens (tetanus and diphtheria toxoid) and lymphocytotropic viruses (e.g., HIV, CMV, EBV, HBV, HSV). *For the T cell compartment they include:* delayed-type hypersensitivity reactions checked by means of the multitest Merieux (readings after 30 min, 10, 24, 48, and 72 h (see below). *For phagocytes:* staining of blood smears for myeloperoxidase, tests of chemotaxis, phagocytosis, and bactericidal activity, and evaluation of oxidative burst (nitroblue tetrazolium, dihydrorhodamine assay). *For complement (C'):* total hemolytic C' activity (CH50), C3, C4, and C3d (indicator of increased intravascular C3 turnover).

Before proceeding to any in-depth analysis of immunological markers and functions the clinician can obtain valuable information as to which part of the immune system may be compromised. Recurrent upper and lower respiratory tract infections (possibly with formation of bronchiectasis) clearly point to a defective humoral immunity. Not all Ig classes must be diminished: *IgA and/or IgG2 subclass deficiency* may suffice to cause increased respiratory tract infections. IgA is the major secretory immunoglobulin, and IgG2 is the subclass which comprises mainly antibodies against polysaccharides of encapsulated bacteria (e.g., *Haemophilus influenzae, Streptococcus pneumoniae*). The absence of these two Ig classes readily explains the increased susceptibility to respiratory infections [4]. Similarly, the *association of IgA deficiency and atopic disease* with elevated IgE often causes chronic upper respiratory tract infections. *Severe hypogammaglobulinemia of all Ig classes* tends to be associated not only wiht respiratory infections but also with GI problems (mild diarrhea, lambliasis), skin infections, and development of malignancies. Underlying diseases may include non-Hodgkin lymphoma, Bence-Jones myeloma, renal or enteric protein loss, and protein-caloric malnutrition. Alternatively, hypogammaglobulinemia may be a sign of primary immunodeficiency such as X-linked congenital agammaglobulinemia (Bruton's disease: lack of peripheral B cells) or CVID, which after selective IgA deficiency is the second most frequent primary immunodeficiency syndrome in adults [5]:

Definition: early- or late-onset idiopathic hypogammaglobulinemia due to variable T and/or B cell disturbances

Inheritance: unclear, autosomal recessive

Clinical findings and prognosis: upper and lower respiratory tract infections (100 %), GI tract infections, gardiasis (50 %), nodular lymphoid hyperplasia or skin infections (20 %) autoimmune phenomena (30 %), and malignancies (20 %)

Prognosis: good if treated regularly by intravenous IgG, 300 mg/kg every 3–6 weeks

Occurrence of typical opportunistic infections such as *Pneumocystic carinii* pneumonia, chronic candidiasis, chronic diarrhea due to cryptosporidiosis, toxoplasmosis, atypical mycobacterial infections, reactivation of latent CMC and HSV infections clearly indicate a *compromised T cell compartment.* In infants these symptoms point to SCID:

Definition: inborn lack of functional T and B cells

Inheritance: autosomal recessive, or X-linked

Subsets: Reticular dysgenesis, SCID without T and B cells, SCID with B cells (Swiss type), adenosine desaminase or nucleoside phosphorylase deficiency, MHC class II deficiency

Clinical findings and prognosis: respiratory infections, diarrhea, dermatitis, candidiasis, infection from bacille Calmette-Guérin, septicemia, failure to thrive, onset around the 3rd month, death within 1–2 years unless treated by haplo/identical bone marrow transplantation.

In adults primarily HIV infection must be considered. According to the Center of Disease Control (CDC) the stages in classifying HIV-associated diseases are the following:

Stage I: acute mononucleosis like disease followed by seroconversion

Stage IIA: asymptomatic

Stage IIB: pathological laboratory values (thrombocytopenia, lymphopenia, CD4/CD8 ratio diminished, anergy)

Stage IIIA: generalized lymphadenopathy

Stage IIIB: pathological laboratory values (see IIB)

Stage IVA: general symptoms: weight loss over 10 %, fever lasting more than 1 month, diarrhea lasting more than 1 month

Stage IVB: neurological complications: dementia, myelopathy, progressive multifocal leukencephaloplakia, peripheral neuropathy

Stage IVC1: opportunistic infections: *Pneumocystic carinii,* cryptosporidiosis, toxoplasmosis of CNS, candidiasis, atypical mycobacteriosis, extrapulmonary tuberculosis, strongyloidiasis, recurrent salmonellosis, disseminated HSV, CMV retinitis

Stage IVC2: oral hairy leukoplakia, multidermatomal HSV, norcardiosis, *Candida* stomatis

Stage IVD: malignant tumors: Kaposi's sarcoma, non-Hodgkin's lymphoma, CNS lymphoma

Stage IVE: other symptoms: lymphoid interstitial pneumonia, Hodgkin's lymphoma, other tumors

Frequent skin infections from staphyloccoci suggest a *defect in granulocyte/macrophage function*. Recurrent neisserial infections are sometimes found in association with *defects in the late complement components (C5–C9)*. Overwhelming infections with encapsulated bacteria (pneumococci, meningococci, *Haemophilus influenzae*) are often encountered in splenectomized patients (overwhelming postsplenectomy infections). *Defects in the early complement components (C1–C4)* are regularly seen in collagen vascular diseases.

A particularly useful screening of immune functions in vivo is provided by the *Multitest Merieux*. The test antigens consist of tetanus toxoid, diphtheria toxin, streptococcal antigen, tuberculin (PPD), glycerine (control), candidin, trychophytin, and proteus antigen. Itching and flaring within 20–30 min suggest an IgE-mediated type I response. Positive skin reactions at 12–24 h point to the presence of precipitating IgG antibodies (type III or Arthus reaction). A positive reaction at 48–72 h is indicative of a delayed-type hypersensitivity or type IV reaction, according to Coombs and Gell. Over the age of 10 years the sum of the diameters of all positive type IV reactions normally exceeds 15 mm in men and 12 mm in women, with at least three out of seven positive reactions (Fig. 1). Frequent infections in conjunction with hypo- or dysgammaglobulinemia and/or an abnormal Multitest Merieux call, in our clinical practice, for the performance of a numerical and functional analysis of the peripheral T, B, and NK cell compartents (*cellular immune status*). Taking as examples SCID, CVID, and acquired immunodeficiency syndrome (AIDS), we outline the principles below of a basic test program for the detection of clinically relevant immunodeficiencies.

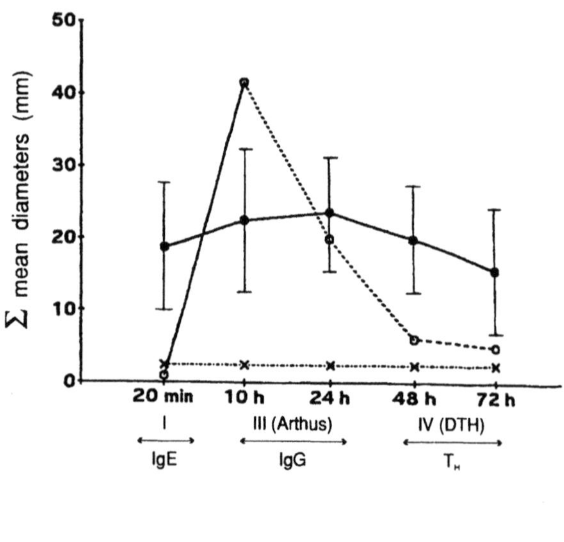

Fig. 1. Skin reactions obtained with Multitest Merieux in a group of 15 healthy male individuals (●—●), one patient with HIV infection CDC III (O—O), and one patient patient with CVID (x—x). The latter patient was totally anergic. The HIV patient exhibited a strong Arthus reaction (type III) after 24 h, while his delayed-type reaction (*DTH*) after 48 h (type IV) was negative due to impaired T cell immunity

Cellular Immune Status

The aim of any cellular in vitro testing is the development of reproducible in vitro correlates for immunodeficiency. Modern leukocyte phenotyping by cytofluorometry (FACS) and tests for lymphoproliferation, Ig synthesis, and cytotoxicity have proven to be reasonable in vitro correlates for disturbances of the peripheral T, B, and NK cell compartments, respectively. Some of the measurable abnormalities are so typical for certain immunodeficiencies that they are indispensable for the establishment of diagnosis.

Phenotyping of Lymphocyte Surface Markers

Although less sophisticated phenotyping may be performed with small whole-blood samples, the most frequently used technology involves isolation of peripheral blood mononuclear cells (PBL) by Ficoll-Hypaque gradient followed by double fluorescent staining with monoclonal antibodies specific for distinct surface markers and subsequent FACS analysis. Up to 100 surface markers have now been classified in "clusters of differentiation" (CD) [6], allowing the identification of many lymphocyte subpopulations. Table 1 summarizes normal ranges (percentage of PBLs) of CD markers that are

Table 1. Useful CD marker combinations in the diagnosis of immunodeficiencis: normal values (n=40)

Antigen detected	First marker (PE)		Second marker (FITC)		Double positive (%)
	Marker	%	Marker	%	
Isotype control	IgG2a	0	IgG1	0	0
Gate control	CD2	72–96	CD14	<2	<5
Ts/Th	CD8	14–45	CD4	35–72	<2
Naive CD4	CD45RA	22–58	CD4	35–72	14–43
Memory CD4	CD29	35–84	CD4	35–72	11–38
Homing CD4	Leu8	44–87	CD4	35–72	28–60
Activated T	CD3	69–93	HLA-DR	5–24	1–11
IL-2 receptor T	CD3	69–93	CD25	1–8	1–7
TCRαβ	CD3	69–93	TCRαβ	51–88	51–88
IL-2 receptor B	CD20	1–12	CD25	1–8	0–2
Autoreactive B	CD20	1–12	CD5	63–93	0–2
NK cells	CD3	69–93	CD16	4–20	<1
NK subtype	CD8	14–45	CD16	3–31	2–16
T suppressor	CD8	14–45	CD57	1–25	3–17
Immature B	sIg	1–20			
Mature B	cIg	1–5			

Percentage of gated lymphocytes staining positively with the respective markers; the ranges indicate the highest and lowest values in a group of 40 healthy controls aged from 21 to 57 years. PE, Phycoerythrin; FITC, fluorescein isothiocyanate; IL-2, interleukin-2; TCRαβ, T cell receptors α, β.

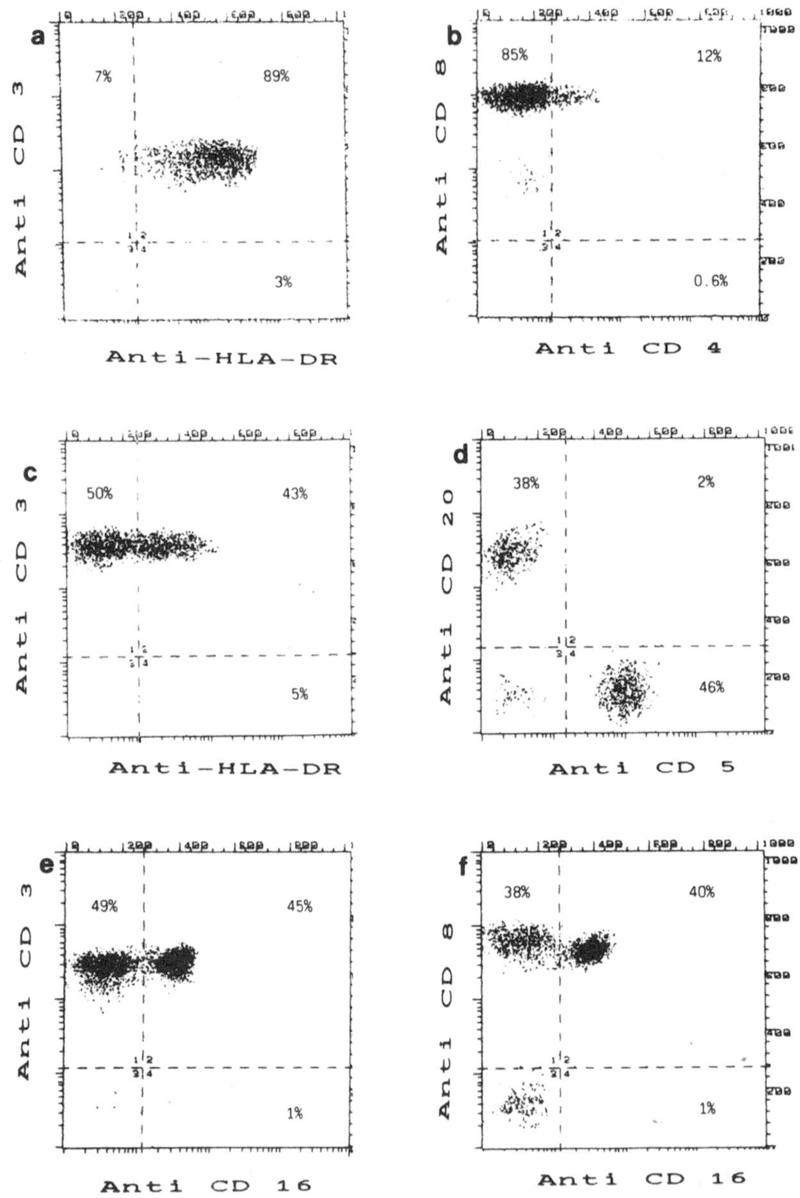

Fig. 2a–f. Highly abnormal blood lymphocyte phenotypes in patients with SCID, CVID, and AIDS. **a, b** Maternofetal graft-versus-host reaction in a 2-month-old infant with SCID. Virtually all T cells express CD8 and HLA-DR, indicating a population of highly activated cytotoxic T cells. Lymphoproliferation was completely negative (data not shown). **c** A 55-year-old female with CVID. Note the high proportion of activated HLA-DR^+, $CD3^+$ T cells (43 %; upper control limit 11 %). **d** A 45-year-old patient with a different type of CVID. Note the high percentage of 38 % $CD20^+$ B cells (upper normal limit 12 %). **e, f** A 46-year-old HIV-positive patient (stage CDC IVC1) with an exceptionally high proportion of $CD3^+$ $CD8^+$ $CD16^+$ T cells, considered as "aged killer cells" (normal <1 %)

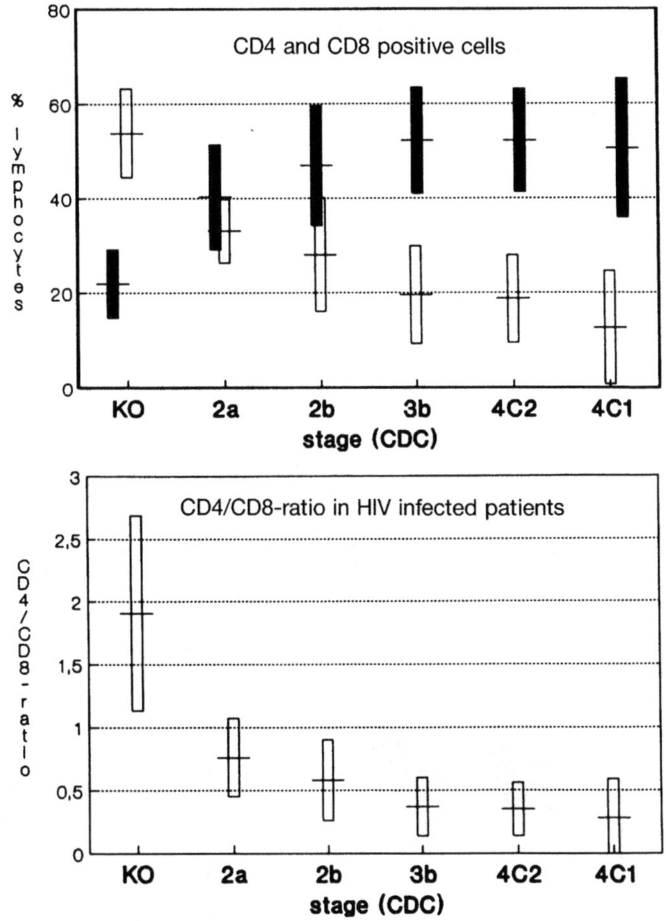

Fig. 3a, b. **a** Stage (CDC) dependent changes in $CD4^+$ (*white bars*) and $CD8^+$ (*black bars*) T lymphocytes in HIV-infected patients (n=91). **b** Concomitant changes in the CD4/CD8 ratio

currently used in our laboratory for the analysis of patients with immunodeficiencies. Besides the single markers, normal ranges of double positive cell populations are also given. Some typical phenotyping results of patients suffering from SCID, CVID, or AIDS are shown in Fig. 2. Lymphocyte phenotype changes occur during progression of AIDS (Fig. 3) or may be used to classify subtypes of CVID and SCID (Figs. 4, 5) [7].

Of considerable relevance is lymphocyte analysis in tissues. Notably, immunohistochemistry of gut biopsies obtained from CVID patients provides interesting insights into the pathophysiology of this diesease. Besides nodular lymphoid hyperplasia, seen in 40 %–50 % of these patients, most of them completely lack IgA producing plasma cells in their lamina propria (Table 2; Fig. 6). This finding may explain the great susceptibility to mucosal infections in CVID.

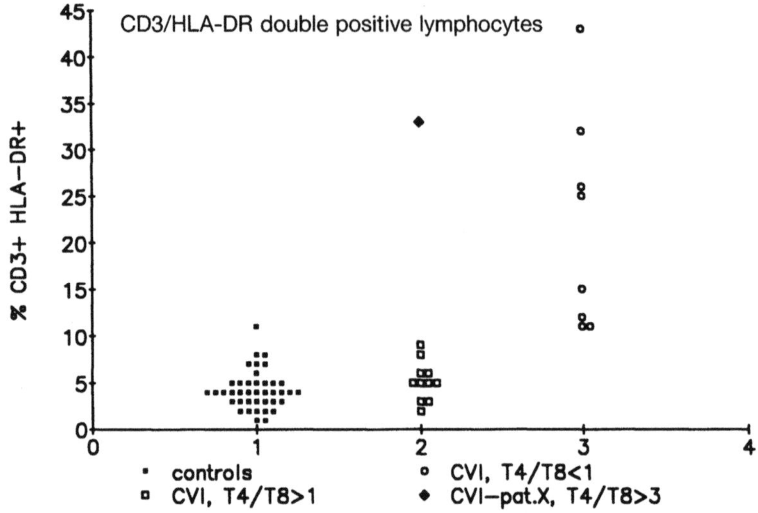

Fig. 4. Classification of CVID patients. The group with low CD4/CD8 ratio tended to have high proportions of activated $CD3^+$ HLA-DR^+ T cells; they were often anergic on the Merieux Multitest and presented with more severe disease. One patient (◆) with an exceptionally high CD4/CD8 ratio and 34 % of $CD3^+$ HLA-DR^+ T lymphocytes belonged to a CVID subgroup with sarcoidlike lesions in liver and bone marrow [12]

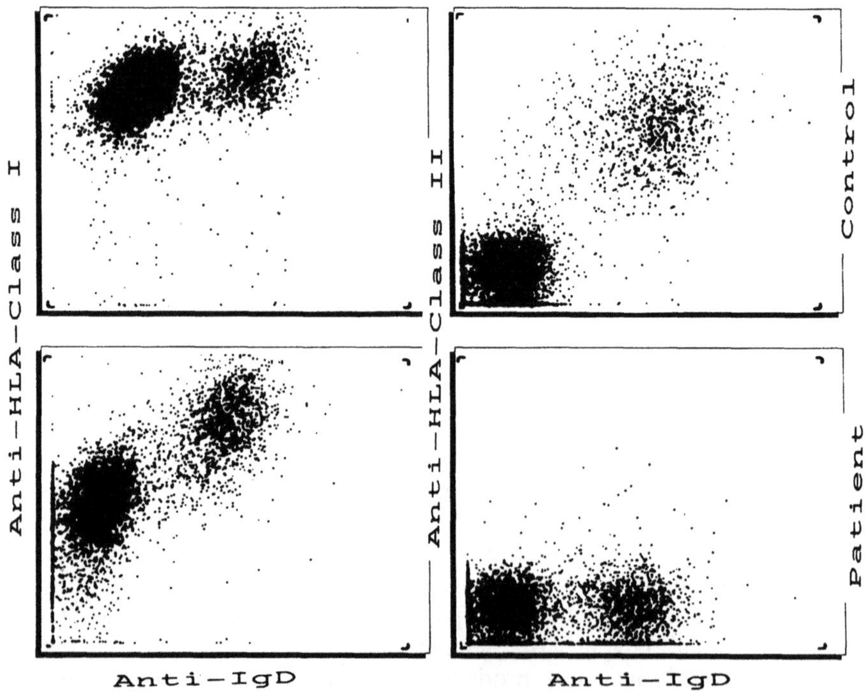

Fig. 5. Double-marker FACS analysis of lymphocytes from an infant with MHC class II deficiency (kindly donated by Dr. M. Hadam, Med. Hochschule Hannover)

Table 2. Percentage of plasma cells in gut biopsies of patients with CVID

Patient no.	Serum Ig (g/l)			Gut plasma cells (%)					
	IgG	IgA	IgM	IgA1	IgA2	IgM	IgG	J	S
1	2.0	0.3	0.2	0[§]	0	1	5	10	++
2	5.0	0.3	0.9	0	0	4	3	4	+
3	5.5	0.4	1.2	13	9	5	9	11	++
4	4.2	1.3	0.4	11	7	11	10	13	+++
5	4.8	0.3	0.3	0	0	14	13	0	++
6	1.8	0.3	0.3	0	0	0	2	8	+
7	2.9	0.3	0.3	0	0	3	6	nt	0
8	4.6	0.4	0.2	0	0	0	4	3	+++
9	4.9	0.4	1.0	12	3	8	4	2	+
10	1.2	0.3	0.2	0	0	10	4	4	++
Controls (range)	8–18	0.5–4.5	0.6–2.8	25–50	nt	3–20	4–18	25–100	+

[§] Percentage of positive cells of 200 counted mononuclear cells in the lamina propria of small intestine biopsies. J, J-chain; S, secretory component in epithelial cells of the gut; nt, not tested.

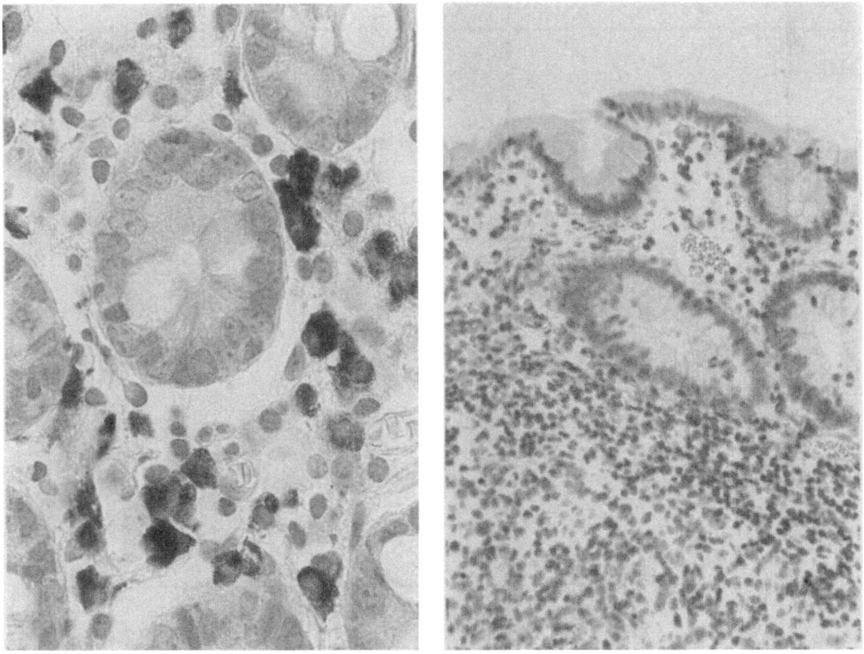

Fig. 6a, b. **a** IgA1-producing plasma cells in a duodenal biopsy of a healthy person. **b** Complete absence of these cells in a patient with CVID and nodular lymphoid hyperplasia; note the lymphoid infiltration of the lamina propria and the atrophy of the villi

Lymphocyte Proliferation

Proliferative responses in vitro to mitogens, antigens, and allogeneic cells (mixed lymphocyte culture) are typical features of immunocompetent, lymphokine-producing T cells. Therefore, any severe T cell deficiency is detected by this method, which is based on [^{3}H]thymidine uptake by 3- or 6-day-old mitogen- or antigen-driven lymphocyte cultures, respectively [3]. Subtle T cell defects may still respond normally to T cell mitogens, while being

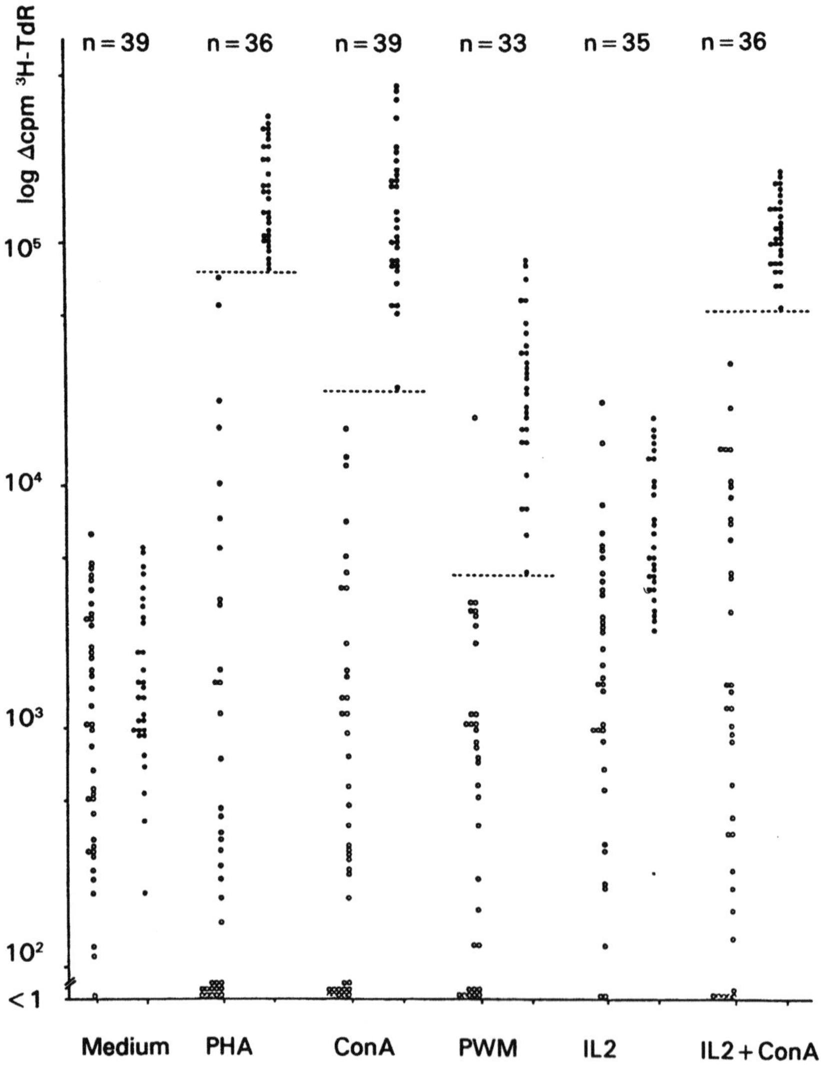

Fig. 7. Impaired lymphoproliferation of blood lymphocytes from SCID infants (—○—; n=39) compared to healthy control persons (—●—; n=31). *PHA*, phytohemagglutin; *ConA*, concanavalin A; *PWM*, pokeweed mitogen; IL2, interleukin-2

unresponsive to antigens. A complete or nearly complete failure of T cells to respond to mitogens is the diagnostic hallmark of SCID (Fig. 7). T cell hyporesponsiveness is also seen in advanced AIDS, severe chronic infections, lymphomas, leukemias following aggressive cytostatic or radiation therapy and in some patients with CVID. Prolonged periods of reduced T cell responsiveness always signify a poor prognosis.

Natural Lymphoytotoxicity

Spontaneous, non-MHC restricted killing of various tumor cell lines has been identified as a distinct feature of NK cells [8]. This "third population" of lymphocytes accounts for less than 10% of PBL. It is heterogeneous with regard to surface markers; the majority of NK cells carry CD2, CD16, CD56, and low CD8, and a subpopulation express CD57. An antigen receptor has so far not been identified, nor is the in vivo function of these cells evident. They seem to play a role in controlling extramedullary hematopoiesis and metastatic tumor cell spread. Cytotoxic activity is measured in a short-term ^{51}Cr release assay which involves the killing of the erythroleukemia cell line

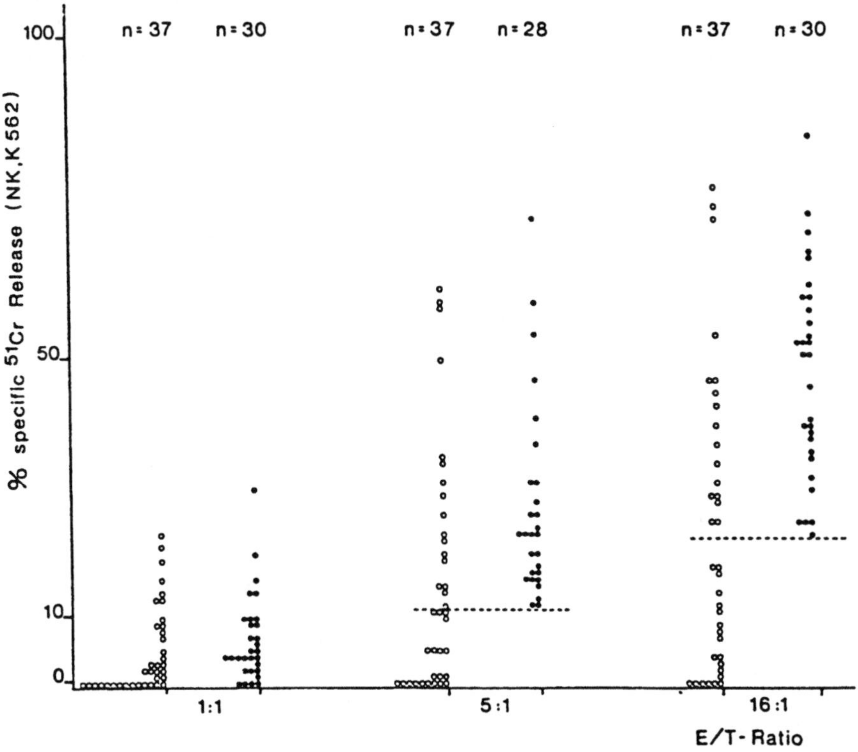

Fig. 8. NK cell activities in SCID infants (—●—) and healthy control persons (—○—). Half of the patients exhibit impaired NK cell activity

K562 at an increasing effector/target ratio. In some immunodeficiencies NK cell activity is depressed or absent. Notably, half of the SCID infants lack NK cell function (Fig. 8) [9]; similarly, in advanced AIDS, in disseminated malignancies and in patients with chronic parasitic disease NK cell function is usually depressed.

Ig Synthesis In Vitro

PBLs stimulated with pokeweed mitogen or staphylococcal Cowan I lysate for 9 days produce great amounts of IgG, IgM, and IgA due to polyclonal plasma cell differentiation. A substantial proportion of patients with CVID or other types of immunodefiency fail to produce any immunoglobulins in vitro (Fig. 9); some CVID patients' lymphocytes manage to produce still low amounts of IgM. CVID patients are currently being classified according to their capacity to produce IgG and IgM in vitro following stimulation with anti-IgM and IL-2 [10] (Table 3). Patients in group A fail to produce Ig with any stimulant used, those in group B produce IgM but no IgG, and those in group C show no defect of their in vitro Ig production but fail to produce Ig in vivo. A similar grading is achieved by stimulating PBL from CVID patients with staphylococcal Cowan I lysate and pokeweed mitogen (Fig. 9) [11]. So far there is no clearcut correlation between the CVID classification based on T cell surface markers (Fig. 4) [12] and Ig synthesis in vitro (Table 3; Fig. 9).

Table 3. Classification of CVID patients (n=52) by production of immunoglobulins in vitro using anti-IgM and interleukin-2 (from [10])

Group	Ig production in vitro	*n*
A	B cells unable to produce IgG and IgM	20
B	B cells able to produce IgM	14
C	B cells able to produce IgG and IgM	13
D	no B cells present in blood	5

Conclusions

Diagnosis of immunodeficiency has gained increasing importance in daily clinical practice. Therefore, performing a rational diagnostic work-up of patients suspected of suffering from immunodeficiency is no longer the domain of a few highly specialized experts. Here we outline a clinical and laboratory procedure designed to identify numerical and functional abnormalities in blood and tissue lymphocyte compartments of three specific immune defects – SCID, CVID, and AIDS. Whereas lymphocyte phenotyping by FACS analysis has reached a high degree of sophistication and reliability,

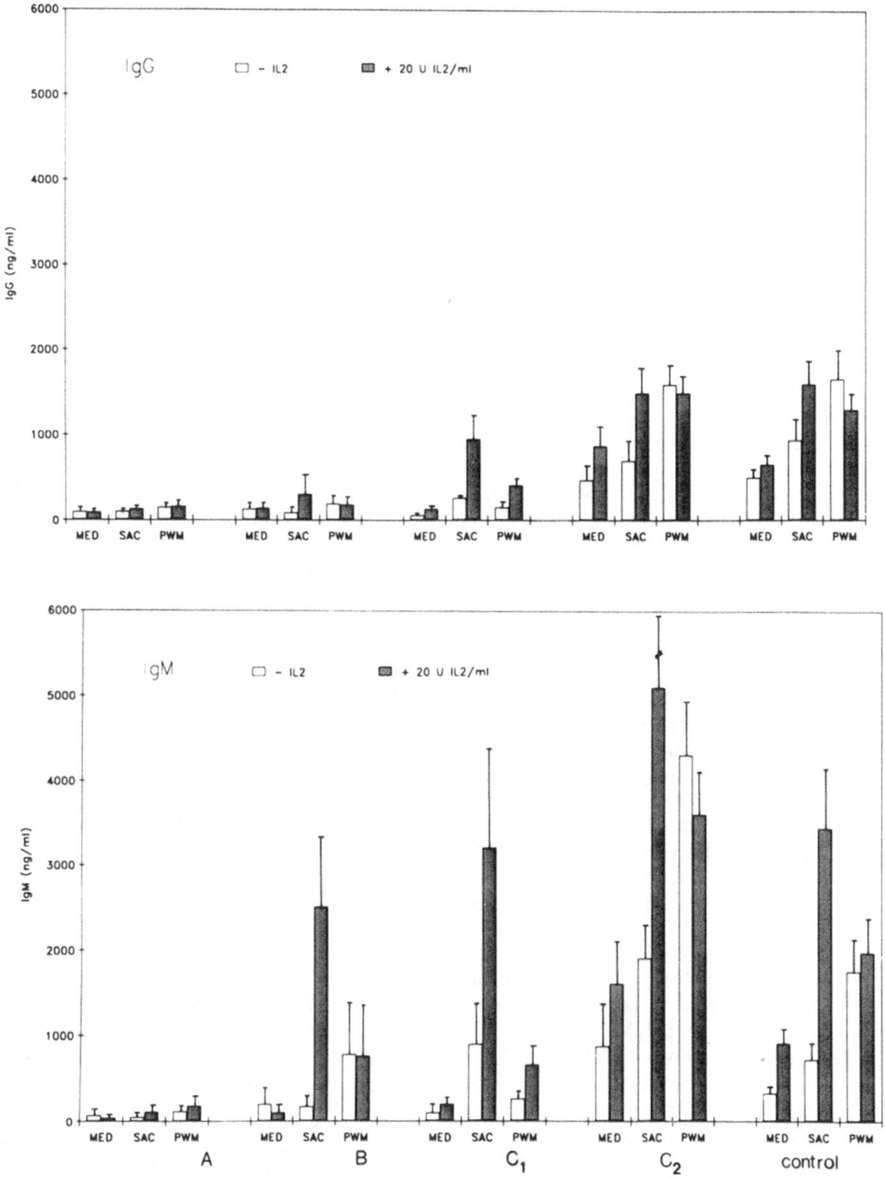

Fig. 9. IgM and IgG production in vitro by PBL from 25 CVID patients and 10 healthy controls following stimulation with medium (*MED*), *Staphylococcus aureus* Cowan I (*SAC*), or pokeweed mitogen (*PWM*) in the presence or absence of exogenous interleukin-2 (IL2; 20 U/ml). Cumulative IgM and IgG concentrations (ng/ml) were measured in 9-day culture supernatants by enzyme-linked immunosorbent assay. Patients were classified according to a modified scheme of Bryant et al. [10] (see Table 8): *A*, no IgM or IgG synthesis irrespective of stimulant and IL2 (n=9); *B*, normal IgM but no IgG synthesis (n=4); C_1, normal IgM and IgG synthesis only after exogeneous IL2 substitution (n=5); C_2, normal IgM and IgG synthesis after PWM stimulation without IL2 substitution (n=7). Results are expressed as mean ± SEM [11]

functional assays such as those for T and B cell proliferation, NK cell activity, and Ig production in vitro still suffer from technical drawbacks, making these tests less than perfectly comparable from one laboratory to another. However, as long as more sophisticated, molecular methods are not yet available, functional in vitro tests are indispensable for the diagnosis of primary immunodeficiencies.

Acknowledgements. This research was supported by Deutsche Forschungsgemeinschaft grant Pe 151/9-3.

References

1. WHO Meeting Report (1989) Primary immunodeficiency diseases. Immunodefic Rev 1:173–205
2. Hitzig WH, Griscelli C (1986) Pädiatrische Immunologie – Angeborene und erworbene Immundefekte. Thieme, Stuttgart
3. Schlesier M, Dräger R, Wolff-Vorbeck G, Peter HH (1991) Methoden zur Abklärung der Immundefizienz. Klinische Immunologie, vol 9, chap 8., Urban and Schwarzenberg, Munich (in press)
4. Hanson LÄ, Söderström T, Oxelius VA (1986) Immunoglobulin subclass deficiencies. Monographs in allergy, vol 20. Karger, Basel
5. Cunningham-Rundles C (1989) Clinical and immunologic analysis of 103 patients with common variable immunodeficiency. J Clin Immunol 9: 22–33
6. Knapp W, Dörken B, Rieber EP, Stein H, Gilks WR, Schmidt RE, Von dem Borne AEGKr (eds) (1989) Leukocyte typing: IV white cell differentiation antigens. Oxford University Press, Oxford
7. Wright JJ, Wagner DK, Blaese RM, Hagengruber C, Waldmann TA, Fleisher TA (1990) Characterization of common variable immunodeficiency: identification of a subset of patients with distinct immunophenotypic and clinical features. Blood 76: 2046–2051
8. Hersey P, Bolhuis R (1987) Nonspecific, MHC unrestricted killer cells and their receptors. Immunol Today 8: 233–239
9. Peter HH, Kliche A, Dräger R, Schlesier M, Vaith P, Blütters-Sawatzki R, Ebell W, Friedrich W (1986) NK cell function in SCID: possible relevance for classification and prognosis. In: Griscelli C, Vossen J (eds) Progress in immunodeficiency research and therapy II. Elsevier, Amsterdam, pp 287–295
10. Bryant A, Calver NC, Toubi E, Webster ADB, Farrant J (1990) Classification of patients with common variable immunodeficiency by B cell secretion of IgM and IgG in response to anti-IgM and interleukin-2. Clin Immunol Immunopathol 56: 239–248
11. Rump JA, Jahreis A, Schlesier M, Dräger R, Melchers I, Peter HH (1992) Possible role of IL-2 deficiency for hypogammaglobulinemia in patients with common variable immunodeficiency. Clin exp Immunol 89: 204–210
12. Baumert E, Wolff-Vorbeck G, Schlesier M, Peter HH (1992) Immunophenotypical alterations in a subset of patients with common variable immunodeficiency (CVID). Clin exp Immunol 90: 25–30.

Bone Marrow Transplantation in the Treatment of Congenital T Cell Disorders

W. Friedrich, C. Knobloch, and *W. Hartmann*

Introduction

Bone marrow transplantation (BMT) plays a central role in the management of congenital immunodeficiencies characterized by profound abnormalities of the T cell system [10, 14, 19]. This heterogeneous group of disorders may be corrected by the establishment of a new, donor-dependent immmune system. BMT in these disorders also represents a unique model to study and to define cellular interactions which are operative in the functional reconstitution of the lymphohemopoietic system in man.

There are several specific aspects to BMT in the therapy of congenital immunodeficiency disease as compared to other disorders. Since the hemopoietic system is usually intact, and since there is a diminished or even absent potential for graft rejection, significant modifications of the transplant procedure may be possible. Since BMT represents, with few exceptions, the only therapeutic alternative in these otherwise lethal disorders, and since it is exceptional to have an HLA-compatible donor, transplant attempts using alternative donors habe been extensively explored. Recently, broad experience has been gained in the use of T cell depleted BMT using HLA-haploidentical parents as donors [3, 15].

Here we review current experience of the use of BMT in particular in patients with severe combined immunodeficiency (SCID), with an emphasis on the use of HLA-nonidentical donors and several of the issues related to this approach.

BMT in Severe Combined Immunodeficiency

General aspects

SCID represents a group of disorders characterized by profound abnormalities of both T and B cell mediated immunity. Although clinically fairly homogeneous, with early onset of serious infections and, if unrecognized, rapid clinical detoriation and death within the first 2 years of life, affected infants nevertheless constitute a heterogeneous group of patients with variable immunological, genetic, and pathological findings as well as a heterogeneous pathogenic basis of the underlying immunological defect [1,

19, 21]. The first successful BMT in a SCID patient was performed in 1968, and this patient has reached adulthood by now [9]. Results of BMT have been reviewed periodically, documenting continued progress with a overall success rate now exceeding 80 % when using HLA-compatible donors [1, 3, 4, 13]. This improvement also reflects important advances in supportive care. Effective treatment and prevention of infections such as pneumonia from *Pneumocystis carinii* and fungal disease are possible now. Severe nutritional deficiencies secondary to chronic intestinal infections can usually be controlled by prolongued use of total parenteral nutrition. Full compensation of humoral immunodificiency can be achieved by providing intravenous immunoglobulins in high amounts. Also, better knowledge and awareness of these rare disorders has led to earlier recognition and referral of affected infants.

HLA-Identical BMT

While only rarely an option – in our experience only 6 of 55 patients with SCID had a compatible sibling – HLA-identical BMT has become almost a standard procedure. The rate of complications from graft-versus-host disease (GvHD) has been remarkably low, with almost no documented cases in the literature of severe chronic GvHD. Most importantly, HLA-identical BMT from sibling donors is performed without the use of conditioning treatment. Following infusion of marrow cells, previously absent cellular immune functions develop rapidly within a few weeks, presumably reflecting engraftment of an expanding pool of postthymic T cells contained in the marrow graft. The reconstitution by T cells derived from lymphoid precursor cells following passage through the host thymus apparently is slow, as is evidenced by the gradual appearance of radiologically visible thymic tissue after BMT.

At the time of the development of cellular immunity, the patient may occasionally develop florid symptoms from existing, previously more silent infections, reflecting the capacity to mount an inflammatory response. In a rare patient, this may lead to a dramatic clinical detoriation, as we have observed in a child suffering from previously controlled mycobacterial infection caused by bacille Calmette-Guérin.

A majority of patients with SCID have circulating, nonfunctioning B lymphocytes detectable at diagnosis. Interestingly, the reconstitution of humoral immunity has been shown to result from the functional maturation of these B cells [11]. In patients lacking B cells (patients B – SCID), humoral immune reconstitution, on the other hand, has been noted to be more variable. The particular transplant approach in SCID, with no cytoreductive conditioning used prior to BMT, leads to a unique state of lymphohemopoeitic chimerism, with T cells derived from the donor and all other blood elements remaining of host type.

BMT from HLA-Nonidentical Donors

HLA-nonidentical BMT in SCID, as in any other disorder, has been associated with an unacceptably high rate of severe, usually uncontrollable complications from GvHD [10, 13]. By removing mature T cells from the marrow graft, the risk of this complication can be significantly reduced. This approach was successfully introduced in the treatment of SCID in 1982 by Reisner et al., using HLA-haploidentical parents as donors [18]. A number of studies have subsequently confirmed the usefulness of this strategy [3, 4, 7, 8, 15], and T cell depleted BMT has opened now the possibility of curative treatment in each newly diagnosed patient regardless of the availability of a matched donor.

Several important issues, however, have emerged with extended experience of HLA-haploidentical BMT. While complications of GvHD are prevented to a large extent, the course and outcome of these transplants may vary significantly. Most importantly, when performed in a conventional way, i.e., without using cytoreductive conditioning prior to BMT, immunological reconstitution may not develop to the same extent as observed in HLA-matched BMT. This is also demonstrated by our own experience in 24 infants with SCID transplanted from HLA-haploidentical parents. Of these, 12 patients (50%) developed normal T cell functions, while in the others reconstitution either failed completely (six cases) or remained subnormal. Furthermore, the process of Tcell reconstitution by donor cells is slow, usually extending over the course of several months, as is demonstrated in Fig. 1.

Another unexpected observation – again one that is in contrast to the common experience in HLA-identical BMT – is that B cells in patients with B^+ SCID frequently fail to maturate fully in spite of normal functions of donor-derived T cells. Furthermore, in our experience, patients lacking autologous B cells (B^- SCID) have remained severely hypogammaglobuli-

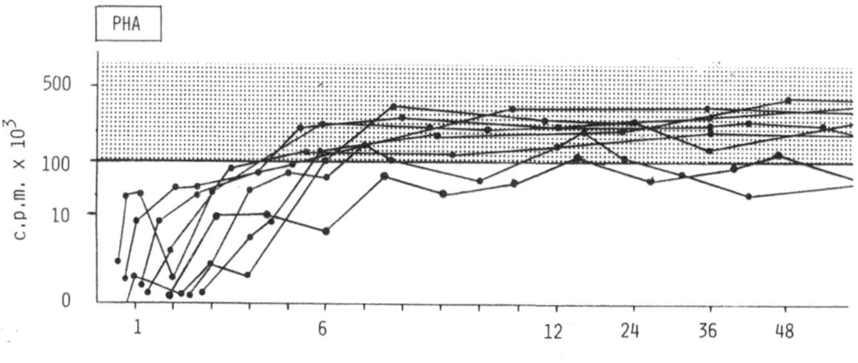

Fig. 1. The course of Tcell reconstitution as determined by sequential phytohemagglutinin mitogen responsiveness in eight patients with SCID following HLA-haploidentical BMT without conditioning

nemic. No engraftment of donor B cells has been observed in these cases. The basis of this unexpected outcome with insufficient B cell reconstitution by host B cells and failure of donor B cell engraftment remains poorly understood. Even with extended observation times of several years after BMT and stable, normal reconstitution of T cell immunity, humoral immune functions have remained insufficient in most patients studied by us (see Fig. 2).

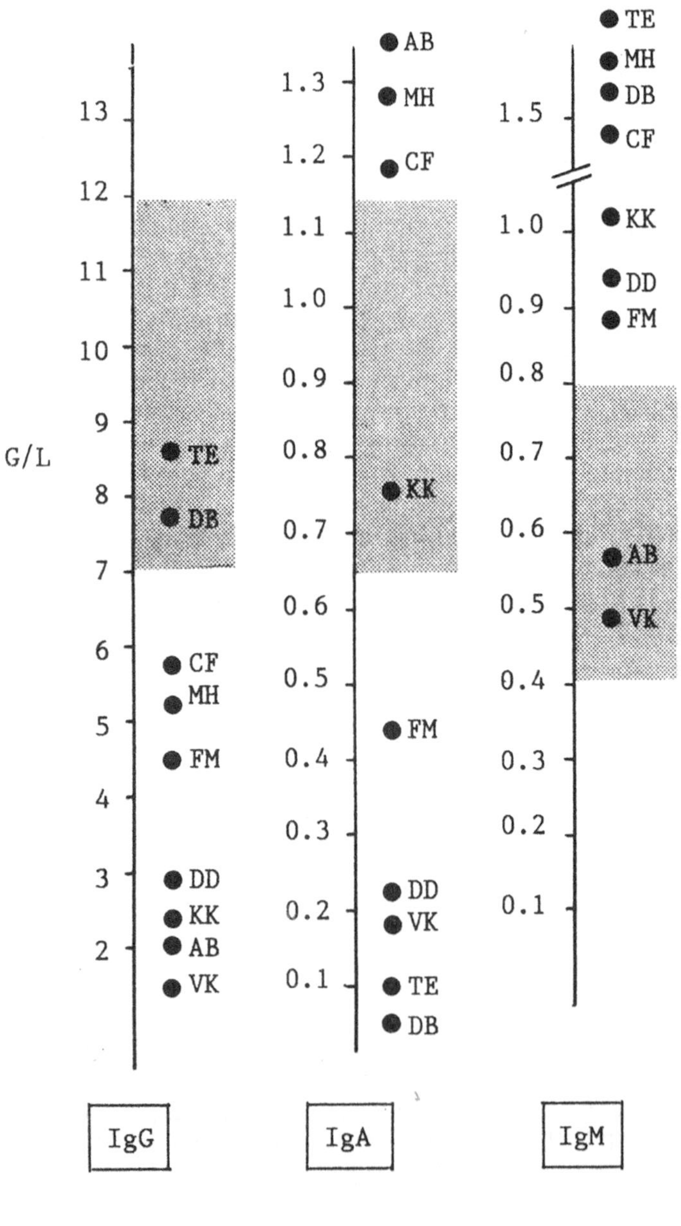

Fig. 2. Immunoglobulin serum levels in nine patients with B^+ SCID after HLA-haploidentical BMT. All patients had normal T cell immunity and were between 4 and 7 years after BMT. *Shaded area*, normal ranges (2 SD) in age-matched controls

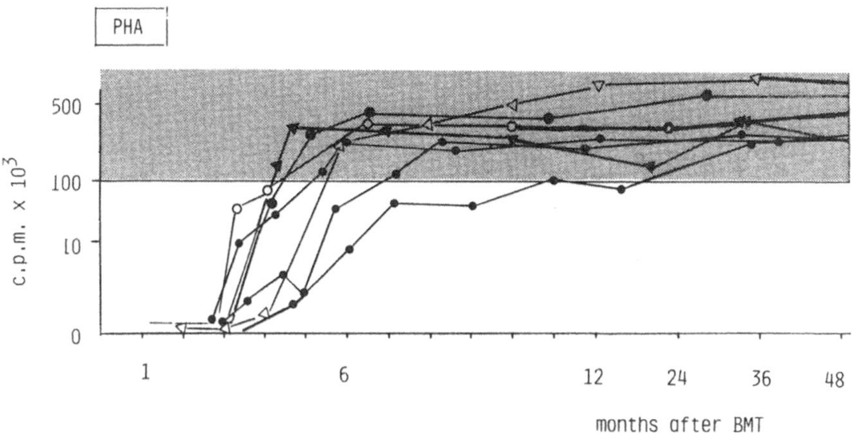

Fig. 3. The course of T cell reconstitution in seven patients with SCID following BMT with prior cytoreductive conditioning. *Open bars*, two patients who had failed previous transplants attempts

To improve donor cell engraftment and immunological reconstitution, cytoreductive conditioning prior to BMT has been introduced. Figure 3 demonstrates the course of T cell reconstitution as observed in a group of patients following BMT with conditioning. Of note, the time course to develop normal T cell immunity was comparable to that of patients shown in Fig. 1, with a similar delay of several months, reflecting the slow maturation of lymphoid precursor cells. The use of conditioning also markedly improved the outcome in regard to humoral immune reconstitution, as is shown in Fig. 4.

Not unexpectedly, the use of conditioning unfortunately may induce complications from toxicity, which in our experience have occasionally been severe and lethal. Also, for undetermined reasons, the incidence and severity of complications from GvHD have been noted to be more significant in this group as compared to non-conditioned patients in spite of the same protocol used for T cell depletion. According to our experience (and as shown in Fig. 5), for these reasons, the overall survival in conditioned patients has not been better as compared to non-conditioned patients.

The usefulness of pretransplant conditioning to improve donor cell engraftment indicates that host-mediated cellular resistance, which is susceptible to suppression by chemotherapy, is central to the observed graft failure in SCID. In several variants of the disorder, such as in SCID with adenosine deaminase deficiency and in SCID with nonfunctional host T cells, BMT without the use of conditioning has only rarely been successful. In addition, evidence has been obtained that natural killer (NK) cell activity, which is preserved in a substantial number of patients, may be involved in graft failure [6, 15]. Although direct demonstration of such a mechanism is lacking, we and others have noted some, but not an absolute, correlation of NK cell activity at diagnosis with graft failure. More recently, we have also obtained evidence

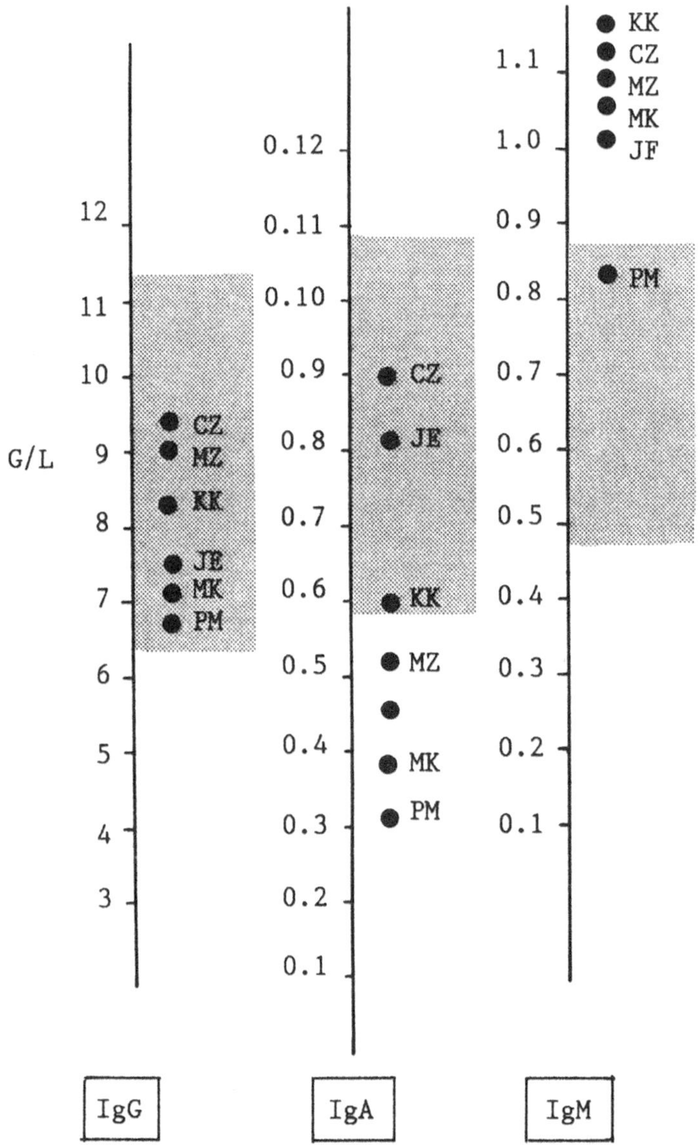

Fig. 4. Immunoglobulin serum levels in six SCID patients transplanted with the use of prior conditioning

that positive NK cell functions are frequently associated with congenital engraftment of low numbers of maternally derived Tcells originating from an intrauterine maternofetal transfusion [17]. According to an ongoing prospective study performed by us, using sensitive methods to detect maternally derived cells, such an engraftment has been found in a majority of patients and likely represents an important basis for graft failure.

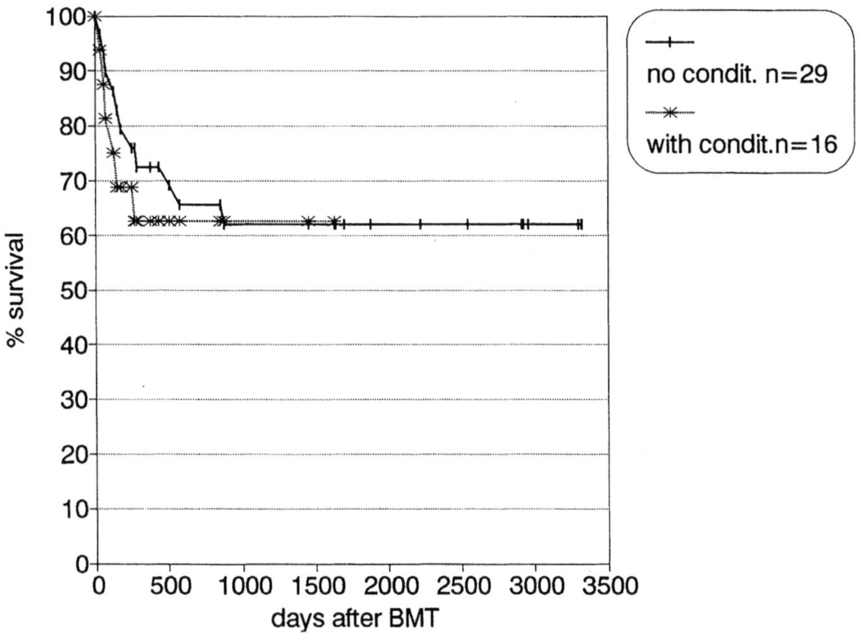

Fig. 5. Survival in 45 patients with SCID following HLA-haploidentical BMT without or with the use of pretransplant conditioning

Presently, most transplant centers in Europe which treat patients with congenital immunodeficiency disorders take part in coordinated, prospective studies to explore and optimize transplant modalities, in particular in regard to conditioning regimen. Obviously the use of cytotoxic agents in small infants prior to BMT has significant drawbacks, and it will be critical to develop the least toxic regimen to overcome the problem of graft resistance.

BMT in Wiskott-Aldrich Syndrome

Wiskott-Aldrich syndrome (WAS) is another immunological disorder that is a formidable candidate for curative treatment by BMT [16]. With the use of HLA-identical siblings as donors, results have been excellent [12, 14]. In our own experience, all eight boys with WAS are long-term survivors with normal immunological and hematological functions. Included are two more recently treated patients who received grafts from unrelated, HLA-matched donors. The use of HLA nonidentical donors is currently being explored. With standard conditioning, which in WAS involves busulfan in combination with cyclophosphamide, graft failure has again been a significant problem.

Currently explored conditioning protocols thus include more intensive myeloablative and immunosuppressive agents and early results are promising [5, 20].

Conclusions

Primary T cell disorders have contributed significantly to our understanding of the human immune system. Furthermore, because of their extremely dismal prognosis, therapeutic strategies aimed at immunological reconstitution have always been intensively explored. The advanced stage of clinical BMT, as used in a variety of disorders, in part reflects this. The majority of patients affected with severe congenital immunodeficiencies can now be treated effectively, with a high chance to permanently reverse the disorder.

References

1. Bortin MM, Rimm RA (1977) Severe combined immunodeficiency: characterization of the disease and results of bone marrow transplantation. JAMA 238: 591–608
2. Buckley H, Schiff SE, Sampson HA, Schiff RI et al. (1986) Development of immunity in human severe primary T cell deficiencies following haploidentical bone marrow transplantation. J Immunol 136: 2398–2407
3. Fischer A, Friedrich W, Levinsky R, Vossen J et al. (1986) Bone marrow transplantation for immunodeficiencies and osteopetrosis: European survey 1968–1985. Lancet II: 1080–1083
4. Fischer A, Landais P, Friedrich W, Morgan G et al. (1990) European experience of bone-marrow transplantation for severe combined immunodeficiency. Lancet II: 850–854
5. Fischer A, Friedrich W, Fasth A, Blanche S et al. (1991) Reduction of graft failure by a monoclonal antibody (anti-LFA-1 CD11a) after HLA nonidentical bone marrow transplantation in children with immunodeficiencies, osteopetrosis and Fanconi's anemia: a European Group for Immunodeficiency/European Group for Bone Marrow Transplantation Report. Blood 77: 249–256
6. Friedrich W, Peter HH, Blütters-Sawatzki R, Ebell W (1986) Analysis of the immunoreconstitution in 19 patients with severe combined immunodeficiency after HLA haploidentical bone-marrow transplantation. In: Vossen J, Griscelli C (eds) Progress in immunodeficiency research and therapy II. Experta Medica, Amsterdam, pp 351–359
7. Friedrich W, Goldmann SF, Vetter U, Fliedner TM et al. (1984) Immunological reconstitution in severe combined immunodeficiency after transplantation of HLA haploidentical, T cell depleted bone-marrow. Lancet I: 761–764
8. Friedrich W, Goldmann SF, Ebell W, Blütters-Sawatzki R et al. (1986) Severe combined immunodeficiency: treatment by bone-marrow transplantation in 15 infants using HLA haploidentical donors. Eur J Pediatr 144: 125–130
9. Gatti RA, Meeuwissen HJ, Allen HD, Hong R, Good R (1968) Immunologic reconstituion of sex linked lymphopenic immunodeficiency. Lancet II: 1366–1369
10. Good RA, Kapoor N, Pahwa RN Wert A, O'Reilly RJ (1980) Current approaches to the primary immunodeficiencies In: Fougereau M, Dausset J (eds) Progress in immunology IV. Academic, London

11. Griscelli C, Durandy A, Virelizier JL, Ballet JJ et al. (1978) Selective defect of precursor T cells associated with apparently normal B lymphocytes in severe combined immunodeficiency. J Pediatr 93: 404–411
12. Kapoor N, Kirkpatrick D, Blaese RM, Oleske J et al. (1981) Reconstitution of normal megakaryocytopoiesis and immune functions in Wiskott-Aldrich syndrome by marrow transplantation following myeloablation and immunosuppression with busulfan and cyclophosphamide. Blood 57: 692–699
13. Kenny AB, Hitzig WA (1979) Bone marrow transplantation for severe combined immunodeficiency. Eur J Pediatr 131: 155–177
14. O'Reilly RJ, Brochstein J, Dinsmore B, Kirkpatrick (1984) Marrow transplantation for congenital disorders. Semin Hematol 21: 188–213
15. O'Reilly J, Keever CA, Small TN, Brochstein J (1990) The use of HLA-nonidentical T-cell depleted marrow transplants for correction of severe combined immunodeficiency disease. Immunodefic Rev 1: 273–309
16. Parkman R, Rappaport D, Geha R, Cassady R et al. (1978) Complete correction of Wiskott-Aldrich syndrome by allogeneic marrow transplantation. N Engl J Med 298: 921–927
17. Pollak MS, Kirkpatrick D, Kapoor N, O'Reilly (1982) Identification by HLA typing of intrauterine-derived maternal T cells four patients with severe combined immunodeficiency. N Engl J Med 307: 662–666
18. Reisner Y, Kapoor N, Kirpatrick D, Cunningham-Rundels S et al. (1983) Transplantation for severe combined immunodeficiency with HLA A, B, C, DR incompatible paternal marrow fractionated by soybean agglutination and sheep red blood cells. Blood 61: 341–348
19. Rosen FS, Cooper MD, Wegewood RJP (1984) The primary immunodeficiencies. N Engl J Med 311: 235–242; 300–310
20. Rumelhart SL, Trigg ME Horowitz SD, Hong R (1990) Monoclonal antibody T-cell-depleted HLA-haploidentical bone marrow transplantation for Wiskott-Aldrich syndrome. Blood 75: 1031–1035
21. World Health Organization (1983) Primary immunodeficiency disease (Report prepared for the WHO by a scientific group on immunodeficiencies). Clin Immunol Immunpathol 28: 450–447

Investigation of Immune Responses After Vaccination in Immunocompromised Populations

M.M. Eibl and *H.M. Wolf*

Introduction

While primary immunodeficiency disorders are rare diseases with well-defined immunological abnormalities, secondary immunodeficiencies affect a large and growing population and are heterogeneous in nature. Secondary immunodeficiencies are known to occur in patients with malignancies associated with the disease itself (e.g., lymphoid malignancies) and/or with cytotoxic or radiation treatment. Improved therapeutic regimens bring about cure and allow long-term disease-free survival of patients with certain forms of cancer, thus increasing the size of the immunocompromised population with this disease.

Much more commonly, however, secondary immunodeficiencies arise in the course of bacterial, viral, and parasitic infections. During the past decade, human immunodeficiency virus (HIV) infection has led to a rapid increase in the immunocompromised population worldwide. Recent reports estimate the total number of HIV-infected individuals to be 10 million, with 1 million in the United States and 500000 in Europe. Infection with HIV often leads to destruction of the immune system, with subsequent development of acquired immunodeficiency syndrome (AIDS). Cohort studies show that over a 10-year period approximately 30 % of infected persons develop symptoms characteristic of AIDS, while 70 % remain free from disease during this time. Most infected individuals, however, exhibit some functional impairment of the immune system. Patients with AIDS develop a number of opportunistic infections as a consequence of severe depletion of CD4 T lymphocytes [1–5]. However, a functional impairment of T helper cells has been detected in HIV-infected individuals without a critical reduction in CD4 cells (absolute number of CD4 positive cells > 400/μl) [6–11]. One of the early defects in these persons is a selective loss of T helper function, measured by in vitro testing of proliferation to recall antigens, while the response to mitogens and alloantigens is normal. Although this early immunodeficiency is not associated with pathological susceptibility to opportunistic infections, there is evidence suggesting that it might be a predictor for progression towards AIDS [12].

The classical and most commonly used indicator of protective immunity to pathogens has been the presence and titer of binding and neutralizing antibodies. More recently, however, the importance of cell-mediated immunity, including immunological memory, has been emphasized. T cell reactivity to recall antigens is an important measure of immunological memory and can be taken as one of the indications of an individual's ability to develop protective immunity to pathogens.

Cellular Immune Responses in Immunocompromised Populations

Cellular Immune Responses to Recall Antigens (TT_{Al}, TBEV) in Members of Groups at Risk for HIV Infection

Abnormalities of humoral and cellular immunity have been described in members of groups at risk for HIV infection (homosexuals, drug addicts, hemophiliacs), both in the absence and in the presence of HIV infection [6, 13–19]. To assess cellular immune reactivity to recall antigens in an immunocompromised population we first studied lymphocyte proliferative responses following stimulation with aluminum-adjuvanted tetanus toxoid (TT_{Al}) in members of groups at risk for HIV infection and in asymptomatic HIV-infected individuals. Only subjects who had received their last tetanus booster immunization within 10 years before the study (i.e., who were vaccinated according to the regular regimen) were included. Healthy adult volunteers were examined as controls.

Mononuclear cells were isolated from the peripheral blood by buoyant density gradient centrifugation. The cells were than incubated at 1×10^5 cells/well in 96-well flat-bottomed microtiter plates for 7 days in the presence or absence of TT_{Al} (2.5 Lf and 0.5 Lf/ml). The resulting lymphocyte proliferation was assessed by measuring [^{3}H] thymidine incorporation, and the peak response of the two concentrations was used to evaluate the cells' capacity to respond to antigen. The results depicted in Fig. 1 indicate that asymptomatic HIV-positive individuals with decreased numbers of CD4-positive cells (CD4 counts below 400/µl) show a markedly decreased TT_{Al}-specific lymphocyte response compared to HIV-negative heterosexual controls. However, even HIV-positive drug addicts and HIV-positive homosexuals with CD4-positive T cells over 400/µl show a significantly decreased lymphocyte response following stimulation with AlOH-adjuvanted tetanus toxoid (TT_{Al}). This indicates that the CD4-positive T cell (which is the principal cell responding to recall antigen) is functionally impaired in HIV-infected individuals even before CD4 depletion occurs. In contrast to the HIV-infected individuals studied, the capacity of the lymphocytes to respond to TT_{Al} was comparable in HIV-negative members of risk groups for HIV infection and HIV-negative controls.

To investigate the immune response of asymptomatic HIV-positive individuals without a severe depletion of CD4-positive T cells to a recall antigen of viral origin, we examined lymphocyte proliferative responses to tick-borne encephalitis virus (TBEV) in HIV-infected individuals with a history of previous TBE vaccination within the preceding 3 years. Antigen-specific

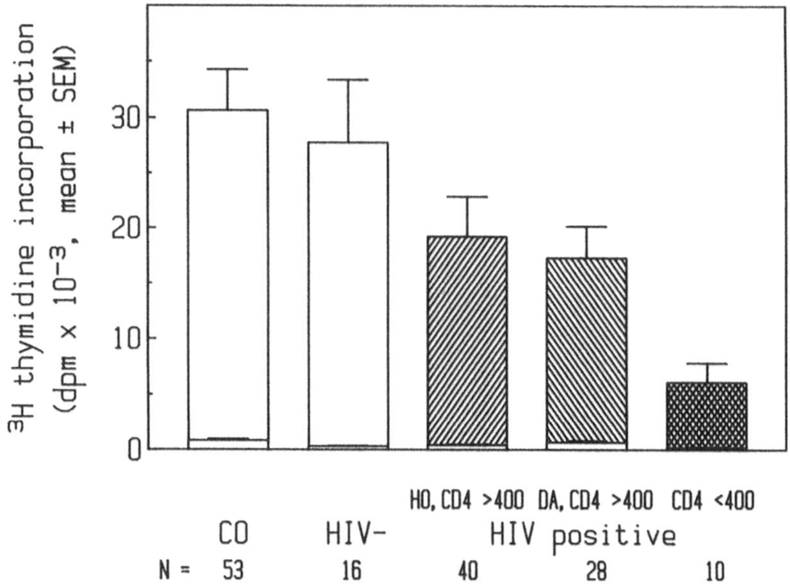

Fig. 1. HIV-positive members of risk groups for HIV infection (homosexuals, drug addicts) show a decreased proliferative response of mononuclear cells following stimulation with AlOH-adjuvanted tetanus toxoid. Mononuclear cells were purified from the peripheral blood of HIV-positive and HIV-negative members of risk groups for HIV infection (*HO*, homosexuals; *DA*, drug addicts) and healthy heterosexual controls (*CO*). Antigen-specific proliferative responses of lymphocytes were examined by measuring [^{3}H] thymidine incorporation after incubation of the cells for 7 days in the presence of aluminum-adjuvanted tetanus toxoid. The HIV-positive individuals (HO or DA) were assigned to different study groups according to their absolute number of CD4-positive peripheral blood Tcells (CD4 above or below 400/μl). Results are given as dpm [^{3}H] thymidine incorporation (mean ± SEM of the respective study group), with the number of individuals in the respective study group shown at the bottom of the figure. Mean proliferative responses of the cells in the absence of antigen (medium control) were always below 1000 dpm (data not shown). Statistically significant differences as calculated by the Mann-Whitney *U* test: controls versus HIV-positive homosexuals with CD4 counts above 400/μl, $p = 0.0082$; controls versus HIV-positive drug addicts with CD4 counts above 400/μl, $p = 0.0133$; controls versus HIV-positive members of risk groups (both HO and DA) with CD4 counts below 400/μl, $p = 0.0009$

lymphocyte proliferation was measured as described for TT_{Al} using inactivated purified TBEV at 1.0 and 0.2 μg/ml. Reliable information about the time of TBEV immunization in the HIV-negative controls could not be obtained due to technical reasons. This might explain the lower level of MNC proliferation observed in the controls after stimulation with TBEV compared with TT_{Al}. As can be seen in Fig. 2, the levels of TBEV-specific lymphocyte proliferative responses were significantly lower in HIV-positive members of risk groups than in the controls ($p=0.024$, Mann-Whitney *U* test), although all HIV-positive individuals studied for TBEV-specific MNC proliferation had CD4 counts above 400/μl (data not shown).

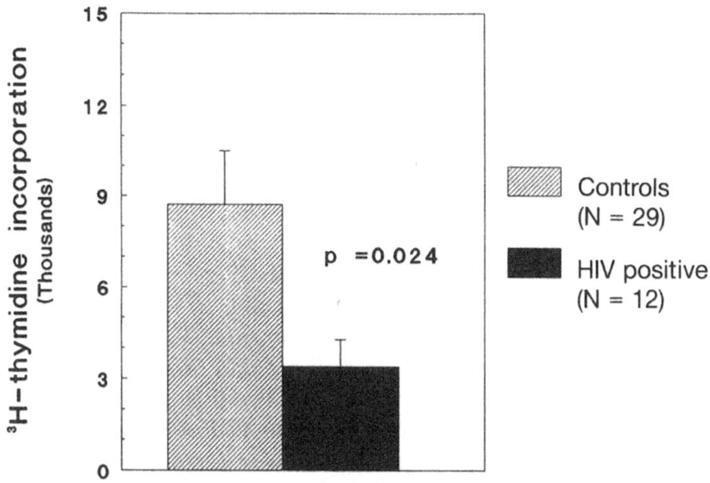

Fig. 2. Decreased proliferative responses of mononuclear cells to a viral antigen (TBEV) in asymptomatic HIV-positive individuals despite normal numbers of CD4-positive T cells. Mononuclear cells were purified from the peripheral blood of asymptomatic HIV-positive members of risk groups for HIV infection (homosexuals and drug addicts). Healthy heterosexual volunteers were included as controls. All HIV-positive individuals shown had a history of previous TBEV vaccination within the previous 3 years before the study. Antigen-specific proliferative responses of lymphocytes were examined by measuring [^{3}H] thymidine incorporation after incubation of the cells for 7 days in the presence of inactivated purified TBEV. TBEV was used at 1.0 and 0.2 μg/ml; the peak response of the two concentrations was employed to evaluate cellular reactivity against TBEV. Results are given as dpm [^{3}H] thymidine incorporation (mean ± SEM of the respective study group). Statistically significant difference between HIV-infected individuals and HIV-negative controls: $p = 0.024$, Mann-Whitney *U* test

Cellular Immune Response After TBE Vaccination in HIV-Positive and HIV-Negative Hemophiliacs

A decreased capacity of T cells in HIV-infected individuals to respond to a viral antigen (TBEV) was further confirmed by studies on T cell responses after primary and secondary TBE vaccination in hemophiliacs. Four clinically asymptomatic HIV-positive hemophiliacs, 12 HIV-negative hemophiliacs, and 16 healthy volunteers were vaccinated with a commercially available TBE vaccine (Immuno, Vienna, Austria). TBEV-specific T cell responses were examined before the first vaccination, 1 month after the first vaccination, and 1 and 7 months after the second vaccination. T cells were purified from peripheral blood mononuclear cells by rosetting with sheep erythrocytes. The purity of the T cell population was higher than 90%. TBEV-specific T cell proliferative responses were examined by incubating T cells (1×10^5/well) in the presence of autologous monocytes (1×10^4, purified from peripheral blood mononuclear cells by adherence to plastic) and purified inactivated

TBEV (1.0 and 0.2 μg/ml final concentration) in 96-well flat-bottomed microtiter plates for 7 days in a CO_2 incubator. T cell proliferation was then assessed by measuring [^{3}H] thymidine incorporation. Results (peak responses of the two concentrations, represented by mean ± SEM of the respective study group) are expressed as net dpm after subtraction of the background (cell proliferation in the presence of medium alone).

The first TBE vaccination induced low TBEV-specific T cell responses in both healthy controls and HIV-negative hemophiliacs, and a second vaccination significantly increased TBEV-specific T cell proliferative responses in these two study populations (Fig. 3). At any time after the first and the second vaccinations, levels of TBEV-specific T cell proliferation were comparable in HIV-negative hemophiliacs and healthy controls. However, the T cells of clinically asymptomatic HIV-positive hemophiliacs displayed a markedly decreased capacity to respond to TBE vaccination (Fig. 3). Only one of four HIV-positive hemophiliacs showed a significant T cell proliferative response following the first TBE vaccination, and this response was short-lived. After the second TBE vaccination, virtually no TBEV-specific T cell proliferation was seen in the HIV-positive patients. Examination of

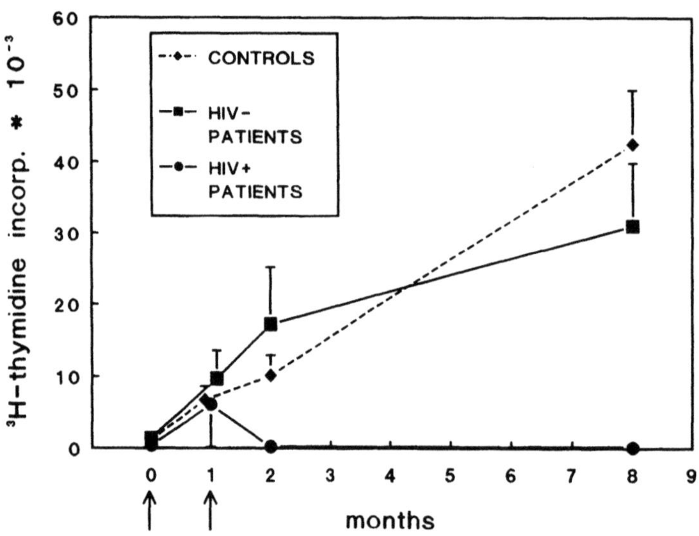

Fig. 3. TBE vaccination induces T cell responses in HIV-negative hemophiliacs and healthy controls, but not in HIV-positive hemophiliacs. Twelve HIV-negative hemophiliacs, four HIV-positive asymptomatic hemophiliacs, and 16 healthy controls were vaccinated twice against TBE (two vaccinations with a 4-week interval; *arrows*). T cell proliferative responses were examined at the indicated times following the first and second vaccinations. T cells were purified from peripheral blood mononuclear cells by rosetting with sheep erythrocytes, and the cells were then incubated for 7 days in the presence of purified inactivated TBE virus (1.0 and 0.2 μg/ml) and autologous monocytes (purified by adherence to plastic surfaces). T cell proliferative responses were assessed by measuring [^{3}H] thymidine incorporation. Results (peak responses of the two concentrations) are given as net dpm (mean ± SEM of the respective study group) after subtraction of the background proliferation of cells in the presence of medium alone

TBEV-specific responses at a later time (7 months after the second TBE vaccination) showed that the response to booster immunization in the HIV-positive hemophiliacs was absent, and not merely delayed, since their T cells failed to proliferate in response to TBEV at that time as well. A decreased cellular response following TBE vaccination in HIV-positive hemophiliacs was also observed after a second booster immunization administered 19 months after primary immunization [20].

Protective Effect of Vaccination in Immunocompromised Populations

The results outlined above confirm previous reports on a functional T cell defect in HIV-infected individuals without a concomitant marked decrease in their number of CD4-positive T cells [6–11]. Our results indicate that the defect in antigen-specific response in HIV-infected individuals with CD4 cells over 400/μl is comparable in the different risk groups and with different antigens (bacterial versus viral origin).

Several mechanisms have been proposed to account for similar findings, as a direct correlation between the impairment of T helper cell function and the decline in CD4 counts has never been established [11, 12]. One of the mechanisms proposed to account for loss of T helper cell function and subsequently responsible for CD4 depletion is programmed cell death or apoptosis [21]. Inappropriate stimulation of T cells could render these cells vulnerable and susceptible to death upon a second stimulation. In this case, deletion of T cells expressing common Vβ genes would be expected, as has recently been described in HIV-infected individuals [22]. Furthermore, recent evidence suggests that asymptomatic HIV-infected individuals with a functional T helper cell defect show faster depletion of CD4 cells than those without such a defect [23].

Another possible cause of the functional defect in T helper cells could be autoimmunity. Viral glycoproteins with homology to MHC might induce autoimmune reactivity [24, 25], and the anti-MHC antibodies could then be responsible for cell depletion or could inhibit antigen-induced T cell proliferation by interrupting the interaction of T cells and antigen-presenting cells. Even though this possibility had been mentioned some time ago, convincing evidence of its relevance has still to be provided.

In addition to the T cell defects described in HIV-infected individuals, several studies have shown that antibody response to primary immunization is suboptimal in this immunocompromised population. Impaired antibody production has been observed in asymptomatic HIV-positive hemophiliacs following primary immunization with hepatitis B vaccine [26–28] as well as in AIDS patients after primary vaccination with the protein neoantigen keyhole limpet hemocyanin [19]. However, the results of studies reporting on the antibody response after immunization with T-independent antigens such as pneumococcal polysaccharides and/or after booster immunization with tetanus toxoid or influenza virus have been inconclusive. Impaired antibody response after vaccination with pneumococcal polysaccharides has been described by Klein et al. [29] and Janoff et al. [30], while Huang et al. [31] have shown that antibody responses to a recall antigen, influenza virus, after booster immunization were normal in HIV-positive homosexual men (asymptomatic or with PGL). Opravil et al. [14] showed a decreased IgG response to tetanus booster immunization. The impairment observed in the antibody response correlated with the severity of the patients' immune defect (as assessed by measuring CD4 cell counts and PHA or PWM lymphoproliferative responses). Significantly decreased antibody responses were also described in asymptomatic HIV-positive risk group members after vaccination with influenza vaccine [32].

The apparent discrepancies in the results of studies on antibody response to recall antigens might be explained by differences among the study populations with regard to their preexisting immunity to antigen, their levels of immunocompetence, and/or the time of primary immunization. It is generally agreed that protection from disease after vaccination against TBEV or tetanus toxoid correlates with antibody titers. We therefore addressed the question of whether the percentage of vaccinated persons in immunocompromised populations producing protective levels of antibodies is comparable to the corresponding percentage in a normal population, and whether antibody levels produced in the immunocompromised are comparable to the levels observed in healthy individuals. The answers to these questions should be of practical importance for vaccination strategies in the different immunocompromised populations.

Frequencies of Protective Antibody Titers in HIV-Infected Individuals with a History of Previous Tetanus or TBE Vaccination

To study the protective effect of vaccination in immunocompromised populations we investigated antibody titers against tetanus toxoid and TBEV in HIV-negative members of risk groups and HIV-infected individuals who had been vaccinated against tetanus or TBE prior to the study according to the recommended vaccination schedule. Healthy heterosexual controls vaccinated against tetanus within the past 10 years or against TBE within the past 3 years were included as controls. Assays for tetanus antibody were performed according to a standard procedure [33]. Antibodies against TBEV were measured using a hemagglutination inhibition assay [34].

The data presented in Table 1 indicate that over 95% of the examined members of a risk group for HIV infection had protective levels of tetanus antibodies (i.e., > 0.02 IU/ml), irrespective of their HIV antibody status. This is in contrast to the functional defect in the T cell response to tetanus toxoid and TBEV that was observed in the HIV-positive study groups. Among HIV-positive homosexuals the number of individuals with low protective

Table 1. Frequencies of protective antibody titers in individuals with a history of previous tetanus vaccination

Study group	*n*	Tetanus antitoxin serum titers					
		Below protective levels (< 0.02 IU/ml)		Low protective levels (0.02–1.0 IU/ml)		High protective levels (> 1.0 IU/ml)	
		n	%	*n*	%	*n*	%
No risk group for HIV infection (controls)	22	1	5	1	5	20	91
Risk group for HIV infection							
HIV-negative	15	0	0	3	20	12	80
HIV-positive							
Homosexuals	47	1	2	12	26	34	72
Drug addicts	36	1	3	4	11	31	86

Chi-square analysis of 4 × 3 contingency table, $p = 0.369$.

tetanus antitoxin levels (0.02–1.0 IU/ml) was slightly higher than among controls; in comparison to HIV-negative heterosexual controls, however, this difference did not reach statistical significance (Table 1).

To investigate protective immunity after vaccination against a viral pathogen, TBE antibodies were assessed in individuals who had received their last TBE booster vaccination within 3 years before the study. While members of a risk group for HIV infection (homosexual men and intravenous drug users) had normal levels of tetanus antitoxins, only 60 % of the HIV-negative and 41 % of the HIV-positive members of risk groups showed protective TBEV antibody levels in the hemagglutination inhibition assay. In contrast, about 90 % of controls had protective TBE antibodies, and the difference between the HIV-positive individuals and the controls was highly significant (Table 2).

Our results point to a discrepancy observed in the antibody response after vaccination against two different antigens (tetanus toxoid and TBEV) in risk groups for HIV infection. The discrepant results may be due to differences in the nature of the antigen (viral versus bacterial origin) and/or the time of primary immunization with the respective antigen. The individuals in this study most likely received primary immunization against tetanus toxoid early in life (probably at preschool age), while primary immunization against TBEV occurred at adult age.

Table 2. Frequencies of protective TBEV antibody levels (≥ 1:10) in individuals with a history of previous TBE immunization

Study group	*N*	Protective TBE antibody levels *n*	%
No risk group for HIV infection (controls)	28	25	89
Risk group for HIV infection			
HIV-negative	15	9	60
HIV-positive	29	12	41

Chi-square analysis of 3 × 2 contingency table, $p = 0.001$. Controls versus HIV-negative members of risk group, Fisher exact test, $p=0.034$; controls versus HIV-positive members of risk group, Fisher exact test, $p < 0.001$.

Antibody Response After TBE Vaccination in Hemophiliacs in the Presence or Absence of HIV Infection

Results described above demonstrated that Tcells of HIV-positive hemophiliacs fail to respond to TBE vaccination. Studies of the protective antibody responses after TBE vaccination in the same patient population revealed that HIV-positive hemophiliacs also displayed a decreased ability to produce antibodies in response to TBE vaccination, while HIV-negative hemophiliacs responded normally [20]. Sixteen hemophiliacs (12 HIV-negative, 4 HIV-positive) and 12 controls were vaccinated against TBEV. TBEV antibodies were examined before and 1 month after primary TBE immunization; 1, 7, and 12 months after the second TBE vaccination, which was given 1 month after primary immunization; and before and 1 and 2 months after the second booster vaccination (administered 19 months after primary immunization). After the second booster, TBE antibodies were examined in eight HIV-negative and four HIV-positive hemophiliacs and in nine controls. Six HIV-negative patients, four HIV-positive subjects, and two controls were examined 1 and 2 months after the second booster. Serum antibody titers were comparable on the two occasions after the second booster, and results were combined for the final evaluation. Results are expressed as mean ± 1 SEM of reciprocal serum titers in each study group (as determined by hemagglutination inhibition assay).

While antibody titers were comparable in HIV-negative hemophiliacs and controls at each time after primary or booster immunization, HIV-positive hemophiliacs displayed a decreased antibody response. None of four HIV-positive subjects produced a significant TBEV antibody titer after the first vaccination. Only two out of four HIV-positive patients showed antibody levels considered to be protective (TBE antibody titer in the hemagglutination inhibition assay ≥ 1:10) after the second vaccination, and they lost their TBE antibodies soon afterwards. Following a second booster vaccination,

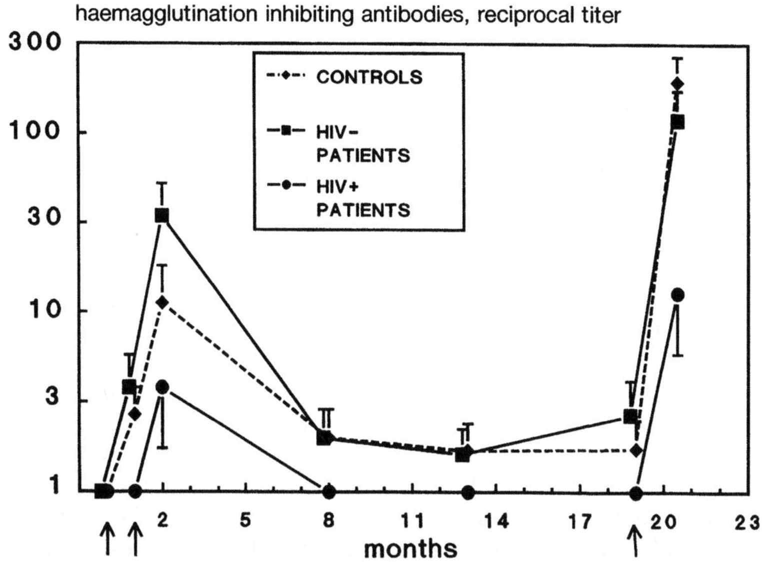

Fig. 4. Serum TBEV antibodies following immunization of HIV-negative and HIV-positive hemophiliacs and controls with TBE vaccine. TBEV antibodies were examined before and 1 month after primary TBE immunization, 1, 7, and 12 months after the second TBE vaccination, and before and 1 and 2 months after the second booster vaccination. Eight HIV-negative and four HIV-positive hemophiliacs and nine controls were examined after the second booster. Six HIV-negative patients, four HIV-positive subjects, and two controls were examined 1 and 2 months after the second booster. TBEV antibodies were determined by hemagglutination inhibition assay, and results are expressed as mean ± SEM of the log-transformed reciprocal serum titers (geometric mean). After the second booster immunization, TBEV antibody titers were significantly lower in the HIV-positive patients than in the controls (one-way analysis of variance, $p < 0.005$; Student's t test of log-transformed values, $p < 0.005$)

three HIV-infected patients developed protective TBEV antibody titers, but the levels of serum antibodies after the second booster immunization were significantly lower in the HIV-positive subjects than in the healthy population ($p < 0.005$; Fig. 4). Thus it appears likely that protective immunity is of shorter duration.

Antibody Responses After Primary Immunization in Patients with Malignancies

The question of protection from disease after vaccination has also been addressed in another immunocompromised population, patients with malignancy. As various forms of malignancy may influence immunocompetence to different extents, we chose patients with breast cancer as our first target group. Breast cancer is the most frequent malignancy in women; thus the total population is sizable and relevant. Furthermore, patients with breast cancer receive different modes of treatment: surgery alone, surgery plus irradiation, or surgery plus chemotherapy, depending on the stage of the disease at diagnosis. This situation makes it possible to study the effect of different treatment regimens as well.

We investigated the antibody response after vaccination against hepatitis B virus in 32 women with breast cancer who had undergone surgical treatment and then received adjuvant radiotherapy or chemotherapy when indicated [35]. After surgical therapy with or without adjuvant therapy, breast cancer patients were vaccinated with a commercially available hepatitis B vaccine (aluminum-adsorbed hepatitis B surface (HBs) antigen; HB-Vax, Merck, Sharp & Dohme) according to the recommended vaccination schedule. Seven healthy age-matched women (controls) were vaccinated in parallel. All patients and controls were negative for HBs antigen and for antibodies against both HBs and hepatitis B virus core antigen. The patients were immunized for the first time either 3 months after surgery (if they received no adjuvant treatment, n=10), 3 months (n=8) or 6 months (n=7) after adjuvant radiotherapy, or following the last course of adjuvant chemotherapy (n=7). HBs antibodies in serum were examined 2, 4, and 8 weeks after the second vaccination and 4 and 8 weeks after the third vaccination. Antibody determinations were performed using a commercially available radioimmunoassay (Immuno, Vienna, Austria).

As can be seen in Fig. 5, the magnitude of antibody response after the second vaccination was significantly lower in breast cancer patients than in the controls. This difference was most significant 4 weeks (p = 0.0007, Mann-Whitney U test) and 8 weeks (p = 0.0036) after the second vaccination. While there was no correlation between the treatment that the patients received and their antibody response, HBs antibody responses were lower in patients with an advanced stage of the disease (as assessed by tumor grading, data not shown). The impairment of the patients' immune system in mounting a sufficient antibody response after primary immunization was overcome in the course of further booster immunizations. After completion of the three-dose HBs immunization regimen 4 and 8 weeks after the third vaccination, HBs antibody levels were comparable in patients and controls. However, patients with adjuvant irradiation still had slightly lower antibody titers 8 weeks after the second booster vaccination than did the controls, suggesting a trend that will have to be confirmed in studies with larger groups of patients (HBs antibody titers, mU/ml, mean ± SEM: patients vaccinated 3 months after adjuvant irradiation, 541 ± 481, n=8; controls, 1138 ± 996, n=7).

Decreased primary antibody responses in patients with breast cancer were also demonstrated after vaccination with another viral antigen (TBEV) [36]. All patients in this study had undergone radical mastectomy or quadrantectomy and were immunized with TBE vaccine after the start of adjuvant chemotherapy (cylophosphamide, methotrexate and 5-fluorouracil). The schedule for the vaccinations followed the recommended regimen of two consecutive vaccinations 4 weeks apart. Six patients received the first

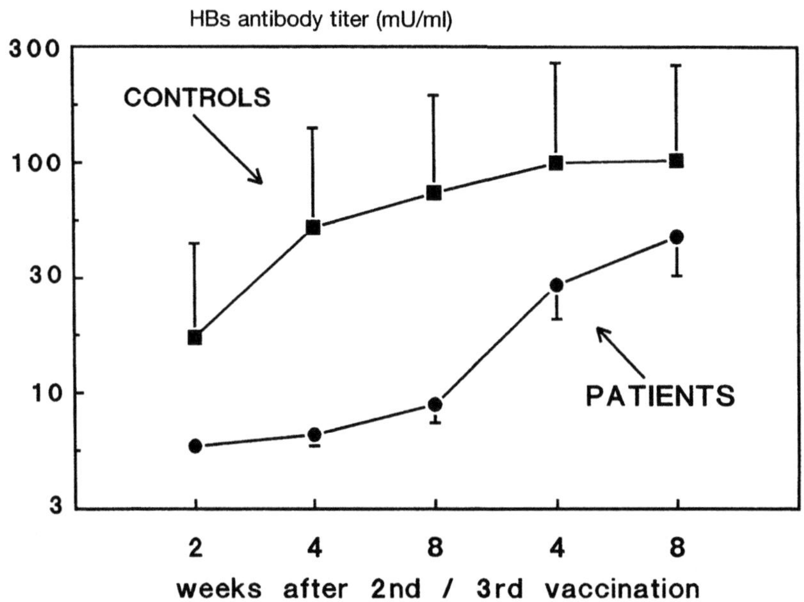

Fig. 5. HBs antibody titers in patients with breast cancer and healthy controls following the second hepatitis B vaccination (1 month after primary vaccination) and the third vaccination (6 months after primary vaccination). Serum antibody titers against HBs antigen were examined using a commercially available radioimmunoassay (Immuno, Vienna, Austria) at the indicated intervals (2, 4, and 8 weeks) after the second and third vaccinations in patients with breast cancer (n=32) and healthy age- and sex-matched volunteers (n=7). Results are expressed as mean ± SEM of the log-transformed values (geometric mean). Statistical evaluation of differences between patients and controls (Mann-Whitney U test): after the second vaccination: 2 weeks, $p = 0.0783$; 4 weeks, $p = 0.0007$; 8 weeks, $p = 0.0036$; after the third vaccination: 4 weeks, $p = 0.1378$; 8 weeks, $p = 0.1880$

vaccination on day 14 of the second CMF course and the second vaccination on day 14 of the third course. Nine patients received the first TBE vaccination 6–12 months after termination of adjuvant CMF therapy. Seven healthy female age-matched volunteers were vaccinated in parallel (controls). All patients and controls were negative for TBEV antibodies prior to the study, indicating that they had never had contact with the virus or been vaccinated against TBE before. The data shown in Table 3 indicate that only 2 out of 15 patients with breast cancer responded with protective TBEV antibody levels 4 weeks after the second TBE vaccination (i.e., TBEV antibody titer of ≥ 1:10 in the hemagglutination inhibition assay). In contrast, all seven controls developed protective TBEV antibodies after the booster immunization. Quantitative analysis of TBEV antibodies with a commercially available enzyme-linked immunosorbent assay (Enzyquick FSME, Immuno, Vienna) confirmed that breast cancer patients undergoing adjuvant chemotherapy have a markedly decreased capacity to produce antibodies after TBE vaccination (Table 3).

Table 3. TBE antibody titers 4 weeks after the second vaccination in breast cancer patients undergoing adjuvant chemotherapy

Study group		HIA (≥ 1:10)		ELISA (VIEU/ml)	
	n	*n*	%	Geometric mean	SD
Controls	7	7	100	295	2.22
Patients vaccinated during CMF chemotherapy	6	1	17[a]	15[c]	2.68
Patients vaccinated 6–12 months after CMF chemotherapy	9	1	11[b]	23[c]	3.89

HIA, hemagglutination inhibition assay; ELISA, enzyme-linked immunosorbent assay; CMF, cyclophosphamide, methotrexate, 5-fluorouracil.
[a]$p = 0.0047$, Fisher's exact test (as compared to controls).
[b]$p = 0.0007$, Fisher's exact test (as compared to controls).
Chi-square analysis of 3 × 2 contingency table: $p = 0.001$.
[c]$p < 0.001$, Student's t-test of the log-transformed values (as compared to controls). VIEU, Vienna units.

Conclusions

In cancer patients, optimal vaccination strategies will have to be developed. These strategies must take into consideration the fact that various forms of cancer and different modes of treatment may have dissimilar effects on the immune system. In HIV-infected populations, investigations of the immune response after vaccination are necessary for the design of improved vaccination strategies, for recommendation of adequate prophylactic measures against infections, and perhaps also as indicators for progression of infection and disease.

Our investigations indicate that different vaccination strategies are required to achieve protection against diseases preventable by vaccination in these populations. The percentage of vaccine responders among members of immunocompromised populations is significantly lower than in the healthy population. The degree of functional impairment is different for humoral and cellular responses and may vary depending on the nature of the antigen (e.g., tetanus toxoid or TBEV). Protective immunity in those who respond is achieved at a later time. While healthy individuals usually express protective antibody levels after the second vaccination, members of an immunocompromised population (e.g., patients with malignancies) are more likely to be protected only after the third vaccination. Even after booster vaccinations, however, antibody levels achieved are often lower in the immunocompromised individuals, and thus the protective immunity is of shorter duration. As a consequence, determination of antibody titers may be necessary to decide whether vaccination has been effective and/or to estimate the duration of the protective response.

References

1. Masur H, Michelis MA, Greene JB, Onorato I, Stouwe RAV, Holzman RS, Wormser G, Brettman L, Lange M, Murray HW, Cunningham-Rundles S (1981) An outbreak of community-acquired Pneumocystis carinii pneumonia: initial manifestation of cellular immune dysfunction. N Engl J Med 305:1431–1438
2. Siegal FP, Lopez C, Hammer GS, Brown AE, Kornfeld SJ, Gold J, Hassett J, Hirschman SZ, Cunningham-Rundles C, Adelsberg BR, Parham DM, Siegal M, Cunningham-Rundles S, Armstrong D (1981) Severe acquired immunodeficiency in male homosexuals, manifested by chronic perianal ulcerative herpes simplex lesions. N Engl J Med 305:1439–1444
3. Gottlieb MS, Schroff R, Schanker HM, Weisman JD, Fan PT, Wolf RA, Saxon A (1981) Pneumocystis carinii pneumonia and mucosal candidiasis in previously healthy homosexual men: evidence of a new acquired cellular immunodeficiency. N Engl J Med 305:1425–1431
4. Fahey JL, Prince H, Weaver M, Groopman J, Visscher B, Schwartz K, Detels R (1984) Quantitative changes in T helper or T suppressor/cytotoxic lymphocyte subsets that distinguish acquired immune deficiency syndrome from other immune subset disorders. Am J Med 76:95–100
5. Goedert JJ, Biggar RJ, Melbye M, Mann DL, Wilson S, Gail MH, Grossman RJ, DiGioia RA, Sanchez WC, Weiss SH, Blattner WA (1987) Effect of T4 count and co-factors on the incidence of AIDS in homosexual men infected with human immunodeficiency virus. JAMA 257:331–334
6. Mannhalter JW, Zlabinger GJ, Ahmad R, Zielinski CC, Schramm W, Eibl MM (1986) A functional defect in the early phase of the immune response observed in patients with haemophilia. Clin Immunol Immunopathol 38:390–397
7. Hoy JF, Lewis DE, Miller GG (1988) Functional versus phenotypic analysis of Tcells in subjects seropositive for the human immunodeficiency virus: a prospective study of in vitro responses to Cryptococcus neoformans. J Infect Dis 158:1071–1078
8. Mannhalter JW, Wolf HM, Pum M, Banekovich M, Hutterer J, Brandstätter R, Eibl MM (1988) Identification of individuals at increased risk for AIDS among clinically asymptomatic homosexuals and abusers of intravenous drugs. Immunol Invest 17:147–157
9. Shearer GM, Clerici M (1991) Early T-helper cell defects in HIV infection. AIDS 5:245–253
10. Giorgi JV, Fahey JL, Smith DC, Hultin LE, Cheng HL, Mitsuyasu RT, Detels R (1987) Early effects of HIV on CD4 lymphocytes in vivo. J Immunol 138:3725–3730
11. Miedema F, Petit AJC, Terpstra FG, Schattenkerk JK, de Wolf F, Al BJ, Roos M, Lange JM, Danner SA, Goudsmit J et al. (1988) Immunological abnormalities in human immunodeficiency virus (HIV) infected asymptomatic homosexual men. HIV affects the immune system before $CD4^+$ T-helper cell depletion occurs. J Clin Invest 82:1908–1914
12. Clerici M, Stocks NI, Zajac RA, Boswell RN, Lucey DR, Via CS, Shearer GM (1989) Detection of three distinct patterns of T-helper cell dysfunction in asymptomatic, human immunodeficiency virus-seropositive patients. J Clin Invest 84:1892–1899
13. Ragni MV, Ruben FL, Winkelstein A, Spero JA, Bontempo FA, Lewis JH (1987) Antibody responses to immunization of patients with hemophilia with and without evidence of human immunodeficiency virus (human T-lymphotropic virus type III) infection. J Lab Clin Med 109:545–549
14. Opravil M, Fierz W, Matter L, Blaser J, Lüthy R (1991) Poor antibody response after tetanus and pneumococcal vaccination in immunocompromised, HIV-infected patients. Clin Exp Immunol 84:185–189
15. Mahir WS, Millard RE, Booth JC, Flute PT (1988) Functional studies of cell-mediatd immunity in haemophilia and other bleeding disorders. Br J Haematol 69:367–370

16. Madhok R, Gracie JA, Smith J, Lowe GDO, Forbes CD (1990) Capacity to produce interleukin 2 is impaired in haemophilia in the absence and presence of HIV 1 infection. Br J Haematol 76:70–74
17. Madhok R, Gracie A, Lowe GDO, Burnett A, Froebel K, Follett E, Forbes CD (1986) Impaired cell mediated immunity in haemophilia in the absence of infection with human immunodeficiency virus. BMJ 293:978–980
18. Lane HC, Depper JM, Greene WC, Whalen G, Waldmann TA, Fauci AS (1985) Qualitative analysis of immune function in patients with the acquired immunodeficiency syndrome. N Engl J Med 313:79–84
19. Lane HC, Masur H, Edgar LC, Whalen G, Rook AH, Fauci AS (1983) Abnormalities of B-cell activation and immunoregulation in patients with the acquired immunodeficiency syndrome. N Engl J Med 309:453–458
20. Wolf HM, Pum M, Jáger R, István L, Mannhalter JW, Eibl MM (1992) Cellular and humoral immune responses in haemophiliacs after vaccination against tick-borne encephalitis. Br J Haematol 82: 374–383
21. Ameisen JC, Capron A (1991) Cell dysfunction and depletion in AIDS: the programmed cell death hypothesis. Immunol Today 12:102–105
22. Inberti L, Sotini A, Bettinardi A, Puoti M, Primi D (1991) Selective depletion in HIV infection of T cells that bear specific T cell receptor Vβ sequences. Science 254:860–862
23. Lucey DR, Melcher GP, Hendrix CW, Zajac RA, Goetz DW, Butzin CA, Clerici M, Warner RD, Abbadessa S, Hall K et al. (1991) Human immunodeficiency virus infection in the US Air Force: seroconversions, clinical staging and assessment of T helper cell functional assay to predict change in $CD4^+$ T cell counts. J Infect Dis 164:631–637
24. Golding H, Robey FA, Gates FT, Linder W, Beining PR, Hoffman T, Golding B (1988) Identification of homologous regions in human immunodeficiency virus I gp41 and human MHC class II β domain. J Exp Med 167:914–923
25. Golding H, Shearer GM, Hillman K, Lucas P, Manischewitz J, Zajac RA, Clerici M, Gress RE, Boswell RN, Golding B (1989) Common epitope in human immunodeficiency virus (HIV) 1-gp41 and HLA class II elicits immunosuppressive autoantibodies capable of contributing to immune dysfunction in HIV-1-infected individuals. J Clin Invest 83:1430–1435
26. Zanetti AR, Mannucci PM, Tanzi E, Moroni GA, De Paschale M, Forfini M, Carnelli V, Tirindelli MC, De Biasi R, Ciavarella N, De Rosa V, Rodeghiero F, Colombo M (1986) Hepatitis B vaccination of 113 hemophiliacs: lower antibody response in anti-LAV/HTLV-III-positive patients. Am J Hematol 23:339–345
27. Drake JH, Parmely RT, Britton HA (1987) Loss of hepatitis B antibody in human immunodeficiency virus-positive hemophilia patients. Pediatr Infect Dis J 6:1051–1054
28. Chan W, Petric M, Wang E, Koren G, Read S, Blanchette V (1990) Response to hepatitis B immunization in children with hemophilia: relationship to infection with human immunodeficiency virus type 1. J Pediatr 117:427–430
29. Klein RS, Selwyn PA, Maude D, Pollard C, Freeman K, Schiffman G (1989) Response to pneumococcal vaccine among asymptomatic heterosexual partners of persons with AIDS and intravenous drug users infected with human immunodeficiency virus. J Infect Dis 160:826–831
30. Janoff EN, Douglas JM, Gabriel M, Blaser MJ, Davidson AJ, Cohn DL, Judson FN (1988) Class-specific antibody response to pneumococcal capsular polysaccharides in men infected with human immunodeficiency virus type 1. J Infect Dis 158:983–990
31. Huang K, Ruben FL, Rinaldo CR, Kingsley L, Lyter DW, Ho M (1987) Antibody responses after influenza and pneumococcal immunization in HIV-infected homosexual men. JAMA 257:2047–2050
32. Miotti PG, Nelson KE, Dallabetta GA, Farzadegan H, Margolick J, Clements M (1989) The influence of HIV infection on antibody responses to a two-dose regimen of influenza vaccine. JAMA 262:779–783

33. Europäisches Arzneibuch, Österreichische Ausgabe, (1982) pp 259–262
34. Clarke DH, Casals J (1958) Techniques for hemagglutination and hemagglutination-inhibition with arthropod-borne viruses. Am J Trop Med Hyg 7:561–573
35. Rosen HR, Stierer M, Wolf HM, Eibl MM (1992) Impaired primary antibody responses after vaccination against hepatitis B in patients with breast cancer. Breast Cancer Res Treat 23: 233–240
36. Zielinski CC, Stuller I, Dorner F, Pötzi P, Müller C, Eibl MM (1986) Impaired primary, but not secondary, immune response in breast cancer patients under adjuvant chemotherapy. Cancer 58:1648–1652

Symposium in Immunology II
Autoimmunity – Basic and Clinical Aspects

Immunologic Basis of Autoimmunity

Structure and Function of MHC Class I Molecules

H. G. Rammensee

Introduction

The immune system consists of various, rather heterogeneous components with a wide spectrum of complexities. Some of the components are rather simple devices, such as the barrier functions exerted by skin or by gastric fluid. Others are more sophisticated, as exemplified by the presence of lysozyme in secretory fluids, resulting in the selective destruction of bacterial cell walls. The complement cascade is among the more complex components of the immune system, whereas its adaptive parts, the T cell and B cell compartments with their accessories, are the most sophisticated of all.

The special ability of the B and T cell compartments is to distinguish between self and nonself, and to mount a vigorous and specific response against structures recognized as foreign, even against synthetic molecules never occurring in nature. Having now some insight into the ways in which self/nonself discrimination is achieved, it appears that the most challenging task of the immune system is not to mount a specific response against a structure never heard of before but rather to avoid attacking self structures. This decision-making process is centrally regulated by trimolecular complexes consisting of T cell receptors, MHC molecules, and antigenic fragments (peptides). MHC molecules select a limited number of samples derived from both self and foreign molecules occurring intracellularly and present these samples to T cells. The latter then react against those antigenic samples that they have never seen before, that is, against foreign structures. The subject of this chapter is to discuss structure and function of one of the two MHC classes (class I), the one expressed on most somatic cells.

Overview of MHC Research

Early in this century, E. E. Tyzzer and others observed that tissue grafted between unrelated mice was usually rejected, whereas grafts exchanged between highly inbred mice were usually accepted. Analysis of the genetic traits governing acceptance or rejection of a graft led C. C. Little to the hypothesis that not a single but rather a large number of genes must be involved. G. Snell introduced the term "histocompatibility" to describe these genes. The first histocompatibility (H) gene was identified by P. Gorer in

1936, which was called H-2, taking into account that the respective gene product had been known earlier as the serologically detectable blood group antigen number 2 of the mouse (reviewed in [1]).

Minor and Major Histocompatibility Genes

Starting in the 1940s, Snell introduced a new approach to study the genetics (and later the function) of histocompatibility genes [2]. He bred congenic pairs of mouse strains differing at individual H genes but being otherwise identical. Using this approach, he and his coworkers described a large number of additional H genes, numbered H-1, H-3, H-4, and so forth. (To date, the numbering has arrived at H-48 [3]). Studying the traits of all these H genes, it soon emerged that H-2 was special. Grafts exchanged across strains with different H-2 alleles were rejected much more rapidly than those across non-H-2 incompatibilities. This difference caused Snell and coworkers in 1954 to term all members of the increasing number of non-H-2 genes collectively as "minor H genes" [4], as opposed to the "strong" H-2, which was now also called "major histocompatibility complex" [1]. "Complex" rather than "gene" or "locus" was introduced to account for the fact that H-2 was not a single locus but rather a group of loci on chromosome 17 coding for similar gene products.

Vigorous graft rejection was not the only outstanding feature of H-2. Foreign H-2 products expressed on grafted tissues or cell suspensions also induced a strong humoral response; confrontation of lymphocytes (T cells) with cells expressing foreign H-2 products resulted in strong T cell activation, a phenomenon termed alloreactivity. H-2 genes were found to be extremely polymorphic, that is, the species mouse expresses a couple of hundred alleles at a given H-2 locus [1].

Discovery of the Human MHC

Using sera of multiparous women containing antibodies against polymorphic antigens expressed on the offspring's leukocytes, Dansset, Pagne, and van Rood discovered H-2-like gene products in humans. These molecules were termed human leukocyte antigens (HLA). As a general name for H-2-like genes in all species, MHC was adapted [1].

Early Indications of MHC Function

Until the 1960s, MHC genes and their products appeared to be a bizarre phenomenon without any obvious function. All the traits studied so far were either artifactual (as consequences of transplantation) or appeared useless (antibodies of mothers against their offspring). Then, two traits pointing to a physiological function of MHC molecules were discovered. First, the so-called "immune response genes," governing response or nonresponse of a given mouse strain to a given antigen (such as the copolymer GAT) could be mapped within the MHC-region [5]. Second, T cells specific for foreign antigen, such as ovalbumin or viral antigen, were found to recognize the respective antigen only in context of a self MHC molecule, a phenomenon called MHC restriction [6, 7]. Thus, it emerged that MHC molecules have something to do with the normal immune response against environmental antigens. Today it is generally accepted that MHC molecules act as peptide receptors in that they present peptide fragments of antigens to T cells.

Class I and Class II

The "C" in the symbol MHC stands for "complex," reflecting the large number of loci found in the MHC regions of various species, as well as the large number of different alleles found for individual MHC loci. According to their traits, Klein grouped MHC genes into two classes, I and II [8]. This classification, established before the function of MHC molecules was really known, turned out to be very useful since the functions of the two classes of molecules are quite different: class II gene products present peptides derived from proteins occurring in the endocytic compartment of cells, whereas class I molecules can present peptides from every protein synthesized by a cell.

Mouse MHC: H-2

Most mouse MHC loci are on chromosome 17, with the exception of the β_2-microglobulin gene, which is on chromosome 2. The mouse MHC (H-2) contains the genes for the heavy chains of class I molecules, such as H-2 K, D, or L. The β_2-microglobulin is the light chain of class I molecules. H-2 also contains loci for several class II α and β genes, which are located between K and D class I genes. In addition, there are several dozen "class I-like" genes on chromosome 17, whose function is not yet understood, as well as a couple of other genes whose functions may or may not be related to the immune system.

Human MHC: HLA

The human MHC is called HLA, for human leukocyte antigen. Human class II genes and class I heavy chain genes are on chromosome 6; β_2-microglobulin is on chromosome 15. The gene order is different from that in the mouse; all class II genes – HLA-DR, DQ, and DP – are centromeric of the class I heavy chain genes B, A, and C.

Polymorphism

MHC genes of humans and mice are extremely polymorphic, that is, each species has many alleles per locus, and the sequences of individual alleles differ substantially from each other. MHC class I alleles of the more commonly used inbred mouse strains are H-2K^b, K^d, K^k, K^s, or D^b, D^d, and so on. The array of alleles expressed by the different MHC loci of an individual chromosome is called haplotype; mice of the haplotype H-2^b, for examle, express H-2K^b, $A_\alpha{}^b$ $A_\beta{}^b$, and D^b. Frequent human HLA alleles are HLA-A2, A1, A3, or HLA-B7 and B27. These allelic forms have been determined serologically and may split up into different subtypes. For example, sequencing of HLA-A2 genes from different individuals has indicated the existence of natural A2 variants differing in a few amino acid residues but indistinguishable by serology. To account for such natural variants, a nomenclature consisting of a combination of letters and numbers was introduced. HLA-A*0201, for example, is the most frequent A2 allele, whereas A*0205 is one of the natural A2 variants occurring at lower frequency, differing from A*0201 at four amino acids [9].

Structure of MHC Class I Molecules

Sequencing of MHC proteins and genes followed by X-ray analysis of MHC crystals allowed determination of the three-dimensional structure. The structure of HLA-A2, the first one to be described by Bjorkman and colleagues [10], is shown in Fig. 1. The A2 heavy chain (ca. 300 amino acids) contains three extracellular domains, α1, α2, and α3, a transmembrane stretch, and a cytoplasmatic tail at the C-terminus. The light chain, β_2-microglobulin, is noncovalently attached to α3. The α1 and α2 domains form a groove about 25 Å long and 10 Å wide, bordered by two alpha-helixes on the sides and a beta-pleated sheet structure on the ground. The groove of the A2 crystal contained material not belonging to the A2 sequence. This "contamination" was interpreted as bound peptides, or as the natural ligands of MHC molecules, a notion finally confirmed today [11, 12].

MHC Class I Molecules Are Peptide Receptors

The Antigens Naturally Presented by MHC Molecules Can Be Mimicked by Synthetic Peptides

T helper cells do not recognize native protein antigens; rather, they require fragments of antigens which have been processed by antigen-presenting cells and are presented to T cells in the context of MHC class II molecules [13]. Similarly, cytotoxic T lymphocytes (CTL) recognize fragments of viral protein in the context of class I molecules of infected cells. This has been

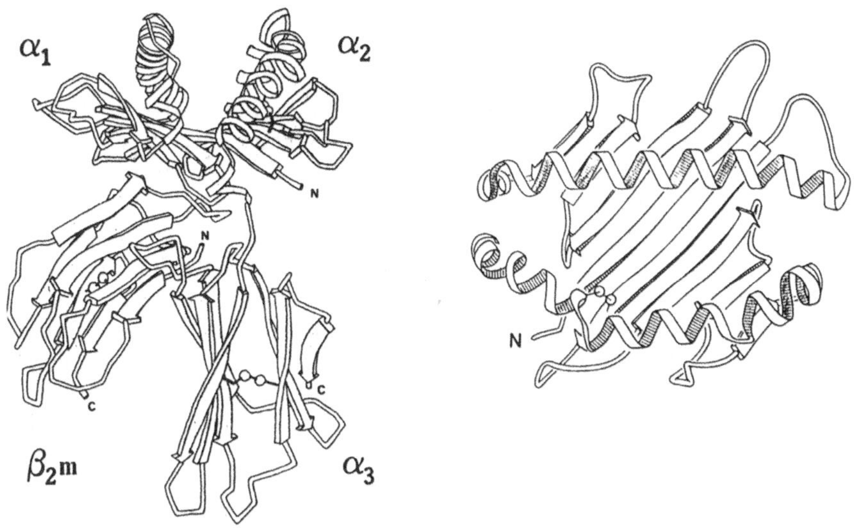

Fig. 1. Structure of the HLA-A2 molecule (adapted from [10]). *Left*, side view of the part of the molecule outside the cell. The transmembrane region and the cytoplasmic tail would continue at the bottom (C-teminal end). Above, the peptide binding site, between the two alpha-helices. *Right*, top view into the peptide binding groove, which is made up of a beta-pleated sheet and two alpha-helices

deduced from observations that virus-specific CTL can recognize not only virus-infected cells but also cells transfected with genes coding for only small parts of viral proteins [14]. In addition, virus-specific CTL have been found to recognize noninfected target cells expressing the correct MHC molecules, if these target cells have been preincubated with synthetic peptides made according to partial sequences of viral proteins [15, 16]. Thus, the peptide-like material found in the MHC class I groove by crystallographic analysis was easily interpretable as peptides similar to those recognized by class I restricted T cells.

Identification of Naturally Presented Viral Peptides

Influenza-specific CTL from C57BL/6 mice (H-2^b) were shown by Townsend and colleagues to recognize a synthetic peptide according to influenza nucleoprotein (NP) amino acids 365–380 (IASNENMETMESSTLE), in the context of the D^b-molecule [16]. Similarly, influenza-specific CTL from BALB/c mice (H-2^d) have been found to recognize another synthetic NP peptide, 147–158 (TYQRTRALVRTG), in the context of the K^d molecule [17].

Acid extraction of naturally processed peptides from virus-infected cells, detection by CTL, and comparison of these peptides to the above-mentioned synthetic peptides indicated that the natural peptides were different [18]. Sequence analysis of the respective natural peptides revealed nonapeptides in both case (ASNENMETM and TYQRTRALV). Thus, only one single species of peptides was produced by virus-infected cells to be recognized by a given virus-specific CTL. ASNENMETM could be extracted only from infected $H\text{-}2^b$ cells, not from $H\text{-}2^d$ cells. In contrast, TYQRTRALV was found only in $H\text{-}2^d$, and not $H\text{-}2^b$ cells. These results suggested strongly that the peptides isolated from whole infected cells were MHC associated. Indeed, a naturally processed peptide from vesicular stomatitis virus nucleocapside protein was eluted from purified K^b molecules isolated from VSV-infected cells [19]. Thus, it emerged that virus-infected cells indeed produce peptides from viral proteins and present these peptides on MHC class I molecules for recognition by T cells.

Isolation of Naturally Processed Minor Histocompatibility Peptides

The observation that virus-specific CTL recognize fragments of proteins synthesized in a cell rather than complete proteins led to the hypothesis [14] that CTL generally may recognize peptides derived from cellular proteins. Accordingly, CTL specific for the elusive minor histocompatibility [4] antigens were postulated to recognize MHC class I presented peptides derived from normal cellular proteins [14, 20, 21]. Minor H antigens have been known as a phenomenon since the 1950s (see "Minor and Major Histocompatibility Genes"), when it was observed that incompatibilities at minor H genes between donor and recipient of a graft can lead to graft rejection. The above postulate about the peptidic nature of minor H antigens was confirmed by enzymatic digestion of minor H proteins [22] and by acid extraction of natural minor H peptides from normal cells [23]. Naturally occurring peptides recognized by CTL specific for the minor H antigens $H\text{-}4^b$, the male-specific H-Y antigen, and other minor H antigens were found in acid extracts of male BALB/B mice ($H\text{-}2^b$-, $H\text{-}4^b$- like) but not in female B6 mice ($H\text{-}2^b$, $H\text{-}4^a$). On HPLC gradients, the individual minor H activities eluted as single, sharp peaks, indicating that single peptide species represent individual minor H antigens. Again, minor H peptides were also eluted from the restricting class I molecules. For example, the K^b-restricted $H\text{-}4^b$ peptide was eluted from purified K^b molecules but not from D^b molecules, whereas the D^b-restricted H-Y peptide was found only on D^b and not on K^b molecules [24]. The sequences of such peptides representing classical minor H antigens are not yet known. Minor H antigens known by sequence are the maternally transmitted Mta antigens, encoded for by mitochondrial genes [25] and presented by a "nonclassical" class I molecule, Hmt. In this instance, however, the naturally presented peptide has not been determined.

In conclusion, minor H antigens as recognized by CTL are peptides derived from various polymorphic proteins and presented by class I molecules (other minor H antigens are recognized by class II restricted T cells).

Isolation of Natural Peptides Recognized by Alloreactive T Cells

The trait leading to discovery of MHC in 1936 was the strong rejection of tissue grafted between MHC-incompatible individuals [1]. An in vitro correlation of this phenomenon is the strong polyclonal activation of T cells confronted in miced leukocyte cultures with stimulator cells expressing foreign MHC genes, a phenomenon termed alloreactivity [16]. Peculiarities of alloreactive T cells are:

a) a high frequency of T cells reactive against a given foreign MHC molecule and
b) a strong reaction of unprimed T cells [26].

Several theories have been put forward to explain the phenomenon of alloreactivity. One postulates the recognition of complexes of foreign MHC molecules and their natural ligands (peptides from cellular proteins) [27]. Another theory invokes recognition by T cells of determinants on MHC molecules independent of peptides [28, 29]. Recent experiments indicate that both hypotheses appear to be correct [24]. Whereas it has not been possible to demonstrate formally T cell recognition of MHC molecules in the absence of peptides (although the existence of T cells with this specificity is likely), there is ample evidence for peptide-specific alloreactive T cells (e.g., [30–32]). A recent extensive study on the peptide specificity of alloreactive CTL directed against a single MHC molecule (H-2K^b) indicated a rather complex pattern of peptide involvement [24]. One category of alloreactive CTL requires individual, well-defined peptides produced in cells in absolute dependency of particular MHC molecules, similarly as in the case with virus-specific or minor H specific CTL. Another category, however, can recognize peptides produced in cells independent of MHC molecules, although the natural target antigens recognized by these cells are also MHC bound (see also "MHC Dependency of the Cellular Peptide Pool"). Still another category recognizes MHC molecules occupied with any of a large array of peptides, and for some CTL no peptide dependency has been detected. The latter may recognize "empty" MHC molecules without peptide, although this notion is difficult to prove.

Thus, alloreactive CTL directed against a single foreign MHC class I molecule are rather heterogeneous; many of them see peptides presented by the foreign MHC molecule. Apart from shedding light on the nature of T cell alloreactivity, the analysis of peptides recognized by alloreactive T cells is also useful for addressing general questions concerning antigen processing (as discussed in "How Do cells Produce the Peptides?").

MHC Allele Specific Rules for Peptide Presentation

Comparison of the first identified natural K^d-restricted CTL epitope with synthetic peptides known to contain other K^d-restricted epitopes suggested a common motif for all K^d-presented peptides: all these were suspected to be nonapeptides with tyrosine at position 2 and an aliphatic residue at 9 [33]. This was confirmed when the peptide population naturally associated with K^d molecules was sequenced as a pool. The K^d-specific motif for peptide presentation (not just for peptide binding!) deduced from pool sequencing was similar as suspected, except that phenylalanine was also found at position 2, although at low frequency [34].

The approach of pool sequencing was also applied to several other mouse and human class I molecules [34]. For each individual class I molecule a distinct allele-specific peptide motif was found. These motifs are characterized by allele-specific lengths. Most class I alleles looked at require nonapeptides (for example, HLA-A2, H-$2K^d$, H-$2D^b$), a few require octapeptides (e.g., H-$2K^b$). Each motif defines anchor positions of conserved amino acid occupancy, such as the aromatic residues at position 2 of the K^d motif.

The side chains of these anchor residues protrude into the allele-specific pockets found by analysis of MHC crystals [11]. One of the anchor positions is always at the C-terminus, and is aliphatic in most cases. A compilation of all allele-specific motifs of MHC class I molecules known to date is presented in Table 1. All motifs except that for HLA-B27 have been deduced by pool sequencing of self peptides; the B27 motif was derived by analyzing several individual B27-eluted peptides [35]. Computer modeling and crystallographic analysis of A2 or B27/peptide complexes have indicated the peptides to be in an extended conformation, that is, not as an alpha-helix [11, 12, 36].

Prediction of Naturally Presented Peptides

The allele-specific peptide motifs found for the different MHC class I molecules are not only informative for the nature of peptide-MHC interaction; they are also of practical value for predicting natural T cell epitopes within proteins of pathogen origin or other proteins of immunological interest. Using the K^b motif, for example, the naturally processed peptide from chicken ovalbumin transfected into mouse cells and recognized by K^b-restricted CTL was predicted to be SIINFEKL (F and L would be the K^b-specific anchor residues), a notion confirmed experimentally [37]. Similarly, a natural peptide recognized by K^d-restricted, tumor-specific CTL was predicted and determined to be KYQAVTTTL (Wallny et al. submitted). For a K^d-restricted CTL epitope of lysteriolysine, a protein from *Listeria monocytogenes*, the K^d-specific motif was used to determine the peptide GYKDGNEYI as the natural T cell epitope [38]. Thus, the possibility of determining exactly natural T cell epitopes through MHC allele specific peptide motifs is useful for vaccine development.

Table 1. Peptide motifs of MHC class I molecules

	Position								
	1	2	3	4	5	6	7	8	9
H-2K^d									
Anchor		**Y**							**I**
		(F)							**L**
Strong			N	P	M	K	T		
			I			F	N		
			L						
H-2D^b									
Anchor					**N**				**M**
									I
									(L)
Strong		M	I	K		L			
			L	E		F			
			P	Q					
			V	V					
H-2K^b									
Anchor					**F**			**L**	
					Y			**M**	
								(I)	
								(V)	
Strong			Y						
HLA-A*0201									
Anchor		**L**							**V**
		M							(L)
Strong				E		V		K	
				K					
HLA-B*2705									
Anchor		**R**							
Strong			I	K	G	I	T		K
			Y		E	L	I		R

Data are from [34] for (H-2K^d, D^b, K^b, and HLA-A2) and from [35] for (HLA-B27). "Strong" indicates residues used more frequently than others at the position given.

How Do Cells Produce the Peptides?

The Common View

It is established that plasma membrane inserted MHC class I molecules present peptides, and that these peptides are derived from proteins located in the interior of the cell. All steps in between are more or less elusive. A widely propagated but unproven hypothesis postulates that cytosolic proteins are partically degraded by the enzymatic activity of proteasomes [39]. The resulting peptides are then transported by specific peptide transporter molecules into the lumen of the endoplasmatic reticulum, where association of peptides with MHC class I molecules is believed to take place. This hypothesis, however, does not cover peptides derived from noncytosolic proteins. In addition, the production of the correct peptides by cytosolic proteasomes and peptide transport by the so-called "peptide transporters" has not been demonstrated. However, the products of the "transporter genes" as well as subunits of proteasomes are important for antigen presentation, as shown by reconstitution of mutant cells defective in antigen presentation by some of the above-mentioned genes. These genes are located in the MHC region of both man and mouse. This has been taken as a hint that the resulting gene products may have something to do with MHC function.

Some recent observations, however, do not fit well with above view on MHC class I restricted antigen processing, as discussed below.

MHC Dependency of the Cellular Peptide Pool

Peptides recognized by CTL can be detected in acid extracts produced from whole target cells, as has been shown for various peptides recognized by minor H specific, virus-specific, tumor-specific, or alloreactive CTL. Such peptides are found only in target cells expressing not only the protein of peptide origin, such as viral proteins, but also the correct MHC class I molecule [40, 41]. Informative in this respect are experiments done with K^b-restricted CTL specific for the $H\text{-}4^b$ minor H antigen [42]. Acid extracts prepared from cells expressing both $H\text{-}4^b$ and K^b contain two peptides recognized by an $H\text{-}4^b$-specific CTL clone [41]. One of these peptides (the "$H\text{-}4^b$ main peptide") can be isolated from purified K^b-molecules, the other (the "$H\text{-}4^b$ pre-peak") not [24]. In cells expressing $H\text{-}4^b$ but not K^b, the $H\text{-}4^b$ main peptide is not detectable, even if a large number of cells are used for extraction [42]. The $H\text{-}4^b$ prepeak, in contrast, is found in all cells expressing $H\text{-}4^b$, irrespective of the MHC context [41, 42]. We speculate that the $H\text{-}4^b$-prepeak is a precursor peptide, from which the MHC-dependent $H\text{-}4^b$ main peptide is made, but only after interaction with the K^b molecule. That is, MHC would have an instructive in addition to a selective role in peptide presentation [12, 41, 42]. With other antigenic systems (alloreactive CTL) we have identified similar pairs of MHC-dependent and independent peptides [43].

If, on the other hand, proteasomes should process the correct final-sized peptides, which are then brought into the endoplasmic reticulum lumen by peptide transporters – all without contact to MHC molecules – one should expect to find at least a few copies of the correctly size peptides. Two possibilities may explain the discrepancy between the common view on MHC class I restricted presentation and our observations. Either the peptides correctly processed by the proteasomes are so extremely short-lived that they cannot be detected in cells unless they are protected from further degradation by binding to a fitting MHC class I molecule, or precursor peptides (such as the H-4^b prepeak) are the degradation products produced by proteasomes or other proteases, and only upon contact with the MHC molecule is the precursor peptide trimmed to the final peptide presented at the cell surface (see Fig. 2).

Specificity of Peptide Processing Appears To Be Conserved Between Species

As discussed above (see "MHC Allele Specific Rules for Peptide Presentation), each MHC allele has its own peptide motif, i.e., each of the several hundred alleles expressed in a species presents different peptides from a given protein sequence. All these ten-thousands of different peptides derived from the thousands of self and foreign proteins which might be presented by the different MHC allelic products have somehow to be produced by enzymatic degradation. Since cells identical at all genes but a single MHC gene (such as cells from mutant or recombinant pairs of congenic mouse strains) present entirely different sets of peptides from a given protein sequence, it can be deduced that a given cell can produce all the peptides required by the different MHC molecules occurring in the species. Indeed, the very same minor H peptides are produced by cells from various genetically diverse mouse strains if they share only the restricting MHC allele [41]. Similarly, cells from different tissues but expressing the same MHC can process the very same minor H peptides [42]. Moreover, human cells transfected with a mouse MHC class I gene are apparently able to produce the very same peptide as mouse cells would, and to present this peptide on the mouse-derived MHC molecule [44]. In extrapolation, a single human cell – if we assume the common view of class I restricted antigen processing to be correct – would constantly produce not only all the peptides required by all of the class I molecules in the human species but also all those peptides required by all the mouse class I molecules, not to mention those of all other mammals. From a teleological view, this would appear to be a wasted effort. The model for antigen presentation discussed below would avoid such redundancy.

A Model for MHC Class I Restricted Peptide Production

We have proposed a model for MHC class I restricted antigen processing that accomodates the observations discussed above [12, 34] (Fig. 2): Intracellular proteins are degraded by an enzymatic activity cleaving after aliphatic or charged residues. This would result in peptide precursors whose C-termini fit to all of the class I restricted peptide motifs known to date. Such peptide precursors would then be translocated to the compartment of MHC class I

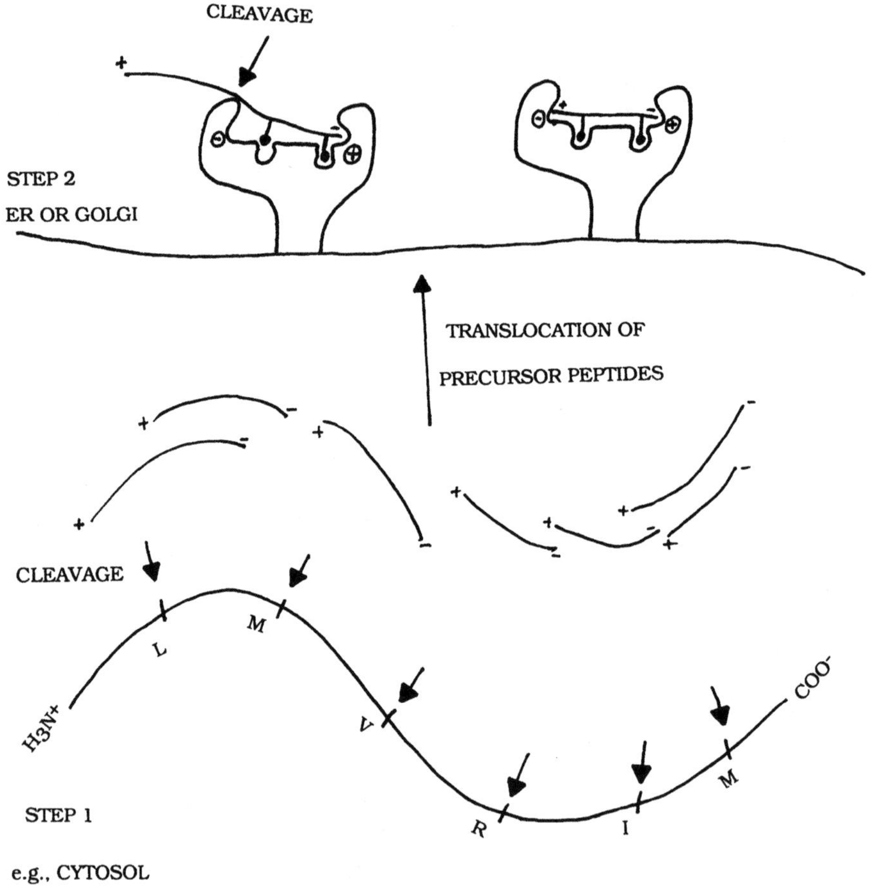

Fig. 2. Hypothetical model for antigen presentation in the MHC class I restricted pathway [12,34]. *Step 1,* a protein is partially degraded by an endopeptidase cleaving after aliphatic or charged residues. The enzymatic activity of cytosolic proteasomes would fit to this specificity; however, step 1 could also occur in other compartments. The resulting precursor peptides are then translocated to the compartment of class I loading (endoplasmic reticulum or early Golgi). The widely postulated peptide transporter gene products might perform this function, although this has not been demonstrated yet. *Step 2,* the precursor peptide binds to a fitting class I molecule, first by an ionic interaction of its positively charged C-terminus with a conserved negatively charged site [11, 36] in the class I groove. After binding, the overhanging N-terminus is trimmed to final length, for example by an exopeptidase. The final sized peptide then fits snugly into the groove. This model ascribes a selective as well as an instructive role to the MHC class I molecule in peptide processing

loading – probably endoplasmic reticulum or early Golgi – and would then bind to the fitting MHC molecule. The "overhanging" N-terminus would then be trimmed by amino peptidase or endopeptidase activity to its final size, which is determined individually by each MHC molecule. This model would explain that MHC molecules determine the peptide content of cells, and also would be consistent with the observation that processed peptides presented by a given class I molecule are obviously identical in cells of different tissues and of different species.

Implication for Self Tolerance and Autoimmunity

The recent insights into MHC class I restricted processing and peptide presentation allow some implications for self tolerance. First, only those self peptides which are actually processed and presented by MHC molecules are relevant for induction of self tolerance. This notion has been confirmed experimentally. It is known that many peptides not conforming at all to MHC specific peptide motifs may still bind to MHC (remember that the above motifs reflect the outcome of the entire processing mechanism and are not just binding motifs). Such peptides – binding to MHC but not naturally presented by MHC molecules – from a self protein of C57BL/6 mice were shown to be recognized by syngeneic T cells [45]. Thus, in extrapolation, T cells are not tolerant to those self peptide sequences which are not actually presented by MHC molecules.

One of the alloreactive CTL clones mentioned above ("Isolation of Natural Peptides Recognized by Alloreactive T cells") has a peptide specificity informative for T cell self tolerance. This clone (derived from a mouse expressing the mutant K^{bml} molecule) recognizes a peptide in context of the foreign K^b molecule [24]. The very same peptide is also presented by K^{bml} molecules, that is, by cells syngeneic to – and not recognized by – the CTL [46]. Thus, these CTL recognize this peptide only in the context of the foreign MHC molecule and not in context of the self MHC molecule. This implies that the process of elimination of self-reactive T cells during T cell development requires recognition of combinations of MHC and peptide, and not just peptide alone. Thus, the old notion that self tolerance is MHC restricted [47–49] has been confirmed on the peptide level.

Summary: A Teleological Consideration on the Function of MHC Class I Molecules

Why is antigen recognition by T cells so complicated? Would a much simpler mechanism not have served the same purpose? The following is an attempt to look at T cell recognition of MHC-class I presented antigens in terms of usefulness for the immune system.

The function of the MHC class I restricted antigen-processing system appears to allow the surveillance of T cells for changes in the cellular protein contents. To achieve this, class I molecules constantly shuffle peptides from any protein synthesized in a cell – no matter which compartment it is destined for – to the cell surface, so that the T cells can "see" them. Anything new to the T cells – that is, peptides not encountered during the T cells' differentiation – is recognized as foreign, and the cells expressing the foreign matter can be eliminated. Why is it that MHC I molecules select only peptides meeting very specific requirements, that is only few peptides from a given protein? A possible reason is that T cells probably need 100 or more copies of the same peptide-MHC combination to become activated [33, 50, 51]; this means that the number of efficiently presented peptides per cell is limited by the number of MHC I molecules on the cell surface (in the order of 10^5). Thus, selection of a few epitopes per protein by MHC I molecules could prevent the system from being overloaded with peptides from a few abundant proteins. The extreme polymorphism of MHC, with its consequence that essentially every individual presents different sets of peptides from a given (foreign) protein, could then have been evolved as a measure to counteract adaption of pathogens to avoid attacks by the immune system. A pathogen may be able to change its genes so as to escape presentation of its peptides by the set of MHC molecules of a given individual; it should be almost impossible, however, to escape the many different MHC molecules expressed in an entire species. Thus, the system of MHC class I restricted antigen presentation appears to be able to protect a population from any pathogen replicating intracellularly, although some individuals may be at risk of not being protected against every single pathogen.

Acknowledgements. I thank Jan Klein for support and Alexandra Muhm for preparing the manuscript. The original work from this laboratory mentioned in this paper was supported by the Deutsche Forschungsgemeinschaft (Sonderforschungsbereich 120).

References

1. Klein J (1986) Natural history of the major histocompatibility complex. Wiley, New York
2. Snell GD (1948) Methods for the study of histocompatibility genes. J Genetics 49:87–108
3. Davis AP, Roopenian DC (1990) Complexity at the mouse minor histocompatibility locus H-4. Immunogenetics 31:7–12
4. Counce S, Smith P, Barth R, Snell GD (1956) Strong and weak histocompatibility gene differences in mice and their role in the rejection of homografts of tumors and skin. Ann Surg 144:198–204
5. McDevitt HO, Benacerraf B (1969) Genetic control of specific immune responses. Adv Immunol 11:31–74
6. Kindred B, Shreffler DC (1972) H-2 dependence of co-operation between T and B cells in vivo. J Immunol 109:940–943
7. Zinkernagel RM and Doherty PC (1974) Restriction of in vitro T cell-mediated cytotoxicity in lymphocytic choriomeningitis within a syngeneic or semiallogeneic system. Nature 248:701–702
8. Klein J (1979) The major histocompatibility complex of the mouse. Science 203:516–521
9. Zemmour J, Parham P (1991) HLA class I nucleotide sequences, 1991. Immunogenetics 33:310–320

10. Bjorkman PJ, Saper MA, Samraoui B, Bennett WS, Strominger JL, Wiley DC (1987) Structure of the human class I histocompatibility antigen, HLA-A2. Nature 329:506–512
11. Madden DR, Gorga JC, Strominger JL, Wiley DC (1991) The structure of HLA-B27 reveals nonamer self-peptides bound in an extended conformation. Nature 353:321–325
12. Rötzschke O, Falk K (1991) Naturally occurring peptide antigens derived from MHC class I-restricted processing pathway. Immunol Today 12:447–455
13. Unanue ER, Cerottini J-C (1989) Antigen presentation. FASEB J 3:2496–2502
14. Townsend AR, Gotch FM, Davey J (1985) Cytotoxic T cells recognize fragments of the influenza nucleoprotein. Cell 42:457–467
15. Wabuke-Bunoti MAN, Taku A, Fan DP, Kent S, Webster RG (1984) Cytolytic T lymphocyte and antibody responses to synthetic peptides of influenza virus hemagglutinin. J Immunol 133:2194–2201
16. Townsend AR, Rothbard J, Gotch FM, Bahadur G, Wraith D, McMichael AJ (1986) The epitopes of influenza nucleoprotein recognized by cytotoxic T lymphocytes can be defined with short synthetic peptides. Cell 44:959–968
17. Taylor PM, Davey J, Howland K, Rothbard JB, Askonas BA (1987) Class I MHC molecules rather than other mouse genes dictate influenza epitope recognition by cytotoxic T cells. Immunogenetics 26:267–272
18. Rötzschke O, Falk K, Deres K, Schild H, Norda M, Metzger J, Jung G, Rammensee H-G (1990) Isolation and analysis of naturally processed viral peptides as recognized by cytotoxic T cells. Nature 348:252–254
19. Van Bleek GM, Nathenson SG (1990) Isolation of an immunodominant viral peptide from the class I H-$2K^b$ molecule. Nature 348:213–216
20. Bevan MJ (1987) Antigen recognition. Class discrimination in the world of immunology. Nature 325:192–194
21. Germain RN (1986) The ins and outs of antigen processing and presentation. Nature 322:687–689
22. Wallny H-J, Rammensee H-G (1990) Identification of classical minor histocompatibility antigen as cell-derived peptide. Nature 343:275–278
23. Rötzschke O, Falk K, Wallny H-J, Faath S, Rammensee H-G (1990) Characterization of naturally occurring minor histocompatibility peptides including H-4 and H-Y. Science 249:283–287
24. Rötzschke O, Falk K, Faath S, Rammensee H-G (1991) On the nature of peptides involved in T cell alloreactivity. J Exp Med 174:1059–1071
25. Loveland B, Wang CR, Yonekawa H, Hermel E, Lindahl KF (1990) Maternally transmitted histocompatibility antigen of mice: a hydrophobic peptide of a mitochondrially encoded protein. Cell 60:971–980
26. Fischer Lindahl K, Wilson DB (1977) Histocompatibility antigen-activated cytotoxic T lymphocytes. II. Estimates of the frequency and specificity of precursors. J Exp Med 145:508–522
27. Matzinger P, Bevan MJ (1977) Hypothesis: why do so many lymphocytes respond to major histocompatibility antigens. Cell Immunol 29:1–5
28. Bevan MJ (1984) High determinant density may explain the phenomenon of alloreactivity. Immunol Today 5:128
29. Kaye J and Janeway CA, Jr. (1984) The Fab fragment of a directly activating monoclonal antibody that precipitates a disulfide-linked heterodimer from a helper T cell clone blocks activation by either allogeneic Ia or antigen and self-Ia. J Exp Med 159:1397–1412
30. Heath WR, Hurd ME, Carbone FR, Sherman LA (1989) Peptide-dependent recognition of H-$2K^b$ by alloreactive cytotoxic T lymphocytes. Nature 341:749–752
31. de Koster HS, Anderson DC, Termijtelen A (1989) T cells sensitized to synthetic HLA-DR3 peptide give evidence of continuous presentation of denatured HLA-DR3 molecules by HLA-DP. J Exp Med 169:1191–1196

32. Song ES, Linsk R, Olson CA, McMillan M, Goodenow RS (1988) Allospecific cytotoxic T lymphoocytes recognize an H-2 peptide in the context of a murine major histocompatibility complex class I molecule. Proc Natl Acad Sci USA 85:1927–1931
33. Falk K, Rötzschke O, Deres K, Metzger J, Jung G, Rammensee H-G (1991) Identification of naturally processed viral nonapeptides allows their quantification in infected cells and suggests an allele-specific T cell epitope forecast. J Exp Med 174:425–434
34. Falk K, Rötzschke O, Stevanovic S, Jung G, Rammensee H-G (1991) Allele-specific motifs revealed by sequencing of self-peptides eluted from MHC molecules. Nature 351:290–296
35. Jardetzky TS, Lane WS, Robinson RA, Madden DR, Wiley DC (1991) Identification of self peptides bound to purified HLA-B27. Nature 353:326–329
36. Saper MA, Bjorkman PJ, Wiley DC (1991) Refined structure of the human histocompatibility antigen HLA-A2 at 2.6A resolution. J Mol Biol 219:277–319
37. Rötzschke O, Falk K, Stevanovic S, Jung G, Walden P, Rammensee HG (1991) Exact prediction of a natural T cell epitope. Eur J Immunol 21:2891–2894
38. Pamer EG, Harty JT, Bevan MJ (1991) Precise prediction of a dominant class I MHC-restricted epitope of Listeria monocytogenes. Nature 353:852–855
39. Driscoll J, Finley D (1992) A controlled breakdown: antigen processing and the turnover of viral proteins. Cell 68:823–825
40. Powis SJ, Townsend ARM, Deverson EV, Bastin J, Butcher GW, Howard JC (1991) Restoration of antigen presentation to the mutant-cell line RMA-s by an MHC-linked transporter. Nature 354:528–531
41. Falk K, Rötzschke O, Rammensee H-G (1990) Cellular peptide composition governed by major histocompatibility complex class I molecules. Nature 348:248–251
42. Wallny H-J, Rötzschke O, Falk K, Hämmerling G, Rammensee H-G (1992) Gene transfer experiments imply instructive role of MHC class I molecules in cellular peptide processing. Eur J Immunol 22:655–659
43. Griem P, Wallny H-J, Falk K, Rötzschke O, Arnold B, Schönrich G, Hämmerling G, Rammensee H-G (1991) Uneven tissue distribution of minor histocompatibility proteins versus peptides is caused by MHC expression. Cell 65:633–640
44. Rötzschke O, Falk K, Rammensee H-G (1992) Specificity of antigen processing for MHC class I restricted presentation is conserved between mouse and man. Eur J Immunol 22: 1323–1326
45. Schild H, Rötzschke O, Kalbacher H, Rammensee H-G (1990) Limit of Tcell tolerance to self proteins by peptide presentation. Science 247:1587–1598
46. Falk K, Rötzschke O, Rammensee H-G (1992) A self peptide naturally presented by both H-2K^{b} and H-2K^{bml} molecules demonstrates MHC restriction of self tolerance at the molecular level. Int Immunol 4:321–325
47. Groves E, Singer A (1983) Role of the H-2 complex in the induction of T cell tolerance to self minor histocompatibility antigens. J Exp Med 158:1483–1497
48. Matzinger P, Zamoyska R, Waldmann H (1984) Self tolerance is H-2-restricted. Nature 308:738–741
49. Rammensee HG, Bevan MJ (1984) Evidence from in vitro studies that tolerance to self antigens is MHC-restricted. Nature 308:741–744
50. Vitiello A, Potter TA, Sherman LA (1990) The role of β2-microglobulin in peptide binding by class I molecules. Science 250:1423–1426
51. Christinck ER, Luscher MA, Barber BH, Williams DB (1991) Peptide binding to class I MHC on living cells and quantitation of complexes required for CTL lysis. Nature 352:67–70

T Cell Receptor Variable Region Repertoire in Lymphocytes from Rheumatoid Arthritis Patients

U. Krawinkel and *G. Pluschke*

Introduction

Rheumatoid arthritis (RA) is a disease characterized by chronic inflammation affecting the synovial membranes of articulating joints. T lymphocytes, as regulators of immune responses, are thought to be involved in the initiation and perpetuation of RA (Feldmann et al. 1988).

Supportive evidence for this idea comes from observations that activated T cells represent 10%–15% of the synovial mononuclear cell infiltrate (Burmester et al. 1984; Knobloch et al. 1985), and that RA is strongly associated with the DR4 and DR1 alleles of the class II genes of the major histocompatibility complex (MHC; Gregersen et al. 1987; Todd et al. 1988; Nepom et al. 1989; Wordsworth et al. 1989; Lang et al. 1990). Moreover, elimination or inhibition of T cells by various techniques sometimes leads to an amelioration of RA (Paulus et al. 1977; Herzog et al. 1987; Reiter et al. 1991). In situ activation and clonal expansion of specific T cell populations caused and selected by as yet unknown synovial antigen(s) is suggested by the observation of dominant T cell receptors (TCR) rearrangement patterns in T lymphocytes isolated from synovial tissue and cultured in vitro (Stamenkovic et al. 1988; Chatila et al. 1990; Miltenburg et al. 1990). Direct analyses of the synovial TCR repertoire utilizing the polymerase chain reaction (PCR) did not confirm the existence of a few dominant T cell clones in the synovial fluid. However, the preferential usage of TCR variable region gene families which are rarely used in blood T lymphocytes has suggested a role for superantigen in the pathogenesis of RA (Paliard et al. 1991; Pluschke et al. 1991; Howell et al. 1991).

In summary, although the pathogenesis of RA is complex, there is highly suggestive evidence for the involvement of T lymphocytes stimulated by (auto)antigen(s). In this chapter we summarize our studies pertaining to this point.

Patients and Methods

Synovial fluid lymphocytes were obtained from therapeutic arthrocenteses of four RA patients who fulfilled at least five of the American Rheumatism Association criteria for RA classification (Arnett et al. 1988). Patients 1, 2, and 3 carried the HLA-DR4 subtypes which predispose to RA, and patient 4 was typed DR7-DW7/DRW8.1-DW1 (Becking 1991).

The synovial TCR-Vα repertoire was analyzed utilizing the anchor PCR technique (Pluschke et al. 1991). The synovial and peripheral TCR-Vβ repertoires were analyzed following essentially the PCR protocol of Choi et al. (1989) with the primers described therein. Vβ2DβJβ-junctional sequences were determined on DNA fragments obtained by PCR amplification of mRNA from synovial fluid lymphocytes. The steps involved are the following.

Analysis of the synovial TCR Vα region repertoire

- mRNA is isolated from SFL and cDNA is synthesized with reverse transcriptase.
- A dG tail is added to the 3' end o the cDNA using terminal transferase.
- PCR amplification of tailed cDNA employs a Cα-specific primer and oligo-dC as a nonspecific primer.
- Amplification products of 100- to 500-bp length are purified on a gel.
- Isolated fragments are reamplified using a nested Cα primer and oligo-dC.
- Products of correct size are isolated after gel purification.
- Ligation of amplification products into a plasmid vector, transformation of bacteria, screening of colonies with another nested Cα oligonucleotide; 50 % of the colonies react positively.
- The VJ-junctional nucleotide sequence of cloned TCR Vα regions is determined.

Analysis of the expressed TCR Vβ region repertoire

- mRNA is isolated from SFL and PBL, cDNA-synthesis with reverse transcriptase.
- PCR amplification of cDNA employing a radioactively labeled Cβ-specific primer and 22 family-specific Vβ primers. As internal standard Cα regions are amplified utilizing radioactively labeled Cα primers.
- Vβ and Cα amplification products are separated on a gel, bands are isolated, and the Vβ/Cα ratio is determined by measuring the incorporated radioactivity.

Analysis of transcripts carrying Vβ2 gene segments

- cDNA from SFL is amplified by PCR utilizing a Cβ-specific primer and a Vβ2-specific primer. Both primers carry restriction sites suitable for cloning the resulting PCR products into plasmid vectors.
- Gel-purification of PCR products.
- Vβ2-carrying DNA fragments are cloned in bacteria and the Vβ2DJ-junctional nucleotide sequences are determined.

Results

TCR Vα Region Repertoire

A total of 55 Vα-Jα-Cα transcripts from synovial lymphocytes of RA patients 3 and 4 were characterized as cDNA clones (Pluschke et al. 1991); 51 clones were in-frame and thus should represent functional TCR transcripts. Sequence analysis showed that the synovial T cell population of both patients was essentially polyclonal although two pairs and one triplet of identical Vα-Jα junctionals indicated the clonal expansion of lymphocytes with Vα-segments from families Vα2, VαFR1, and Vα8. In both patients we observed high expression of Vα segments belonging to families Vα2, Vα8, Vα14, Vα15, and VαFR1. T lymphocytes using Vα2- and Vα8-related V segments are frequent in the PBL of healthy individuals, but expression of segments from families Vα14, Vα15, and VαFR1 is rare (Yoshikai et al. 1986; Kimura et al. 1987; Klein et al. 1987; Roman-Roman et al. 1991). The latter families comprise four genes in the germline, i.e., they represent less than 5 % of the entire Vα gene repertoire. In the expressed synovial repertoire of our two RA patients, however, 30 %–35 % of all TCR α-chain transcripts carried Vα14–, Vα15-, and VαFR1-related sequences (amino acid sequences are given in the one-letter code).

SFL of patient 3

Vα14 —— Jα (4/39)
YFCA ———— **SSGYST**LTF-Cα
YFCA ——— **YRSI**QGAQKLAF-Cα
YFCA ——— **YT**DTGRRALTF-Cα
YFCA — **YRSS**NYGGSQGNLIF-Cα

Vα15 —— Jα (3/39)
YFCA ———— **ED**AGNMLTE-Cα
YFCA ——— **E**SSSGGSYIPTF-Cα
YFCA ——— **MR**SFNQAGTALIF-Cα

VαFR1 —— Jα (6/39)
YLCA ———— **AVSS**YKLIF-Cα
YLCA ———— **VP**NQAGTALIF-Cα
YLCA ——— **VTLY**NQGGKLIF-Cα
YLCA —— **VRP**EYGSSQGNLIF-Cα
YLCA —— **VLPM**EAAGNKLTF-Cα
YLCA ———— **VM**DSSYKLIF-Cα

SFL of patient 4

Vα14 —— Jα (1/12)
YFCA **YRRGM**YSGGGADGLTF-Cα

Vα15 —— **Jα** (2/12)
YFCA ——— **ER**W**D**NNDMRF-Cα
YFCA —— **E**SI**K**GGGSNYKLTF-Cα

VαFR1 Jα (2/12)
YLCA ——— **VVS**DSGYALNF-Cα
YLCA ——— **VVS**DSGYALNF-Cα

PBL of healthy persons

Vα14Jα	(0/66)
Vα15Jα	(066)
VαFR1Jα	(8/238)

Most interestingly, the respective Vα-Jα-junctional sequences in Vα14, Vα15, and VαFR1 transcripts from these patients share similar structural motives, and the VαFR1 response of patient 4 appears to be oligoclonal. These data support the idea that the synovial T cell response of RA patients is selected by as yet unknown antigen(s). Note, that the patient 4 does not carry MHC class II molecules of the HLA-DR4 subtype which is known to predispose to RA.

TCR Vβ Region Repertoire

The relative expression of Vβ families was assessed in SFL and PBL of three RA patients (Table 1). For comparison, we also analyzed the relative Vβ family expression in PBL of two healthy individuals. It did not differ from that of PBL in patients 1 and 2. The SFL of both patients, however, showed a relative overexpression of the Vβ2 family. Patient 2, in addition to Vβ2, overexpressed families Vβ6 and Vβ8. Patient 3, in contrast, showed no preference for a particular Vβ family in the synovial TCR Vβ-chain response. On the contrary, we could not detect Vα9 transcripts in SFL and PBL. This cannot be attributed to a deletion of structural genes since amplification products of correct size we obtained in the PCR analysis of DNA from patient 3 employing primers complementary to three different regions of the Vβ9 gene (Ginter et al., submitted). The disappearance of Vβ9 expressing T cells from the blood and the synovial fluid of RA patients also has been observed by others (Paliard et al. 1991).

Table 1. Comparison of VB gene expression in SFL and PBL from RA patients

Patient no.	Vβ family	Vβ expression ratio SFL/PBL	VDJ junction	Frequency
1	Vβ2	2.2(13.9%/6.6%)	Vβ2——VPTSVNTEAFFG GTRLTVV-Cβ	4×
			Vβ2——APRRYTDTQYFGPGTRLTVL-Cβ	3×
			Vβ2—ADRRYSGNTIYFGEGTWLTVV-Cβ	1×
	Vβ6	2.2(10.3%/4.6%)		
	Vβ8	2.8(6.3%/2.2%)		
	All others	1.8–0.2		
2	Vβ2	2.6(26.9%/10.4%)	Vβ2——AHRQQDPQHFGDGTRLSIL-Cβ	32×
			Vβ2-VLERGRPQNIQYFGAGTRLSVL-Cβ	4×
			Vβ2—RDRRDGTYEQYFGPGTRLTVT-Cβ	2×
			Vβ2——RQYSGNTIYFGEGTWLTVV-Cβ	1×
3	Vβ9	Not detectable		
	All others	1.5–0.4		

The amino acid sequences of 47 Vβ2-Dβ-Iβ junctions are shown in the one-letter code.

To assess the clonality of the synovial Vβ2 response of patients 1 and 2 we sequenced 47 VDJ junctions in Vβ2-carrying mRNAs. In both patients the Vβ2 response was clearly oligoclonal. Moreover, the VDJ junctions of distinct clones were structurally similar (Table 1). The oligoclonality of the Vβ2 reponse observed in SFL from RA patients supports the conclusion derived from our analysis of the synovial Vα region repertoire: there is evidence for an antigen-driven immune response.

Discussion

Our analysis of the TCR V region repertoire in SFL of RA patients provides evidence that the synovial immune response is selected by antigen(s). Some qualities of this response, namely preferential usage or underrepresentation of distinct V region families and apparent lack of conventional MHC restriction has led some authors to the speculation that bacterial or viral superantigen(s) may be involved (Paliard et al. 1991; Howell et al. 1991). The relative overexpression of families Vα14, Vα15, and VαFR1 im SFL from RA patients that differ in their HLA-DR subtypes, and the relative overexpression of the Vβ2 family or the deletion of Vβ9-carrying T cell clones in some patients, may support this hypothesis. In this context it should be noted that a Vβ2 response can be elicited by M proteins of group A streptococci (Tomai et al. 1991). Such bacteria thus may be involved in the pathogenesis of RA.

It has not been reported as yet that superantigens select the expression of Vα region families. This does not rule out the possibility that Vα elements influence the response to superantigen since superantigen-selected TCR Vβ segments may preferentially pair with specific Vα segments. However, we wish to point out that our results can be sufficiently explained by selection through conventional antigen(s). The involvement of superantigen(s) is possible but not imperative.

A role of genes from families Vα14 and VαFR1 in autoimmune responses is also suggested by the finding that TCR from autoreactive T cell lines use Vα segments belonging to these families. The autoreactive clone UA-S2 (Schlesier et al. 1989) from the synovium of a patient with reactive arthritis expresses a VαFR1-carrying TCRα–chain (Hinkkanen et al. 1989), and two clones reactive against small nuclear riboproteins (autoantigens in mixed connective tissue disease) use Vα14-segments in their TCRs (M. Schlesier, personal communication).

In summary, since individual patients show different patterns of TCR V region expression in their synovial immune response (Sottini et al. 1991; Pluschke et al. 1991; Paliard et al. 1991; Howell et al. 1991; Bucht et al. 1992; van Laar et al. 1992), it is obvious that RA is a disease with a complex pathogenesis. However, there seems to be a role for (auto)antigen-activated T lymphocytes in the sequence of reactions that finally lead to the destruction of joint tissue.

Acknowledgements. We thank H.H. Peter, I. Melchers, and M. Schlesier for discussion, and C. Hoffmann for preparing the manuscript. The work was supported by the Deutsche Forschungsgemeinschaft through grant Pe151/1.

References

Arnett FC, Edworthy SM, Bloch DA, McShane DJ, Fries JF, Cooper NS, Healey LA, Kaplan SR, Liang MH, Lutura HS, Medsger TA, Mitchell DM, Neustadt DH, Pinals RS,

Schaller JG, Sharp JT, Wilder RL, Hunder GG (1988) The American Rheuma Association 1987 revised criteria for the classification of rheumatoid arthritis. Arthritis Rheum. 31:315–324

Becking A (1991) Molekularbiologische HLA-DR Subtypisierung bei Patienten mit Rheumatoider Arthritis. MD thesis, University of Freiburg

Bucht A, Oksenberg JR, Lindblad S, Grönberg A, Steinman L, Klareskog L (1992) Characterization of T cell receptor αβ repertoire in synovial tissue from different temporal phases of rheumatoid arthritis. Scand J Immunol 35:159–165

Burmester GR, Jahn B, Gramatzky M, Zacher J, Kalden JR (1984). Divergence in expression of TAC and Ia antigens in the non-blastoid small T cells of inflammation and normal T cells activated in vitro. J Immunol 133:1230–1234

Chatila MK, Pandolfi F, Stamenkovich I, Kurnik JT (1990) Clonal dominance among synovial tissue infiltrating lymphocytes in arthritis. Hum Immunol 28:252–257

Choi YW, Kotzin B, Herron L, Callahan J, Marrack P, Kappler J (1989) Interaction of Staphylococcus aureus toxin superantigens with human T cells. Proc Natl Acad Sci USA 86:8941–8944

Feldmann M, Londai M, Leech Z, Brennan F, Savill C, Maini RN (1988) Analysis of T-cell clones in rheumatoid arthritis. Springer Semin Immunopathol 10:157–167

Gregersen PK, Silver J, Winchester RJ (1987) The shared epitope hypothesis. An approach to understanding the molecular genetics of susceptibility to rheumatoid arthritis. Arthritis Rheum 30:1205–1213

Herzog C, Walker C, Pichler W, Aeschlimann A, Wassmer P, Stockinger H, Knapp W, Rieber EP, Müller W (1987) Monoclonal anti CD4 in arthritis. Lancet II:1461–1462

Hinkkanen A, Steimle V, Schlesier M, Peter HH, Epplen JT (1989) The antigen receptor of an autoreactive T-cell clone from human rheumatic synovia. Immunogenetics 29:131–133

Howell MD, Diveley JP, Lundeen KA, Esty A, Winters ST, Carlo DJ, Brostoff SW (1991) Limited T cell receptor β-chain heterogeneity among IL2 receptor positive synovial T cells suggests a role for superantigen in rheumatoid arthritis. Proc Natl Acad Sci USA 88:10921–10925

Kimura N, Toyonaga B, Yoshikai Y, Du RP, Mak TW (1987) Sequences and repertoire of the human T cell receptor α and β chain variable region genes in thymocytes. Eur J Immunol 17:375–383

Klein MH, Concannon P, Everett M, Kim LDH, Hunkapiller T, Hood L (1987) Diversity and structure of human T cell receptor α-chain variable region genes. Proc Natl Acad Sci USA 84:6884–6888

Knobloch C, Schlesier M, Dräger R, Gärtner M, Peter HH (1985) Quantitative absorption of interleukin2 by peripheral blood and synovial fluid lymphocytes from patients with rheumatoid arthritis. Rheumatol Int 5:133–139

Lang B, Melchers I, Urlacher A, Tanzi-Fetta RF, Kohlbrenner S, Tongio MM, Peter HH (1990) HLA-DR1 and DRw6 association in DR 4 negative rheumatoid arthritis patients. Rheumatol Int 10:171–175

Miltenburg AMM, van Laar JM, Daha MR, DeVries RR, van der Elsen PJ, Breedveld FC (1990) Dominant T-cell receptor β-chain gene rearrangements indicate clonal expansion in the rheumatoid joint. Scand J Immunol 31: 121–126

Nepom GT, Byers P, Seyfried C, Healey LA, Wilske KR, Stage D, Nepom BS (1989) HLA genes associated with rheumatoid arthritis. Arthritis Rheum 32 (1):15–21

Paliard X, West SG, Lafferty JA, Clements JR, Kappler JW, Marrack P, Kotzin BL (1991) Evidence for the effects of a superantigen in rheumatoid arthritis. Science 253:325–329

Paulus HE, Machleder HI, Levine S, Yu DTY, MacDonald NS (1977) Lymphocyte involvement in rheumatoid arthritis. Arthritis Rheum 20:1249–1262

Pluschke G, Ricken G, Taube H, Kroniger S, Melchers I, Peter HH, Eichmann K, Krawinkel U (1991) Biased T cell receptor Vα region repertoire in the synovial fluid of rheumatoid arthritis patients. Eur J Immunol 21:2749–2754

Reiter C, Kakavand B, Rieber EP, Schattenkirchner M, Riethmüller G, Krüger K (1991) Treatment of rheumatoid arthritis with monoclonal CD4 antibody M-T151. Arthritis Rheum 34:525–532

Roman-Roman S, Ferradini L, Azocar J, Genevée C, Hercend T, Triebel F (1991) Studies on the human T cell receptor α/β variable region genes. Eur J Immunol 21:927–933

Schlesier M, Ramb-Lindauer C, Dräger R, Urlacher A, Robin-Winn M, Peter HH (1989) Autoreactive T-cells in rheumatic disease. Immunobiology 177:420–427

Sottini A, Imberti L, Gorla R, Cattaneo R, Primi D (1991) Restricted expression of T cell receptor Vβ but not Vα genes in rheumatoid arthritis. Eur J Immunol 21:461–466

Stamenkovic I, Stegagno M, Wright KA, Krane SM, Amento EP, Colvin RB, Duquesnoy RJ, Kurnick JT (1988) Clonal dominance among T-lymphocyte infiltrate in arthritis. Proc Natl Acad Sci USA 85:1179–1183

Todd JA, Acha-Orbea H, Bell JI, Chao N, Fronek Z, Jacob CO, McDermott M, Sinha AA, Timmerman L, Steinman L, McDevitt HO (1988) A molecular basis for MHC class II associated autoimmunity. Science 240: 1003–1009

Tomai MA, Aelion JA, Dockter ME, Majumdar G, Spinella DG, Kotb M (1991) T cell receptor V gene usage by human T cells stimulated with the superantigen streptococcal M protein. J Exp Med 174:285–288

Van Laar JM, Miltenburg AMM, Verdonk MJA, Daha MR, DeVries RRP, van der Elsen PJ, Breedveld FC (1992) T cell β chain rearrangements of T cell populations expanded from multiple sites of synovial tissue obtained from a patient with rheumatoid arthritis. Scand J Immunol 35:187–194

Wordsworth BP, Lanchbury JSS, Sakkas LI, Welsh KI, Panayi GS, Bell JI (1989) HLA DR4 subtype frequencies in rheumatoid arthritis indicate that DRB1 is the major susceptibility locus within the HLA class II region. Proc Natl Acad Sci USA 86:10049–10053

Xoshikai Y, Kimura N, Toyonaga B, Mak TW (1986) Sequences and repertoire of human T cell recepter α-chain variable region genes in mature T-lymphocytes. J Exp Med 164:90–104

Autoantigens and Models of Autoimmunity (Clinical Research)

Transgenic Models to Study Diseases of the Nervous System: An In Vivo Approach to Dissect Complex Pathogenetic Networks

L. Mucke

Introduction

Diseases of the nervous system often pose particular challenges, both in terms of their pathogenetic complexity and their refractoriness to conventional therapeutic strategies. Multiple sclerosis, Alzheimer's disease (AD), and the human immunodeficiency virus 1 (HIV-1) associated cognitive/motor complex dramatically illustrate this point. Because many disease processes that afflict the central nervous system (CNS) evolve slowly, the neuropathologist is often confronted with postmortem material that reflects the intricate combination of causative and compensatory processes. Unfortunately, many features of CNS diseases are also difficult to dissect with in vitro models because of the extensive interactions between different types of predominantly nondividing cells that characterize the adult CNS. Nevertheless, both in vitro models and the pathologic analysis of nervous tissue have provided important leads as to which cellular activities, gene products, infectious agents, or chemical compounds may constitute potential etiologic factors in the development of neurologic illnesses. The association of increased/aberrant expression of major histocompatibility complex (MHC) antigens with autoimmune diseases (for reviews see Bottazzo et al. 1983, 1986; Janeway et al. 1984), of amyloid β protein and α_1-antichymotrypsin (ACT) with AD (for reviews see Selkoe 1991a, b), and of HIV-1 envelope proteins with acquired immundeficiency syndrome (AIDS) dementia (reviewed by Lipton 1992) represent important examples. For the rational design of therapeutic strategies it is, however, often desirable to prove that a suspected pathogenetic factor is sufficient to cause specific disease manifestations in vivo or to define the exact role a protein plays in a multifactorial pathogenetic cascade. This is illustrated, for example, by the disappointing effects that different cytokines had on the course of multiple sclerosis when they were used as therapeutic agents in clinical trials (Knobler et al. 1984; Camenga et al. 1986; Johnson 1988). However, the in vivo analysis and experimental/therapeutic manipulation of cells and chemical factors within the brain parenchyma is complicated by the blood-brain barrier. Direct injections of pathogenetic factors into the parenchyma of the CNS are also problematic. The associated trauma induces a large number of vigorous secondary responses, and the focal concentration of the injected proteins may vary substantially from injection to injection.

Fusion gene constructs expressed in transgenic animals allow the delivery of selected protein factors to specific areas/cells within the intact organism and hence can overcome some of the obstacles outlined above. This chapter provides an outline of how transgenic models may help advance the in vivo analysis of major neurologic diseases.

Expression of Proteins in the CNS of Transgenic Mice

Many excellent reviews have been published on the production and use of transgenic animals (Hogan et al. 1986; Brinster and Palmiter 1986; Gordon 1986; Palmiter and Brinster 1986; Arnold and Hämmerling 1991; Merlino 1991). Mice expressing prion genes (for review see Prusiner 1991) or DNAs encoding the human poliovirus receptor (Ren et al. 1990; Ren and Racaniello 1992) have demonstrated the enormous potential of transgenic models in the analysis of neurologic diseases. The subsequent section summarizes some basic aspects of transgenic technology and points out certain caveats that should be kept in mind when considering this experimental approach.

Basic Principles of Transgenic Technology

Typically, between one and 100 transgene molecules encoding a protein of interest integrate into a random site within the genome when injected into a fertilized egg cell. The integration site of the transgene within the chromatin can dramatically influence its expression (reviewed by Wilson 1990). Because of the randomness of the integration event, transgenic mice that develop from different microinjected zygotes (founders) can show marked differences in the levels and patterns of transgene expression and hence also in their phenotype. Consequently, lines of transgenic mice carrying the same transgene but derived from separate founders may also differ substantially from each other at the expression level. Most founders transmit the transgene to approximately 50 % of their offspring when mated with normal nontransgenic mice. Transgenic mice derived from the same founder usually show very similar levels and patterns of transgene expression.

While the introduction of transgenes into the murine genome has now become a routine procedure in many laboratories, the experimental regulation of the transgene expression continues to be one of the more challenging aspects of transgenic technology. Many features of the fusion gene and of the chromatin surrounding its integration site influence the areas within the body where the transgene encoded protein is expressed, the cell type which produces it, the kinetics of its expression during development, as well as the overall amount and focal concentration of the transgene product (Swain et al. 1987; Brinster et al. 1988; Bonifer et al. 1990; Wilson 1990; Choi et al. 1991; Palmiter et al. 1991). It should also be noted in this context that the expression of fusion genes in cultured cells unfortunately does not reliably predict their expression in vivo (Palmiter et al. 1991, and our own unpublished observations).

Targeting the Expression of Fusion Genes to Specific Cell Types Within the CNS

In the majority of CNS diseases clinical signs and symptoms are related most directly to an impairment of neuronal functions. However, increasing evidence suggests that nonneuronal CNS cells can act as important mediators of neurologic disease processes. Because astrocytes are widely distributed throughout the CNS and participate in diverse biologic processes, including neural-immune interactions (Kimelberg and Norenberg 1989; Frohman et al. 1989; Lieberman et al. 1989), they form excellent targets for the in vivo expression of a number of interesting molecules. Hence, we developed a DNA construct that allows the astrocyte-specific expression of hybrid genes in transgenic mice (Mucke et al. 1991). The regulatory sequences that direct the expression of transgenes in this construct were adopted from the glial fibrillary acidic protein (GFAP) gene. The GFAP gene encodes a relatively abundant intermediate filament cytoskeletal protein (Lewis et al. 1984); Balcarek and Cowan 1985) that is restricted primarily to astroglia (Bignami et al. 1972). Interestingly, the expression of the GFAP gene is upmodulated dramatically by diverse forms of neural injury (Bignami and Dahl 1976; Smith et al. 1983; De La Monte et al. 1987; Delacourte 1990).

A GFAP-*lacZ* fusion gene was constructed (Mucke et al. 1991) by replacing a 50-bp fragment of the first exon of the GFAP gene with the *Escherichia coli lacZ* reporter gene. The *lacZ* gene encodes bacterial beta-galactosidase (β-gal) which can be detected readily in tissue sections by the formation of a blue precipitate upon staining with X-gal (An et al. 1982; Hall et al. 1983; Sanes et al. 1986). The GFAP-*lacZ* fusion gene effectively monitors astrocyte activity in vivo, facilitates the analysis of early astroglial activation events, and demonstrates the characteristic expression pattern directed by our GFAP construct. Germline injection of the GFAP-*lacZ* construct resulted in six separate lines of transgenic mice. In all six lines, the expression of β-gal was restricted to astrocytes. In unmanipulated transgenics, β-gal activity was much more prominent in astrocytes of the hippocampal formation, selected white matter tracts, and glial limitans than in astrocytes of other areas. This expression pattern illustrates the physiologic heterogeneity of astrocytes and likely reflects differences in functional demands placed on these cells in different brain regions. Because astroglial activation is accompanied by an increased expression of the GFAP gene, the expression of the GFAP-*lacZ* fusion gene could be upmodulated experimentally with gliosis-provoking maneuvers such as focal mechanical trauma (Fig. 1). In two lines of GFAP-*lacZ* transgenic mice no β-gal expression was seen in the unmanipulated state, but transgene expression was inducible by focal injury. The ability to focally upmodulate the expression of transgenes at defined time points in

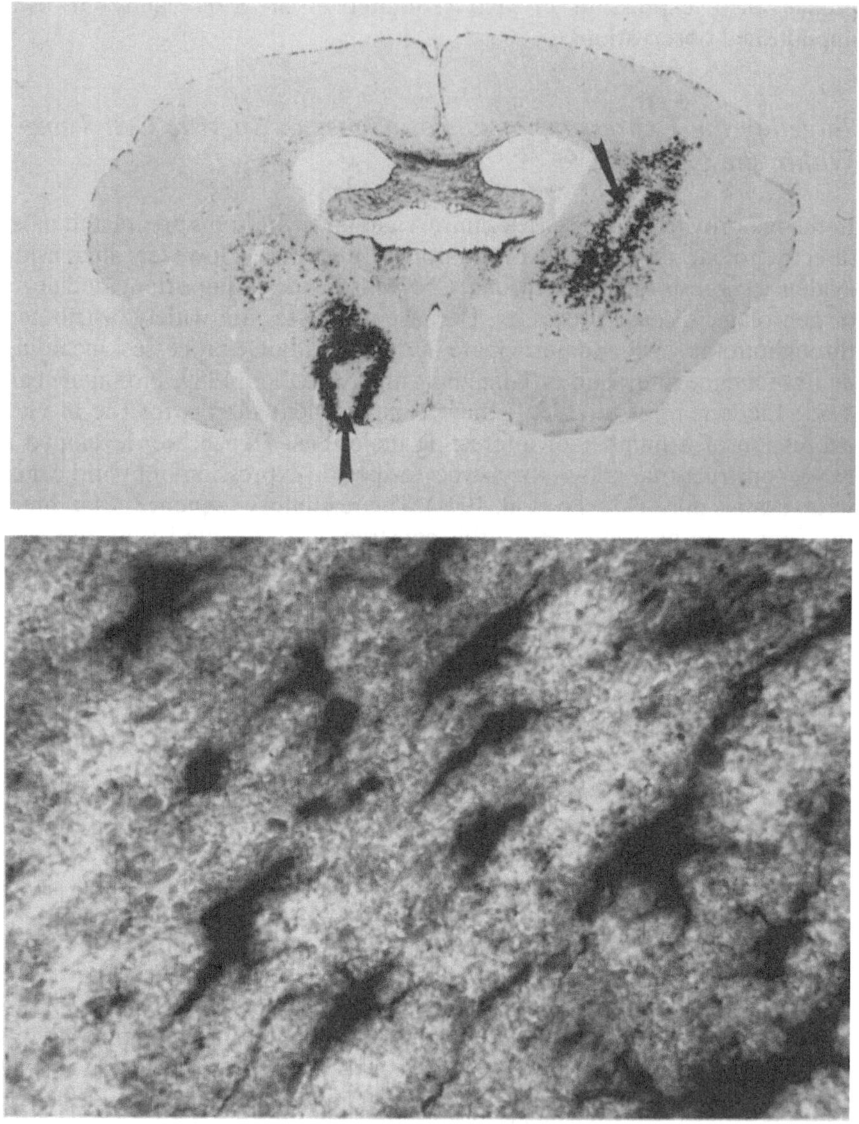

Fig. 1. Hybrid gene expression directed by the GFAP construct. The pattern of hybrid gene expression directed by the modified GFAP gene is revealed in mice transgenic for a GFAP-*lacZ* fusion gene by staining with X-gal (dark precipitate indicates β-gal activity). While in unmanipulated mice hybrid gene expression was seen primarily in the hippocampal formation, major white matter tracts and along the glial limitans, transgene expression could be effectively upmodulated in all brain regions by focal injury. *Upper panel*, frontal brain section (×10; stained with X-gal and eosion) of a GFAP-*lacZ* transgenic mouse showing intense induction of β-gal expression by reactive astrocytes around two foci of mechanically induced tissue necrosis (*arrows*). *Lower Panel*, astrocytes in the fimbria hippocampi of an unmanipulated GFAP-*lacZ* transgenic mouse (×190; stained with X-gal and hematoxylin)

the adult CNS by activation of astrocytes represents a major advantage of the GFAP vector because it allows experimental manipulation of the levels of transgene products in different brain regions of the same animal. In transgenic mice with low baseline expression it also makes it possible to assess detrimental proteins that would be lethal if expressed constitutively at higher levels.

The GFAP vector has already been used successfully to express a variety of biologically active molecules such as MHC antigens, viral products, cytokines and enzymes in astrocytes of transgenic mice (see examples below). These studies are expected to provide insights into the pathogenesis of viral – and immune-mediated neurologic diseases as well as neurodegenerative disorders.

Transgenic Models

Many neurologic disease processes are mediated by proteins derived either from the host (e.g., cytokines and amyloid β protein) or from the environment (e.g., microbial products). While rodent models can probably never faithfully simulate all aspects of a human disease, the expression of potentially pathogenetic factors in the CNS of transgenic mice should

a) help decide whether these factors are sufficient to induce certain disease manifestations or require cofactors,
b) provide valuable general information on their effects within the intact adult CNS,
c) allow the study of interactions between different factors in vivo by crossing lines of transgenic mice that express individual proteins, and
d) facilitate the development of novel therapeutic strategies based on the experimental manipulation of proteins with confirmed pathogenetic activity.

Presentation of Viral Antigens by Transgenic Astrocytes Expressing an MHC Class I Minigene

Abnormal immune responses feature prominently in the pathogenesis of a number of neurologic diseases. Multiple sclerosis, acute disseminated encephalomyelitis and experimental allergic encephalomyelitis are examples of such disorders with a predeliction for the CNS. While the CNS used to be considered an immunologically privileged site, more recent studies have shown that activated T lymphocytes can traverse the blood-brain barrier and migrate through the brain parenchyma (Wekerle et al. 1986, 1987; Hickey et al. 1991). An important prerequisite for the efficient presentation of antigens to T cells is the expression of MHC antigens (Doherty and Zinkernagel 1974; Zinkernagel and Doherty 1974, 1983; Janeway et al. 1984). It has been hypothesized that increased/aberrant MHC expression can intensify immune surveillance and may even be a critical pathogenetic factor in the development of a number of autoimmune diseases (Bottazzo et al. 1983, 1986; Wekerle et al. 1986). While there is little evidence for MHC expression on brain cells in the normal state, a number of factors can upmodulate MHC expression in astrocytes (Wong et al. 1984; Hickey et al. 1985; Massa and ter Meulen 1987; Massa et al. 1987; Suzumura et al. 1986, 1988). Because these findings suggest that antigen presentation within the CNS could be involved in the pathogenesis of immune-mediated neurologic diseases we chose (in collaboration with G. Rall, M. Nerenberg, and M. Oldstone) to assess and manipulate the antigen-presenting capacity of astrocytes in vitro and in vivo.

A minigene encoding the MHC class I antigen D^b was expressed in astrocytes of transgenic C57BL/6(H-2^b) and BALB/c(H-2^d) mice with the help of the GFAP vector (see above). The astroglial expression of a functional MHC class I glycoprotein derived from the GFAP-D^b fusion gene and the antigen-presenting capacity of GFAP-D^b transgenic astrocytes were demonstrated in chromium release assays. Primary astrocytes obtained from transgenic BALB/c mice (H-2^d) expressing the allogeneic D^b molecule were able to present lymphocytic choriomeningitis virus (LCMV) antigens to D^b-restricted, LCMV-primed cytotoxic T cells whereas astrocytes from nontransgenic BALB/c mice (D^b negative) were not. Our data are in agreement with previous reports on the antigen-presenting capacity of astrocytes (Fontana et al. 1984, 1986; Fierz et al. 1985; Male et al. 1987; Skias et al. 1987). Other studies have demonstrated the importance of microglia as antigen-presenting cells in the CNS (Giulian 1987; Lassmann et al. 1991). The proficient antigen presentation by microglia makes the assessment of antigen presentation by astrocytes in explant cultures problematic because such cultures can easily become contaminated with microglia despite vigorous selection methods. However, our GFAP-D^b transgenic BALB/c (H-2^d) mice circumvent this problem because antigen presentation by BALB/c microglia would be H-2^d restricted and could not have contributed directly to the D^b restricted presentation of LCMV antigens in our cultures of GFAP-D^b transgenic BALB/c astrocytes.

The GFAP-D^b transgenic model combines inducibility of transgene expression by focal neurologic injury, mediated through the regulatory sequences adopted from the GFAP gene (see above), with the capacity of transgenic astrocytes to present viral antigens to immune cells. Hence, the model should allow us to assess the combination of aberrant MHC expression and environmental insults, an interaction of potential importance in the pathogenesis of autoimmune diseases.

Transgenic Models to Study the Neurologic Manifestations of Alzheimer's Disease (AD) and HIV-1-Infection

The dementia of AD is accompanied by the cerebral accumulation of abnormal proteins derived from the amyloid β protein precursor (APP).

Increasing evidence suggests that these proteins are detrimental to the surrounding brain cells and may be a major cause of the symptoms seen in AD (for reviews see Selkoe 1991a, b; Yankner and Mesulam 1991). The close association of three different APP point mutations (affecting the same amino acid in the transmembrane domain of the molecule) with early-onset familial AD (Chartier-Harlin et al. 1991; Goate et al. 1991; Murrell et al. 1991) substantiate the suspicion that APP is causally involved in AD.

To test their pathogenetic potential in vivo, mutated and nonmutated forms of human APP were expressed in brains of transgenic mice (in collaboration with S. Forss-Petter and C. Abraham). For expression in neurons, cDNAs encoding full-length human APPs were fused with a vector derived from the neuron-specific enolase (NSE) gene. Four different NSE-APP fusion genes were constructed encoding different forms of either wild-type/nonmutated APP or APP carrying the Val→Ile change found in cases of familial AD (Goate et al. 1991). Fusion genes were injected individually into the germline of mice. Expression of the four NSE-APP constructs was detectable by standard northern and western analysis. Neuronal expression of human APPs was demonstrated by immunostaining of brain sections (fixed in 70% ethanol/0.15 *M* NaCl) with an anti-human APP antibody (αC5) from Athena Neurosciences (San Francisco, CA). For each NSE-APP construct, two to five lines of transgenic mice with clearcut cerebral expression of human APPs were analyzed. Our transgenic models make it possible to quantitate differences in the effects of mutated and nonmutated forms of human APP in vivo.

Within the neuritic plaques of AD, amyloid β protein is closely associated with the serine protease inhibitor ACT (Abraham et al. 1988). It is possible that ACT interacts with a region in the β protein which resembles the active site of a serine protease (C. Abraham, personal communication). ACT could also be indirectly involved in the abnormal proteolytic degradation of APP, by means of inhibiting one or more of the proteases that normally digest it. To assess whether the overproduction of ACT found in AD brains represents a beneficial compensatory response or a detrimental pathogenetic factor, a cDNA-encoding human ACT was fused with the GFAP vector. Six separate lines of GFAP-ACT transgenic mice were established. Expression of human ACT mRNA and protein were demonstrated in the brains of GFAP-ACT transgenic mice by northern and western analyses. To assess the interaction of ACT with APP in vivo, APP/ACT doubly transgenic mice are currently being produced by crossing lines of NSE-APP with GFAP-ACT transgenic mice.

Another devastating dementia that has emerged only recently but is rapidly becoming of major importance is associated with HIV-1 infection (Navia et al. 1986; Navia and Price 1987; Price and Brew 1988). In vitro evidence suggests that the HIV-1 envelope glycoprotein gp120 may be directly or indirectly responsible for the neuronal dysfunction that underlies AIDS dementia (Brenneman et al. 1988; Giulian et al. 1990; Lipton et al. 1991; Lipton 1992). To assess the pathogenetic potential of HIV-1 gp120 in vivo we have produced transgenic mice with either neuronal or astroglial expression of the HIV-1 gp120 molecule. Transgenic models were also established (in collaboration with I. Campbell) to determine the potential contribution of different cytokines to the development of neurologic dysfunction.

It is our hope that the analysis of the transgenic models described above will lead to the identification of novel therapeutic strategies for the treatment and prevention of the neurologic impairment seen in AD and HIV-1 infection.

An Approach to Multifactorial Etiologies

As outlined above, the effects of individual proteins can be assessed in vivo by expressing them in specific cells of transgenic mice. When targeted to the CNS, some factors (e.g. interleukin-6) are sufficient to induce specific neuropathologic and clinical disease manifestations (see Campbell et al. 1992). Other proteins, however, may participate in complex multifactorial pathogenetic networks and require one or more cofactors for the induction of disease. At this point in time, it seems likely that the involvement of amyloid proteins in AD and of MHC molecules in multiple sclerosis will turn out to be examples of such complex scenarios. It is to be hoped that the experimental manipulation of transgenic mice expressing combinations of different fusion genes (see, for example, the NSE-APP/GFAP-ACT doubly transgenic mice above) will facilitate the in vivo analysis of neurologic diseases with multifactorial etiologies.

Acknowledgments. We thank W. Johnson, E. Rockenstein, and J. Price for excellent technical support and G. Rall for helpful comments on the manuscript. This research was supported by the Harry Weaver Neuroscience Scholar Award from the National Multiple Sclerosis Society, Faculty Scholar Award from the Alzheimer's Association, and NIH grant AG-04342.

References

Abraham CR, Selkoe DJ, Potter H (1988) Immunochemical identification of the serine protease inhibitor alpha1-antichymotrypsin in the brain amyloid deposits of Alzheimer's disease. Cell 52:487–501

An G, Hidaka K, Siminovitch L (1982) Expression of bacterial beta-galatosidase in animal cells. Mol Cell Biol 2:1628–1632

Arnold B, Hämmerling GJ (1991) MHC class-I transgenic mice. Annu Rev Immunol 9:297–322

Balcarek JM, Cowan NJ (1985) Structure of the mouse glial fibrillary acidic protein gene: implications for the evolution of the intermediate filament multigene family. Nucleic Acids Res 13:5527–5543

Bignami A, Dahl D (1976) The astroglial response to stabbing. Immunofluorescence studies with antibodies to astrocyte-specific protein (GFA) in mammalian and submammalian vertebrates. Neuropathol Appl Neurobiol 2:99–110

Bignami A, Eng LF, Dahl D, Uyeda CT (1972) Localization of glial fibrillary acidic protein in astrocytes by immunofluorescence. Brain Res 43:429–435

Bonifer C, Vidal M, Grosveld F, Sippel AE (1990) Tissue specific and position independent expression of the complete gene domain for chicken lysozyme in transgenic mice. EMBO J 9:2843–2848

Bottazzo GF, Pujol-Borrell R, Hanafusa T, Feldmann M (1983) Role of aberrant HLA-DR expression and antigen presentation in induction of endocrine autoimmunity. Lancet 2:1115–1119

Bottazzo GF, Todd I, Mirakian R, Belfiore A, Pujol-Borrell R (1986) Organ-specific autoimmunity: a 1986 overview. Immunol Rev 94:137–169

Brenneman DE, Westbrook GL, Fitzgerald SP, Ennist DL, Elkins KL, Ruff MR, Pert CB (1988) Neuronal cell killing by the envelope protein of HIV and its prevention by vasoactive intestinal peptide. Nature 335:639–642

Brinster RL, Palmiter RD (1986) Introduction of genes into the germline of animals. Harvey Lectures Ser 80:1–38

Brinster RL, Allen JM, Behringer RR, Gelinas RE, Palmiter RD (1988) Introns increase transcriptional efficiency in transgenic mice. Proc Natl Acad Sci USA 85:836–840

Camenga DL, Johnson KP, Alter M, Engelhardt CD, Fishman PS, Greenstein JI, Haley AS, Hirsch RL, Kleiner JE, Kofie VY, et al (1986) Systemic recombinant alpha-2 interferon therapy in relapsing multiple sclerosis. Arch Neurol 43:1239–1246

Campbell IL, Oldstone MBA, Mucke L (1992) Neurologic disease induced in transgenic mice by the astrocyte-specific expression of interleukin-6. Soc Neurosci Abstr (in press)

Chartier-Harlin M-C, Crawford F, Houlden H, Warren A, Hughes D, Fidani L, Goate A, Rossor M, Roques P, Hardy J, Mullan M (1991) Early-onset Alzheimer's disease caused by mutations at codon 717 of the beta-amyloid precursor protein gene. Nature 353:844–846

Choi T, Huang M, Gorman C, Jaenisch R (1991) A generic intron increases gene expression in transgenic mice. Mol Cell Biol 11:3070–3074

De La Monte SM, Ho DD, Schooley RT, Hirsch MS, Richardson EPJr (1987) Subacute encephalomyelitis of AIDS and its relation to HTLV-III infection. Neurology 37:562–569

Delacourte A (1990) General and dramatic glial reaction in Alzheimer brains. Neurology 40:33–37

Doherty PC, Zinkernagel RM (1974) T-cell-mediated immunopathology in viral infections. Transplant Rev 19:89–120

Fierz W, Endler B, Reske K, Wekerle H, Fontana A (1985) Astrocytes as antigen-presenting cells. I. Induction of Ia antigen expression on astrocytes by T cells via immune interferon and its effect on antigen presentation. J Immunol 134:3785–3793

Fontana A, Fierz W, Wekerle H (1984) Astrocytes present myelin basic protein to encephalitogenic T-cell lines. Nature 307:273–276

Fontana A, Erb P, Pircher H, Zinkernagel R, Weber E, Fierz W (1986) Astrocytes as antigen-presenting cells. II. Unlike H-2K-dependent cytotoxic T cells, H-2Ia-restricted T cells are only stimulated in the presence of interferon gamma. J Neuroimmunol 12:15–28

Frohman EM, van den Noort S, Gupta S (1989) Astrocytes and intracerebral immune responses. J Clin Immunol 9:1–9

Giulian, D (1987) Ameboid microglia as effectors of inflammation in the central nervous system. J Neurosci Res 18:155–171

Giulian D, Vaca K, Noonan CA (1990) Secretion of neurotoxin by mononuclear phagocytes infected with HIV-1. Science 250:1593–1596

Goate A, Chartier-Harlin M-C, Mullan M, Brown J, Crawford F, Fidani L, Giuffra L, Haynes A, Irving N, James L, Mant R, Newton P, Rooke K, Roques P, Talbot C, Pericak-Vance M, Roses A, Williamson R, Rossor M, Owen M, Hardy J (1991) Segregation of a missense mutation in the amyloid precursor protein gene with familial Alzheimer's disease. Nature 349:704–706

Gordon JW (1986) Transgenic mice in immunology. M Sinai J Med 53:223–231

Hall CV, Jacob PE, Ringold GM, Lee F (1983) Expression and regulation of Escherichia coli lacZ gene fusions in mammalian cells. J Mol Appl Genet 2:101–109
Hickey WF, Osborn JP, Kirby WM (1985) Expression of Ia molecules by astrocytes during acute experimental allergic encephalomyelitis in the Lewis rat. Cell Immunol 91:528–535
Hickey WF, Hsu BL, Kimura H (1991) T-lymphocyte entry into the central nervous system. J Neurosci Res 28:254–260
Hogan B, Costantini F, Lacy E (1986) Manipulating the mouse embryo. A laboratory manual. Cold Spring Harbor Laboratory, Cold Spring Harbor
Janeway CAJr, Bottomly K, Babich J, Conrad P, Conzen S, Jones B, Kaye J, Katz M, McVay L, Murphy DB, Tite J (1984) Quantitative variation in Ia antigen expression plays a central role in immune regulation. Immunol Today 5:99–105
Johnson KP (1988) Treatment of multiple sclerosis with various interferons: the cons Neurology 38:62–65
Kimelberg HK, Norenberg MD (1989) Astrocytes Sci Am 66–76
Knobler RL, Panitch HS, Braheny SL, Sipe JC, Rice GP, Huddlestone JR, Francis GS, Hooper CK, Kamin Lewis RM, Johnson KP, et al (1984) Systemic alpha-interferon therapy of multiple sclerosis. Neurology 34:1273–1279
Lassmann H, Zimprich F, Vass K, Hickey WF (1991) Microglial cells are a component of the perivascular glia limitans. J Neurosci Res 28:236–243
Lewis SA, Balcarek JM, Krek V, Shelanski M, Cowan NJ (1984) Sequence of a cDNA clone encoding mouse glial fibrillary acidic protein: structural conservation of intermediate filaments. Proc Natl Acad Sci USA 81:2743–2746
Lieberman AP, Ptha PM, Shin HS, Shin ML (1989) Production of tumor necrosis factor and other cytokines by astrocytes stimulated with lipopolysaccharide or a neurotropic virus. Proc Natl Acad Sci USA 86:6348–6352
Lipton SA (1992) Models of neuronal injury in AIDS: another role for the NMDA receptor? Trends Neurosci 15:75–79
Lipton SA, Sucher NJ, Kaiser PK, Dreyer EB (1991) Synergistic effects of HIV coat protein and NMDA receptor-mediated neurotoxicity. Neuron 7:111–118
Male DK, Pryce G, Hughes CC (1987) Antigen presentation in brain: MHC induction on brain endothelium and astrocytes compared. Immunology 60:453–459
Massa PT, ter Meulen V (1987) Analysis of Ia induction on Lewis rat astrocytes in vitro by virus particles and bacterial adjuvants. J Neuroimmunol 13:259–271
Massa PT, Brinkmann R, ter Meulen V (1987) Inducibility of Ia antigen on astrocytes by murine coronavirus JHM is rat strain dependent. J Exp Med 166:259–264
Merlino GT (1991) Transgenic animals in biomedical research. FASEB J 5:2996–3001
Mucke L, Oldstone MBA, Morris JC, Nerenberg MI (1991) Rapid activation of astrocyte-specific expression of GFAP-lacZ transgene by focal injury. New Biologist 3:465–474
Murrell J, Farlow M, Ghetti B, Benson MD (1991) A mutation in the amyloid precursor protein associated with hereditary Alzheimer's disease. Science 254:97–99
Navia BA, Price RW (1987) The acquired immunodeficiency syndrome dementia complex as the presenting or sole manifestation of human immunodeficiency virus infection. Arch Neurol 44:65–69
Navia BA, Cho ES, Petito CK, Price RW (1986) The AIDS dementia complex. II. Neuropathology Ann Neurol 19:525–535
Palmiter RD, Brinster RL (1986) Germ-line transformation of mice. Annu Rev Genet 20:465–499
Palmiter RD, Sandgren EP, Avarbock MR, Allen DD, Brinster RL (1991) Heterologous introns can enhance expression of transgenes in mice. Proc Natl Acad Sci USA 88:478–482
Price RW, Brew BJ (1988) The AIDS dementia complex. J Infect Dis 158: 1079–1083
Prusiner SB (1991) Molecular biology and transgenetics of prion diseases. Crit Rev Biochem Mol Biol 26:397–438

Ren R, Racaniello VR (1992) Human poliovirus receptor gene expression and poliovirus tissue tropism in transgenic mice. J Virol 66:296–304

Ren RB, Costantini F, Gorgacz EJ, Lee JJ, Racaniello VR (1990) Transgenic mice expressing a human poliovirus receptor: a new model for poliomyelitis. Cell 63:353–362

Sanes JR, Rubenstein JLR, Nicolas J-F (1986) Use of a recombinant retrovirus to study post-implantation cell lineage in mouse embryos. EMBO J 5:3133–3142

Selkoe DJ (1991a) The molecular pathology of Alzheimer's disease. Neuron 6:487–496

Selkoe DJ (1991b) Amyloid protein in Alzheimer's disease. Sci Am 11:68–78

Skias DD, Kim D-K, Reder AT, Antel JP, Lancki DW, Fitch FW (1987) Susceptibility of astrocytes to class I MHC antigen-specific cytotoxicity. J Immunol 138:3254–3258

Smith ME, Somera FP, Eng LF (1983) Immunocytochemical staining for glial fibrillary acidic protein and the metabolism of cytoskeletal proteins in experimental allergic encephalomyelitis. Brain Res 264:241–253

Suzumura A, Lavi E, Weiss SR, Silberberg DH (1986) Coronavirus infection induces H-2 antigen expression on oligodendrocytes and astrocytes. Science 232:991–993

Suzumura A, Lavi E, Bhat S, Murasko D, Weiss SR, Silberberg DH (1988) Induction of glial cell MHC antigen expression in neurotropic coronavirus infections. Characterization of the H-2-inducing soluble factor elaborated by infected brain cells. J Immunol 140:2068–2072

Swain JL, Stewart TA, Leder P (1987) Parental legacy determines methylation and expression of an autosomal transgene: a molecular mechanism for parental imprinting. Cell 50:719–727

Wekerle H, Linington C, Lassmann H, Meyermann R (1986) Cellular immune reactivity within the CNS. Trends Neurosci 9:271–277

Wekerle H, Sun D, Oropeza-Wekerle RL, Meyermann R (1987) Immune reactivity in the nervous system: modulation of T-lymphocyte activation by glial cells. J Exp Biol 132:43–57

Wilson C (1990) Position effects on eukaryotic gene expression. Annu Rev Cell Biol 6:679–714

Wong GH, Bartlett PF, Clark Lewis I, Battye F, Schrader JW (1984) Inducible expression of H-2 and Ia antigens on brain cells. Nature 310:688–691

Working Group of the American Academy of Neurology AIDS Task Force (1991) Nomenclature and research case definitions for neurologic manifestations of human immunodeficiency virus-type 1 (HIV-1) infection. Neurology 41:778–785

Yankner BA, Mesulam M-M (1991) Beta-amyloid and the pathogenesis of Alzheimer's disease. N Engl J Med 325:1849–1857

Zinkernagel RM, Doherty PC (1974) Restriction of in vitro T cell mediated cytotoxicity in lymphocytic choriomeningitis within a syngeneic or semiallogeneic system. Nature 248:701

Zinkernagel RM, Doherty PC (1983) MHC-restricted cytotoxic T cells: studies on the biological role of polymorphic major transplantation antigens determining T cell restriction-specificity, function, and responsiveness. Adv Immunol 27:51–77

Mechanisms of Extrathymic Tolerance

B. Arnold, G. Schönrich and *G. J. Hämmerling*

Introduction

The central question in immunology is how the immune system can differentiate between self and nonself and thus protect against infections by avoiding autoimmunity. This distinction is based on specific recognition events by receptors on B and T lymphocytes. Since the antigen-specific receptors are generated by random rearrangement of DNA segments, a sufficiently high number of specificities is created to react with any foreign, but also of course with any self structure. Mechanisms must therefore exist ensuring the inactivation of any harmful self-reactive lympocyte.

The repertoire of immunocompetent T lymphocytes is generated by two selection processes within the thymus (von Boehmer 1990). Immature thymocytes which have expressed the T cell receptor (TCR) genes are positively selected for their capacity to bind to self major histocompatibility complex (MHC) molecules (Kisielow et al. 1988 b; McDonald et al. 1988; Blackman et al. 1989). This event is the basis for the finding that mature T lymphocytes recognize antigen (peptides) presented only by self MHC molecules (MHC restriction) (Zinkernagel and Doherty 1974). Simultaneously or subsequently thymocytes are deleted when they encounter MHC molecules along with peptides. By this negative selection self tolerance is achieved (Kappler et al. 1987; Kisielow et al. 1988 a; Murphy et al. 1990). Although the molecular mechanisms dictating whether a thymocyte undergoes positive or negative selection are unknown it is generally thought that cells with high affinity for MHC plus self antigen are deleted whereas those with low affinity for MHC plus self antigen are positively selected. The types of cells presenting the peptide-MHC complex in the thymus may also influence this decision (von Boehmer 1990).

The prerequisite for tolerance induction by negative selection is the presence of the respective self antigen in the thymus. Therefore the question arises as to how tolerance is established to self proteins that are not expressed in the thymus. As mentioned above, TCRs do not react with determinants on the intact three-dimensional protein structure but rather with protein fragments (peptide) bound to class I or class II MHC molecules (Björkmann et al. 1987; Babbit et al. 1985). Accordingly, the definition of an extrathymic protein antigen is hampered by the uncertainty of whether or not antigenic peptides of such proteins can reach the thymus via the blood stream or the lymphatic vessels. Indeed, it has been shown that protein antigens administered intraperitoneally (von Boehmer and Kisielow 1990) or intraveneously (Kyewski et al. 1989) can appear in the thymus in a functional form. However, peripheral proteins which could enter the thymus are exogenously acquired antigens picked up by other cells and therefore presented predominantly by class II molecules. Endogenously synthesized proteins are, in contrast, presented mostly by class I molecules (Braciale et al. 1987). Hence particular endogenous self peptides associated with class I molecules on extrathymic nonrecirculating cells could not be seen as antigenic structures in the thymus and would therefore require extrathymic tolerance induction. However, this objection would be irrelevant if self tolerance must be established only on the pool of $CD4^+$ class II restricted T helper cells, assuming that nearly any T and B cell response is dependent on this subset (Cowing 1985). On the other hand, deletion in the thymus is a stochastic event and probably not always complete. Taken together, there is a need for peripheral tolerance mechanisms.

Furthermore, it is of crucial importance for therapeutic intervention in allograft transplantations and autoimmune diseases whether or not mature peripheral T cells are susceptible for tolerance induction. Assuming that the thymus is the only site of tolerance induction, one must inactivate not only the allograft-specific T cells present at the time of transplantation but also all the T cells with a respective specificity exported from the thymus later in life (Fig. 1, upper panel). Therefore only permanent immunosuppression, with all its side effects, could assure the acceptance of an allograft. If, however, there were central and peripheral tolerance induction, one would have to take into account that mature T cells escaping negative selection in the thymus could be rendered nonresponsive by their first contact with the antigen during their early peripheral circulations (Fig. 1, lower panel). In this case graft rejection would be due to the activation of T cells being in peripheral circulation for a longer time. These cells should therefore be the target cells for any kind of treatment because no further immunosuppression would be needed once these cells have been eliminated. The allograft-specific T cells newly exported from the thymus would undergo peripheral tolerance induction. Thus the strategies to improve immunosuppression in allograft transplantation and autoimmune disease would differ depending on the presence or absence of suitable extrathymic processes leading to self tolerance.

A new field of experimental approaches concerning peripheral tolerance has been opened by the possibility to express a "foreign protein," generally a MHC or a viral protein, under the control of tissue-specific promoter elements in nonthymic cells of transgenic mice. Tolerance to the foreign antigen has been induced in some of these systems (Allison et al. 1988; Sarvetnick et al. 1990; Lo et al. 1988; Morahan et al. 1989). However, the mechanisms of the observed in vivo tolerance have remained unclear, mainly because polyclonal T cell responses were studied. Since the tolerant cells were able to respond to antigen in vitro, nondeletional mechanisms were assumed to operate. However, it could not be excluded that these in vitro responding

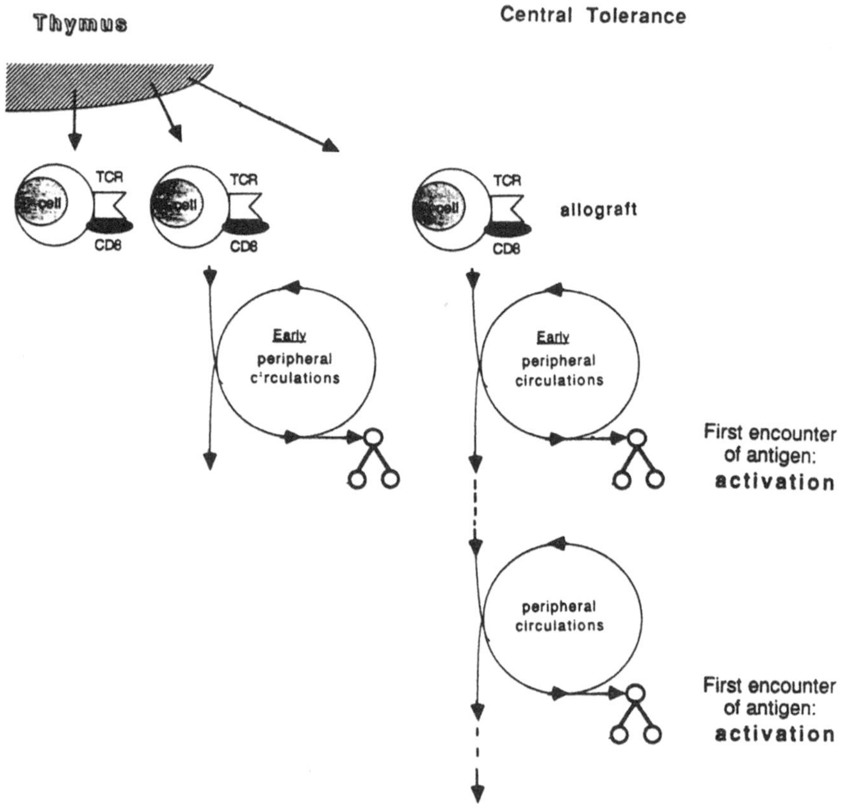

Fig. 1. Models of tolerance induction and their implications for allograft rejection. *Left panel,* tolerance induction occurs only in the thymus. Mature, allograft-specific T cells are activated whenever they encounter the respective antigen for the first time. *Right panel,* since there is in addition to central also peripheral tolerance induction, mature T cells are rendered tolerant whenever they encounter antigen shortly after leaving the thymus. Graft rejection is based on the activation of T cells being longer in peripheral circulations. Elimination of these cells at the time of transplantation should lead to permanent graft acceptance

T cells were of only minor biological relevance, and that the really harmful T cells with high affinity to the respective antigens had been deleted.

Results

The Experimental Approach: Double-Transgenic Mice

To overcome the problem of measuring polyclonal T cell responses we generated two types of transgenic mice. First, the MHC class I gene K^b was expressed under various tissue specific promotor elements on an allogeneic

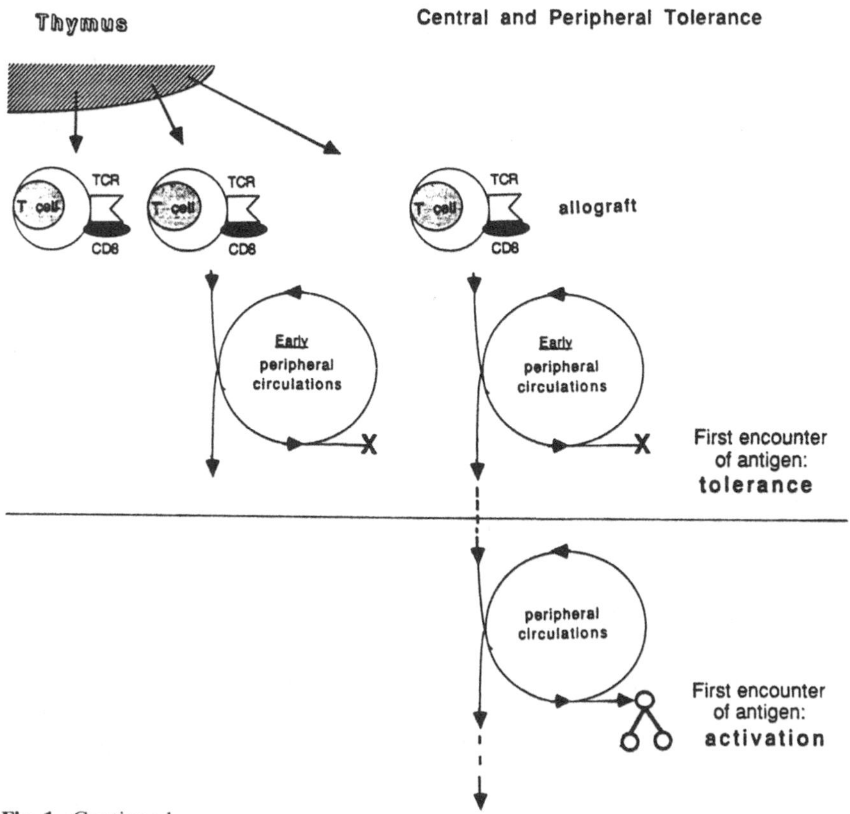

Fig. 1. Continued

background. A class I molecule was chosen as a model antigen because a given TCR recognizes only intact MHC molecules and not degradation products which could migrate to the thymus. Such degradation products would be recognized only as peptides presented by a thymic MHC molecule and would therefore constitute a completely different target structure. In addition, we have recently shown that soluble class I molecules do not induce T cell tolerance for the respective cell-bound class I molecule (Arnold et al. 1990). We used the albumin promoter and the keratin IV promoter for liver-specific and epithelium-specific expression of K^b. The glial fibrillary acidic protein (GFAP) promoter was employed to restrict expression of Kb to cells of neuroectodermal origin. Expression of the transgene was verified on the mRNA level by polymerase chain reaction (PCR) technology using class I allele specific oligonucleotides and on the protein level by immunohistology.

In all three transgenic mouse lines the K^b antigen could be found only in tissue outside the thymus: either only in hepatocytes (albumin promoter) or only in epithelial cells in skin, tongue, and foot pads (keratin promoter) or only in cell types of neuroectodermal origin (GFAP promoter).

Secondly, genes coding for a K^b-specific TCR were introduced into the germline of mice (Schönrich et al. 1991). The respective αβ TCR genes were derived from a K^b-specific and CD8-dependent cytotoxic T cell (CTL) clone isolated from B10.BR(H-2^k) mice (Hue et al. 1990). These TCR transgenic mice were crossed with each of the above K^b transgenic mice. All these mice were tolerant in vivo to K^b as judged by K^b-positive skin graft acceptance and by the growth of K^b-positive tumors (Schönrich et al. 1991). In addition, no signs of autoimmune responses were detectable.

Lack of Tolerance Induction in the Thymus

Although no K^b expression in the thymus of the various transgenic mice was found, it had to be proven that the observed in vivo tolerance was not due to a thymic event. We therefore compared the maturation of T cells in the thymi of the double transgenic mice to the thymocyte development in TCR single transgenic mice using the anti-clonotypic antibody Désiré-1 (Hua et al. 1986). Clonotype$^+$ CD8$^+$ CD4$^-$ mature T cells could be found in normal numbers in the thymus of all these double-transgenic mice, demonstrating that there was no clonal deletion in the thymus (Schönrich et al. 1991, 1992 b). Furthermore, these mature thymocytes could develop into K^b-specific CTL after in vitro stimulation with antigen in the absence of exogenous interleukin 2 and could proliferate in response to anti-clonotypic antibodies. These responses were identical to those of thymocytes from TCR single-transgenic mice.

When we used a 0.8-kb promoter fragment of the keratin IV promoter instead of the 2.4-kb complete promoter (Blessing et al. 1989), we obtained transgenic mice expressing K^b in the thymus on only the fraction of medullary epithelial cells in addition to the extrathymic expression for the 2.4-kb keratin IV-K^b mice described above (Schönrich et al. 1992 a). Despite the K^b expression in the thymic medulla, clonotype$^+$ CD8$^+$ CD4$^-$ thymocytes developed normally in the 0.8-kb keratin IV-K^b mice. However, the mature thymocytes could not be activated by K^b-positive splenocytes regardless of whether interleukin-2 was added and could not proliferate in response to anti-clonotypic antibodies (Schönrich et al. 1992 a). Thus this transgenic mouse line does not only show that expression of the antigen on epithelial cells in the medulla of the thymus can induce anergy, but also that a small alteration in the thymocyte development can be identified by the test system used. It can therefore be concluded that the observed tolerance to K^b in albumin-K^b, GFAP-K^b, and 2.4kb keratin IV-K^b mice is caused by extra-thymic processes.

Distinct Manifestations of Peripheral Tolerance

So far it is unknown which determinants are important for the induction of peripheral tolerance. Two catergories of parameters may be relevant. On the one hand, are determinants concerning the T cell itself, such as affinity of TCR, level of expression of TCR, and accessory molecules and developmental stage of the T cells encountering their antigen. On the other hand, there are the properties of the tissue bearing the target antigen. With our experimental approach we were able to hold all parameters concerning the T cell constant and to examine the toleragenic effects on a well-defined monoclonal T cell population encountering its correspending antigen expressed in different anatomical sites outside the thymus.

Downregulation of TCR and CD8 Molecules on Peripheral T Cells of (TCR×GFAP-K^b)F_1 and (TCR×Albumin-K^b)F_1 Mice

Contact with a K^b antigen in the periphery led to a strong reduction of clonotype$^+$ $CD8^+$ T cells in spleen and lymph nodes of (TCR×GFAP-K^b)F_1 and (TCR×albumin-K^b)F_1 mice in comparison to the numbers found in TCR single-transgenic mice (Fig. 2). This reduction may be caused either by physical elimination of these cells or by modulation of both TCR and CD8 molecules on the cell surface. To distinguish between these two possibilities purified splenic T cells were analyzed by two-color cytofluorometric analysis for the frequency of T cells (as defined by the marker CD2 or Thy-1) lacking the TCR as determined by the presence or absence of the CD3 marker. About 60 % of $CD2^+$ cells showed no expression of CD3 in both double-transgenic animals (Fig. 2, lower part). However, in TCR single-transgenic animals less than 10 % of splenic T cells showed no CD3 expression. These results indicate that the reduction in this cell population determined by disappearance of the cell surface marker (TCR/CD3) is not sufficient evidence to conclude that these cells have been physically eliminated. Apparently, downregulation of TCR and CD8 molecules is one mechanism of peripheral tolerance induction.

Reversal of TCR Downregulation In Vitro

It was now of interest to investigate whether the observed downregulation of TCR and CD8 molecules in vivo can be reversed by stimulation with antigen in vitro. To this end, spleen cells of (TCR×GFAP-K^b)F_1 and (TCR×albumin-K^b)F_1 mice were stained with Désiré 1 and sorted for clonotype$^+$ and clonotype$^-$ cells. The individual cell populations were stimulated with K^b-positive splenocytes in a mixed lymphocyte culture and after 4 days analyzed for clonotype expression and CTL activity. Only clonotype$^-$ cells of (TCR×GFAP-K^b)F_1 mice could develop into clonotype$^+$ cells which could kill K^b-expressing target cells in a clonotype-dependent way. Apparently a small number of CD3/TCR complexes undetectable by cytofluorometric analysis had remained on the cell surface, and antigen-specific stimulation led to upregulation of the CD3/TCR complexes under these in vitro conditions. In contrast, clonotype$^-$ cells of (TCR×albumin-K^b)F_1 mice and of TCR single-transgenic mice did not become clonotype$^+$ after such an in vitro

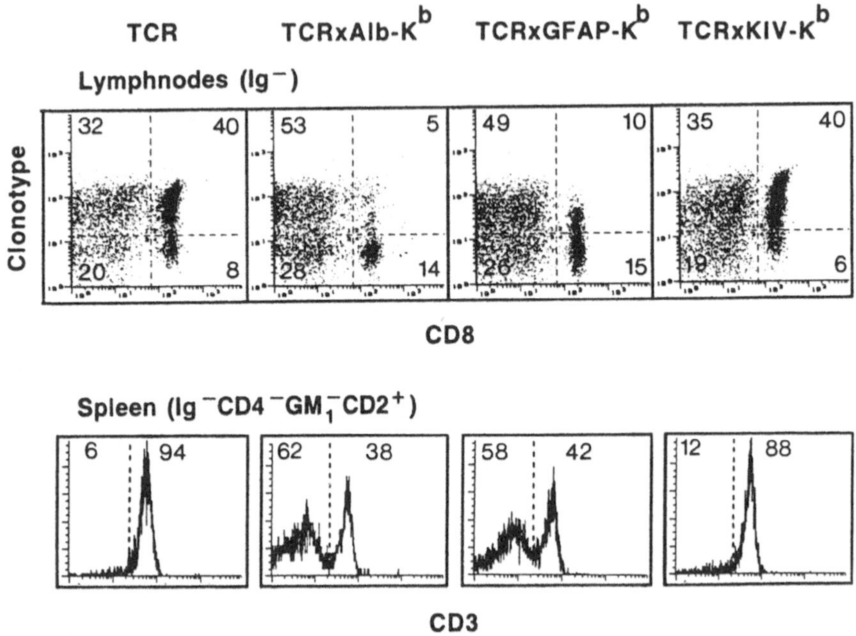

Fig. 2. Cytofluorimetric analysis of clonotype and CD3 expression on peripheral T cells from various transgenic mice of H-2^{dxk} haplotype. *Upper row*, clonotype (fluoroscein isothiocyanate conjugated Désiré-1) is plotted against CD8 (53.6-7 biotinylated plus streptavidin conjugated to peridin chlorophyll). Cells were analyzed on a FACScan. *Lower row*, splenocytes were depleted of B cells, CD4 T cells, and natural killer cells by magnetic cell sorting using the corresponding antibodies and Dynobeads. The CD3 expression (biotinylated 500 A2 plus streptavidin conjugated to peridin chlorophyll) of only $CD2^+$ cells (12.15 A plus fluoroscein isothiocyanate conjugated mouse anti-rat IgG) is shown. *Vertical axis*, relative numbers; *horizontal axis*, fluorescence is plotted on a logarithmic scale. For further details see Schönrich et al. (1992b). Abbreviations indicating the promoter elements used for K^b expression: *Alb*, albumin; *GFAP*, glial fibrillary acidic protein; *KIV*, 2.4 kb keratin IV

stimulation. However, clonotype$^-$ CD3$^-$ T cells of (TCR×albumin-K^b)F_1 mice could be forced to reexpress their TCR by in vitro stimulation with cross-linked anti-CD2 antibodies (Schönrich et al. 1992 b). Thus upregulation of TCR/CD3 complexes in the two types of double transgenic mice required different signals.

Unresponsiveness in (TCR×2.4 kb Keratin IV-K^b)F_1 Mice

In the (TCR×2.4-kb keratin IV-K^b)F_1 animals no phenotypic changes were detected in the peripheral T cell pool. Nevertheless, these mice accepted K^b skin grafts. It has been shown that $CD8^+$ T cells are both necessary and sufficient for rejection of class I allografts (Rosenberg et al. 1986). In addition, we have demonstrated that elimination of $CD4^+$ T cells does not influence the anti K^b response in the TCR single-transgenic mice (Schönrich et al. 1992 b). We therefore conclude that the observed tolerance in these mice is not due to the lack of CD4 T cell help, but that it is based on the induction of nonresponsiveness in the $CD8^+$ T cell compartment. This apparent T cell unresponsiveness was reversible in vitro; K^b-specific clonotype-dependent CTL responses were obtained after antigen stimulation to the same extend as with T cell receptor single transgenic mice.

In summary, in the three transgenic mouse models with extrathymic K^b expression K^b-specific T cells were found to exist at three different levels of tolerance depending on the tissue distribution of the K^b antigen.

Tolerance Induction as a Multistep Process

Assuming that resting T cells can reach different levels of tolerance, it was now of interest to determine whether a tolerant T cell in one stage of tolerance is still susceptible for further signals driving the cell into a deeper tolerance level. In this case T cell tolerance must not necessarily be based on a "single hit" but can rather be the end result of several consecutive steps. We therefore confronted $clonotype^+$ $CD8^+$ T cells which were tolerant in vivo but reacted in vitro again with the K^b antigen and looked for phenotypical and functional changes. The B6bm1 animal differs from a C57BL/6 (H-2b) animal only in three amino acids exchanged in the K^b molecule (Nairn et al. 1980). These bm1 mutations in positions 152, 155, and 156 are very well recognized by T lymphocytes, resulting in rejection of skin grafts between the two types of animals. Our anti-K^b T cell receptor transgenic mice hardly react with the bm1 antigen. Therefore, in contrast to TCR H-2bxk animals, thymic negative selection in TCRbm1$\times$k mice is incomplete. A high number of $CD8^+$ $clonotype^+$ T cells are present in the periphery of TCRbm1$\times$k mice, leading to enlarged lymphoid organs. These T cells with slightly lower CD8 expression do not reject K^b skin grafts. However, anti-K^b CTL responses in vitro are nearly as high as those obtained with TCR H-2dxk mice. The TCRbm1$\times$k animals were injected with 5×10^7 T cell depleted C57BL/6 spleen cells intravenously. After 10 days splenocytes were analyzed for their clonotype and CD8 expression and for their anti-K^b CTL activity in vitro. Although no phenotypical changes were observed, hardly any anti-K^b activity was detectable (Fig. 3). Thus in vivo tolerant T cells which can respond in vitro are apparently still susceptible for further specific tolerance signals in vivo, resulting in non-responsiveness in vitro. This is the first indication that tolerant T cells can be shifted from one tolerance level to another.

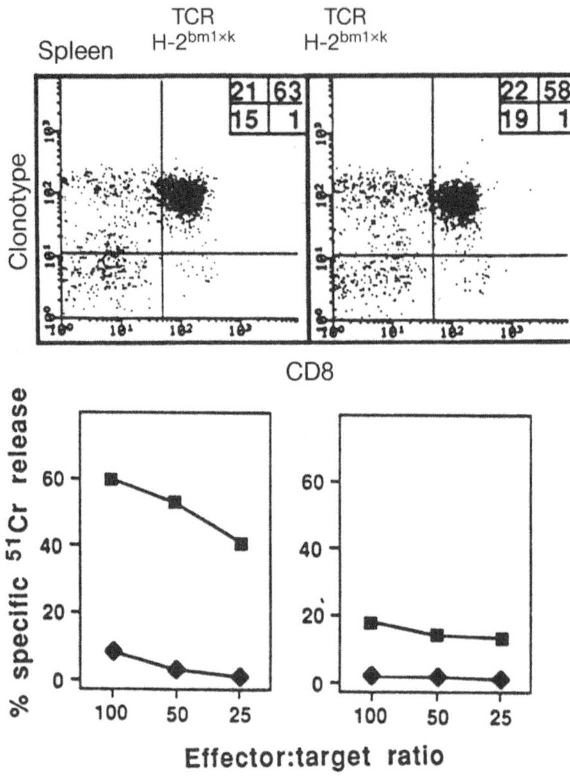

Fig. 3. Phenotype and cytolytic activity of splenocytes from TCR H-$2^{bm1 \times k}$ mice untreated *(left)* and after intravenous injection of 50×10^6 Tcell-depleted C57BL/6 (H-2^b) splenocytes *(right)*. *Upper row,* cytolytic activity of spleen cells stimulated in vitro with irradiated C57BL/6 spleen cells on untransfected fibroblasts (1T22-6; *diamonds*) and fibroblast transfected with the K^b gene (1 T K^b; *squares*). The in vivo tolerant cells are responsive in vitro *(left)*; however, the in vitro acitivity is strongly reduced after injection of K^b positive splenocytes *(right)*

Discussion

Peripheral Tolerance Does Exist

Our data demonstrate that mature Tcells can be rendered tolerant when they encounter antigen in the periphery. There was no sign of any thymic contribution to the observed tolerance in the three transgenic mouse models described. Even if one considers the possibility that undetectable amounts of K^b were present in the thymus of the different transgenic mice, they clearly had no influence on the maturation of precursors into anti-K^b cells in the thymic microenvironment. In addition, peripheral tolerance has also been clearly demonstrated in transgenic mice expressing the influenza hemaglutinin under the rat insulin promoter (Lo et al. 1992). Tolerance has even been demonstrated in chimeric mice which were reconstituted with nontransgenic bone marrow after the transgenic thymus had been replaced by a thymus from a nontransgenis animal. It is indeed remarkable that expression of an extrathymic antigen on very few cells in the body, such as on β islet cells of the pancreas or on cells of neuroectodermal origin such as Schwann's cells in the gut is sufficient to induce tolerance. This points to a rapid and complete circulation and suggests that all T cells meet the transgene product on the various tissues within a relatively short time. This follows from the assumption that these transgenic mice are tolerant only because they express the transgene already early during development. In instances in which transgene expression was observed late during development, autoimmunity instead of tolerance was induced (Adams et al. 1987).

Several important questions concerning peripheral tolerance induction remain. First, why is peripheral tolerance observed only in some experimental systems and not in others? Many investigators have used the rat insulin promoter to direct expression of the transgene product to pancreatic β cells. Ohashi et al. (1991) expressed the glycoprotein of the lymphocytic choriomeningitis virus (LCMV) on islet cells and found no evidence of peripheral tolerance of T cells in these animals. When these mice were crossed with animals expressing a TCR transgene of the respective specificity, LCMV priming induced diabetes within 4 days. This led the authors to the conclusion that antigens on β islet cells are indifferent to T cells inducing neither tolerance nor autoimmunity. On the other hand, transgenic mice expressing the influenza hemaglutinin from A/Japan/305/57 strain in β cells spontaneously developed diabetes, which was interpreted as a result of an autoimmune response (Roman et al. 1990). However, T cell reactivity to the transgene product was not assessed. These four examples of transgene expressions in β islets (Lo et al. 1992; Adams et al. 1987; Ohashi et al. 1991; Roman et al. 1990) show clearly the need for identification of the parameters which control peripheral tolerance induction. One apparent explanation for the different observations in these systems is the variation in the amount of antigen expressed. Recently, a quantitative relationship has been reported between the blood concentration of a self antigen and the state of tolerance for its immunodominant, subdominant, and cryptic peptides at the T cell level (Cibotti et al. 1992).

Secondly, in the case of peripheral tolerance induction it is unclear whether the different manifestations described above are caused by qualitatively distinct signals provided by the respective tissue (e.g., hepatocytes versus keratinocytes or versus cells of neuroectodermal origin) or by different density of the K^b antigen or by different lengths of time of contact between the T lymphocytes and the cells expressing the K^b antigen. We even observed different levels of tolerance in the very same animal. For example, in the (TCR×GFAP-K^b)F_1 mice in addition to cells with downregulated TCR there also exist 1%–2% of clonotype$^+$ CD8$^+$ cells. This is a rather high number of cells with potential reactivity against K^b when compared to a nontransgenic mouse. Nevertheless, these cells failed to cause an autoimmune response and to reject K^b positive tumor cells in vivo. Therefore, in these (TCR×GFAP K^b)F_1 animals we observe induction of unresponsiveness without phenotypical changes and downregulation of TCR and CD8 molecules as the basis for the observed tolerance.

Thirdly, it will be of great importance for any specific immunosuppression to characterize the distinct levels of tolerance to which a resting T cell can be driven and to identify the signals required to shift a T cell from one level to a "deeper" one and finally to deletion. In addition, it will be of interest to determine the life span of unresponsive T cells and to learn whether such cells can regain reactivity in vivo. We have given examples of in vitro reactivity of in vivo unresponsive cells. Learning how to break tolerance in vivo would open new ways to interfere with tumor growth if one considers the possibility that the generally low immune responses to tumors could partially be based on tolerance induction.

Induction of Nonresponsiveness in an Adult Individuum

So far we have discussed tolerance induction to peripheral self antigens constitutively expressed during neonatal life and the possibility that mature T lymphocytes are susceptible to inactivation by antigen for only a short period after exit from the thymus. However, to ensure nonresponsiveness in autoimmune diseases and to transplanted allografts mature T cells must be rendered unresponsive which have been in circulation for a longer time. Up to now inactivation of such T cells has been achieved only by treatment with immunosuppressive drugs or by administration of antibodies directed to CD4, CD8 (Cobbolt et al. 1990). Very recently it has been suggested that tolerance in an adult individuum can occur as a consequence of an immune response. This conclusion was reached when thymectomized adult $Mls1^b$ mice were injected intravenously with $Mls1^1$ lymphoid cells (Webb et al. 1991). Most anti-$Mls1^{1a}$ reactive $V\beta6^+$ $CD4^+$ T cells of the recipient disappeared. However, this disappearance was preceded by a large expansion of these cells. In another study HY-specific $CD8^+$ female T cells were transferred into male nude mice (Rocha and von Boehmer 1991). Again, these potentially autoreactive T cells disappeared after an extensive proliferation phase. If this suggestion is correct, it will be important to identify the distinct signals driving T lymphocytes during an immune response either toward memory or toward nonresponsiveness and/or cell death.

Summary and Conclusions

The studies discussed here show that mature T lymphocytes can be rendered tolerant of antigens expressed exclusively outside the thymus. We analyzed anti-K^b TCR transgenic mice which express the K^b antigen as a second transgene product in extrathymic tissues such as liver, epithelial cells, and cells of neuroectodermal origin. Due to this differential K^b expression anti-K^b reactive T cells were found to exist at three different levels of tolerance. These levels were distinct with regard to downregulation of TCR and CD8 molecules and the requirements for re-expression of TCR in vitro. There is also evidence that even unresponsive T cells in vivo can be shifted to a deeper tolerance level (as judged by in vitro responsiveness) by confronting these cells again with antigen expressed on other cell types. Despite the fact that a detailed knowledge about the mechanisms of peripheral tolerance induction is still lacking, the described observations may be of clinical relevance. Distinct mechanisms of extrathymic tolerance are likely to differ in their efficiency to protect against the breakdown of self tolerance and therefore against autoimmunity. The finding that different tissues can induce different levels of tolerance could explain why some organs are more susceptible to autoimmune diseases than others. Furthermore, strategies to improve immunosuppression in allograft transplantation and autoimmune diseases should concentrate on suitable methods to eliminate the circulating T cell pool which is responsible for graft rejection or the onset of an autoimmune disease. Since allograft specific or autoreactive T cells newly exported from the thymus would undergo peripheral tolerance induction, specific immunosuppression could be achieved this way.

References

Adams TE, Alpert S, Hanahan D (1987) Non-tolerance and autoantibodies to a transgenic self antigen expressed in pancreatic β cells. Nature 325: 223

Allison J, Cambell IL, Morahan G, Mandel TE, Harrison LC (1988) Diabetes in transgenic mice resulting from over-expression of class I histocompatibility molecules in pancreatic β cells. Nature 333: 529

Arnold B, Messerle M, Jatsch L, Kublbeck G, Koszinowski U (1990) Transgenic mice expressing a soluble foreign H-2 class I antigen are tolerant to allogeneic fragments presented by self class I but not to the whole membrane-bound alloantigen. Proc Natl Acad Sci USA 87: 1762

Babbitt BP, Allen PM, Matsueda G, Haber E, Unanue ER (1985) Binding of immunogenic peptides to Ia histocompatibility molecules. Nature 317: 359

Björkman PJ, Saper MA, Samaraoui B, Bennett WS, Strominger JL, Wiley DC (1987) Structure of the human class I histocompatibility complex antigen, HLA-A2. Nature 329: 506

Blackman MA, Marrack P, Kappler J (1989) Influence of the major histocompatibility complex on positive thymic selection of $V_{\beta}17a^+$ T cells. Science 244: 214

Blessing M, Jorcano JL, Franke WW (1989) Enhancer elements directing cell-type-specific expression of cytokeratin genes and changes of the epithelial cytoskeleton by transfections of hybrid cytokeratin genes. EMBO J 8: 117

Braciale TJ, Morrison LA, Sweetser MT, Sambrook J, Gething MJ, Braciale VL (1987) Antigen presentation pathways to class I and class II MHC-restricted T lymphocytes. Immunol Rev 98: 95

Cibotti R, Kanellopoulos JM, Cabaniols J-P, Halle-Panenko O, Kosmatopoulos K, Secarz E, Kourilsky P (1992) Tolerance to a self-protein involves its immunodominant but does not involve its subdominant determinants. Proc Natl Acad Sci USA 89: 416

Cobbold PS, Gilly M, Waldman H (1990) The induction of skin graft tolerance in major histocompatibility complex-mismatched or primed recipients: primed T cells can be tolerized in the periphery with anti-CD4 anti-CD8 antibodies. Eur J Immunol 20: 2747

Cowing C (1985) Does T-cell restriction to Ia limit the need for self-tolerance. Immunol Today 6: 72

Hua C, Boyer C, Buferne M, Schmitt Verhulst AM (1986) Monoclonal antibodies against an H-2Kb-specific cytotoxic T cell clone detect several clone-specific molecules. J Immunol 136: 1937

Hue I, Trucy J, McCoy C, Couez D, Malissen B, Malissen M (1990) A novel type of aberrant T cell receptor alpha-chain gene rearrangement. Implications for allelic exclusion and the V-J recombination process. J Immunol 144: 4410

Kappler JW, Roehm N, Marrack P (1987) T cell tolerance by clonal elimination in the thymus. Cell 49: 273

Kisielow P, Blüthmann H, Staerz UD, Steinmetz M, von Boehmer H (1988 a) Tolerance in T-cell-receptor transgenic mice involves deletion of nonmature $CD4^{+}8^{+}$ thymocytes. Nature 333: 742

Kisielow P, Teh HS, Bluthmann H, von Boehmer H (1988 b) Positive selection of antigen-specific T cells in thymus by restricting MHC molecules. Nature 335: 730

Kyewski BA, Jenkinson EJ, Kingston R, Altevogt P, Owen MJ, Owen JJT (1989) The effects of anti-CD2 antibodies on the differentiation of mouse thymocytes. Eur J Immunol 19: 951

Lo D, Burkly LC, Widera G, Cowing C, Flavell RA, Palmiter RD, Brinster RL (1988) Diabetes and tolerance in transgenic mice expressing class II MHC molecules in pancreatic beta cells. Cell 53: 159

Lo D, Freedman J, Hesse S, Palmiter RD, Brinster RL, Sherman LA (1992) Peripheral tolerance to an islet cell-specific hemagglutinin transgene affects both $CD4^{+}$ and $CD8^{+}$ T cells. Eur J Immunol 22: 1013

McDonald HR, Schneider R, Lees RK, Howe RC, Acha Orbea H, Festenstein H, Zinkernagel RM, Hengartner H (1988) T-cell receptor V beta use predicts reacitivity and tolerance to Mlsa-encoded antigens. Nature 332: 40

Morahan G, Brennan FE, Bhathal PS, Allison J, Cox KO, Miller JFAP (1989) Expression in transgenic mice of class I histocompatibility antigens controlled by the metallothionein promoter. Proc Natl Acad Sci USA 86: 3782

Murphy KM, Heimberger AB, Loh DY (1990) Induction by antigen of intrathymic apoptosis of $CD4^{+}CD8^{+}TCR^{10}$ thymocytes in vivo. Science 250: 1720

Nairn R, Yamaga K, Nathenson S (1980) Biochemistry of the gene product from murine MHC mutants. Annu Rev Genet 14: 241

Ohashi PS, Oehen S, Buerki K, Pircher H, Ohashi CT, Odermatt B, Malissen B, Zinkernagel RM, Hengartner H (1991) Ablation of "tolerance" and induction of diabetes by virus infection in viral antigen transgenic mice. Cell 65: 305

Rocha B, von Boehmer H (1991) Peripheral selection of the T cell repertoire. Science 251: 1225

Roman LM, Simons LF, Hammer RE, Sambrook JF, Gething MJH (1990) The expression of human influenza virus hemagglutinin in the pancreatic β cells of transgenic mice results in autoimmune diabetes. Cell 61: 383

Rosenberg AS, Mizuochi T, Singer A (1986) Analysis of T-cell subsets in rejection of K^{b} mutant skin allografts differing at class I MHC. Nature 322: 829

Sarvetnick N, Shizuru J, Liggitt D, Martin L, McIntyre B, Gregory A, Parslow T, Stewart T (1990) Loss of pancreatic islet tolerance induced by beta-cell expression of interferon-gamma. Nature 346: 844

Schönrich G, Kalinke U, Momburg F, Malissen M, Schmitt-Verhulst AM, Malissen B, Hämmerling GJH, Arnold B (1991) Down-regulation of T cell receptors on self-reactive T cells as a novel mechanism for extrathymic tolerance induction. Cell 65: 293

Schönrich G, Momburg F, Hämmerling GJ, Arnold B (1992 a) Anergy induced by thymic medullary epithelium. Eur J Immunol (in press)

Schönrich G, Momburg F, Malissen M, Schmitt-Verhulst A-M, Malissen B, Hämmerling GJ, Arnold B (1992b) Distinct mechanisms of extrathymic T cell tolerance due to differential expression of self antigen. Int Immunol (in press)
von Boehmer H (1990) Developmental biology of T cells in T cell-receptor transgenic mice. Annu Rev Immunol 8: 531
von Boehmer H, Kisielow P (1990) Self-nonself discrimination by T cells. Science 248: 1369
Webb S, Morris C, Sprent J (1991) Extrathymic tolerance of mature T cells: clonal elimination as a consequence of immunity. Cell 63: 1249
Zinkernagel RM, Doherty PC (1974) Restriction of in vitro T cell-mediated cytotoxicity in lymphocytic choriomeningitis within a syngeneic or semiallogeneic system. Nature 248: 701

Lysosomal Proteins as Autoantigens of Clinical Relevance

W.L. Gross, B.K. Flesch, and *E. Csernok*

Introduction

Ten years ago autoantibodies directed against the cytoplasm of polymorphonuclear leukocytes (PMN) and monocytes were found in a small number of patients with non classified vasculitis [1, 2]. In 1985 a Dutch-Danish collaboration study reported on the high specificity of a subtype of these autoantibodies (anticytoplasmic antibodies, ACPA) for Wegener's granulomatosis (WG) and on the high correlation between ACPA titer and disease activity [3]. These findings were soon corroborated by us [4] and later by other groups and were subsequently extended in a prospective study [5]. ACPA were later redesignated as antineutrophil cytoplasmic autoantibodies (ANCA) because a second fluorescence pattern with association to a morphologically defined subgroup of vasculitis was clearly demonstrated [6]. ANCA screening is routinely performed by indirect immunofluorescence (IIF). Using this technique three different staining patterns can be differentiated: the classic "cytoplasmic" pattern (cANCA), which is preferentially associated with WG; the perinuclear pattern (pANCA), which is associated with necrotizing and crescentic glomerulonephritis; and xANCA, which represents a peculiar mixture of the cANCA and pANCA patterns and is thought to be associated with chronic inflammatory bowel disease [7] (Fig. 1).

Today the various ANCAs serve as useful seromarkers. They can be used (a) as clinical tools to support the diagnosis of WG, vasculitis or glomerulonephritis, and chronic inflammatory bowel disease, and (b) to monitor disease activity. Recent studies support the hypothesis that ANCAs are implicated in the pathogenesis of these diseases.

cANCA and WG

WG was first distinguished as a clinicopathologic entity by Friedrich Wegener in 1936 [8]. He established that this "rhinogenic granulomatosis" preferentially exhibits granulomatous lesions in the respiratory tract. Many other organ systems, including kidneys and lung, may be involved in the disease process. Limited forms of the disorder appear to be more common than first thought, probably because of increased awareness of the disease and its

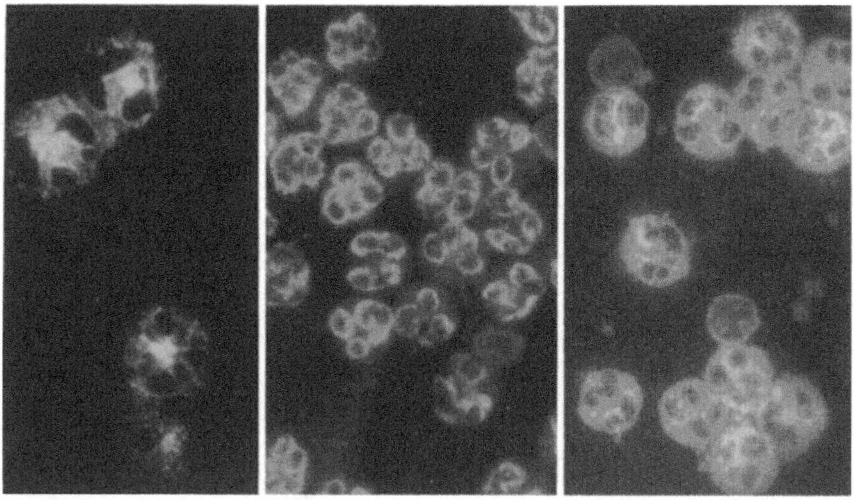

Fig. 1. Different ANCA staining patterns demonstrated by indirect immunofluorescence on ethanol fixed granulocytes

earlier diagnosis (for review see [9]). The upper and lower respiratory tracts seem to be affected first in most patients (initial phase). During this initial phase the peculiar granulomatous inflammation dominates the clinical picture. This process appears to spread continuously from the nasal cavity to the sinuses, pharynx, etc. If untreated, the disease, after a highly variable period of time, can become generalized with various degrees of vasculitis and kidney involvement. In its full-blown phase the disease is life threatening and requires highly aggressive treatment. Diagnosis is based on typical clinical findings and supporting histologic data. In some patients, especially those with limited disease, the diagnosis can be difficult to substantiate. No specific diagnostic laboratory test was available until ANCAs were described. Soon after the first report on the immunodiagnostic importance of ANCAs [4], a number of research projects were started which have dramatically increased both the immunodiagnostic and pathogenetic knowledge of ANCA and WG.

In cooperation with the MAYO Clinic we performed IIF and enzyme-linked immunosorbent assay analyses on 2653 serum samples from 1934 patients, including 277 with WG (222 with biopsy-confirmed disease) (Table 1). Prospective follow-up was documented in 172 WG patients. The specificity of cANCA for WG was 99 % [5]. Sensitivity of cANCA depended on the extent and activity of disease; it was 67 % in patients with active regional symptoms and 32 % in those in full remission after initial regional symptoms. The sensitivity was 96 % in patients with active generalized disease and 41 % in those in full remission after active generalized disease [5].

Table 1. Frequency of positive test results for anticytoplasmic antibodies (cANCA) for patients in the various diagnostic categories of the study population (from [5])

Diagnostic categories	*n*	cANCA Findings	
		IFT	ELISA
Patients with Wegener's granulomatosis			
Biopsy-proven disease	222	168/222	160/222
Clinical diagnosis only	55	35/55	29/55
Control patients			
Normal	319	0/319	0/119
With medical conditions not listed below	714	0/714	1/122
With autoimmune diseases	256	0/171	0/256
Systemic lupus erythematosus	57		
Sjögren's syndrome	24		
Rheumatoid arthritis	109		
Polymyositis or dermatomyositis	11		
Scleroderma	18		
Reiter's syndrome	4		
Primary biliary cirrhosis	3		
Relapsing polychrondritis	1		
Other unclassified forms	29		
With arthritis or arthralgias of unknown origin	14	0/14	1/14
With granulomatous diseases	54	0/54	0/51
Sarcoidosis	34		
Crohn's disease	5		
Tuberculosis	9		
Other diseases	6		
With infections	22	0/22	0/22
With pulmonary diseases	38	0/38	0/34
Idiopathic pulmonary fibrosis	5		
Pneumonia	17		
Primary pulmonary hypertension	1		
Pleurisy	2		
Bronchial carcinomas	6		
Asthma	2		
Histiocytosis X	3		
Alveolitis of indeterminate origin	2		
With lymphoproliferative disorders	9	0/9	0/9
Non-Hodgkin lymphoma	5		
Lymphomatoid granulomatosis	4		
With glomerulonephritis	80	1/80	1/79
With other renal diseases	21	0/21	1/15
Interstitial nephritis	7		
Nephrosclerosis	3		
Pyelonephritis	1		
Other renal diseases	10		
With pulmonary-renal syndromes	7	1/7	1/7
With vasculitis	123	8/123	8/116
Polyarteritis nodosa	20		
Hypersensitivity angiitis	7		

Table 1. Continued

Diagnostic categories	*n*	cANCA Findings	
		IFT	ELISA
Granulomatous vasculitis (Behcet)	26		
Giant cell arteritis	21		
Other unclassified forms	49		

IFT, indirect immunofluorescence technique, ELISA, enzyme-linked immunoadsorbent assay, Number of patients cANCA positive/number of patients tested.

Table 2. Anticytoplasmic autoantibody (cANCA) values, C-reactive protein levels, and erythrocyte sedimentation rates for patients who went into remission (from [5])

Test	Active disease (n=62)	Remission (n=62)	*P* value
cANCA immunofluorescence titer	1:32	1:8	<0.0006
cANCA ELISA value (U/ml)	228	27	<0.0001
C-reactive protein (mg/l)	71	7	<0.0001
Erythrocyte sedimentation rate (mm/h)$^{\alpha}$	79	29	<0.0001

All values are medians.
$^{\alpha}$ Complete data for erythrocyte sedimentation rates were available for only 50 of the 62 patients.

Hence, in active generalized disease cANCA titer correlated well with disease activity (Table 2).

Soon after the immunodiagnostic importance of cANCA was established, many groups began work on identifying the target antigen(s). In 1989 the Groningen group [10] reported on the partial characterization of the cANCA antigen as a diisopropylfluorophosphate-binding serine protease in the primary granules of human neutrophils, which is distinct from neutrophil elastase and cathepsin G. Shortly thereafter [11], we presented data indicating that the cANCA target antigen has biochemical properties identical to those of Proteinase 3 (PR 3), an elastinolytic serine protease of 29 kDa [12] first described by Baggiolini 10 years ago [13]. One year later we decoded PR3 as "Wegener's autoantigen" and extended our previous findings by demonstrating that PR3 is identical to azurophil granule protein (AGP7) [14, 15], p29 [16], and myeloblastin [17]. However, since these terms are also based on the biochemical properties of the same molecule, we prefer the term "Wegener's autoantigen" (WA), which covers both the immunological properties and clinical significance of the cANCA target antigen.

Various functional properties are associated with the cANCA target antigen. Weak antimicrobial activity of AGP7 isolated from PMN against *Escherichia coli* and *Candida albicans* (Table 3) was reported by Gabay et al.

Table 3. Multifunctional properties of "Wegener's autoantigen"

Synonym	Localization/functional characteristics
Proteinase 3	Expression in neutrophil granulocytes and monocytes Degrades matrix proteins as fibronectin, laminin, vitronectin, collagen type IV Is inhibited by α-1AT and α_2-macroglobulin
Myeloblastin	Expression in HL60 promyelocytic cell line and cells from patients with acute myeloid leukemia Downregulated during induced cell differentiation
AGP7	Expression in human PMN Antimicrobial activity against *E. coli* and *C. albicans*

[14]. This effect may be attributed to predicted preferential distribution of positively charged amino acids on the surface of the protein [18]. If cANCA bind to WA (AGP7), it can be speculated that the antimicrobial activity of WA is inhibited by the autoantibodies. This is certainly of interest in a disease which in some features resembles a chronic infectious disease, such as lues.

Myeloblastin, the PR3 homologue isolated from the human leukemia cell line HL-60, is downregulated during induced cell differentiation [17]. Downregulation of myeloblastin expression by an antisense oligodeoxynucleotide stops proliferation of the HL-60 cells and induces differentiation (Table 3). Recently it was demonstrated that myeloblastin mRNA is also expressed in cells from patients with acute myeloid leukemia [19]. It appears possible that inhibition of WA (myeloblastin) by cANCA may also cause changes in granulocyte or monocyte differentiation. The excessive leukocytosis seen in fulminant WG may be the consequence of this autoantibody-induced differentiation process. Experiments using our monoclonal antibodies WGM1, WGM2, and WGM3 (directed against WA) as inducing agents are underway.

Another important feature of WA is its enzymatic activity and substrate specificity. It degrades elastin, hemoglobin [11], fibronectin, laminin, vitronectin, and collagen type IV [20] (Table 3). Furthermore, Kao et al. [12] have shown in an animal model that PR3 (WA) produces emphysema in hamsters, thus demonstrating that in addition to human neutrophil elastase, PMN release a second protease that can cause tissue damage. Moreover, serine proteinases from activated neutrophils, monocytes, and macrophages appear to be at least partially responsible for tissue injury seen in vasculitis and glomerulonephritis. Elastase isolated from experimentally induced granulomas in mice is reported to digest elastic fibers is vessel walls [21]. In man the elastinolytic activity of WA is inhibited by various potent natural inhibitors such as α_1-antitrypsin (α1AT) and α_2-macroglobulin [11]. From the clinical point of view this observation is of interest because α1AT deficiencies are associated with vasculitic processes.

Evidence is accumulating that circulating and deposited lysosomal proteins in WG can be observed in situ [22, 23]. Neutrophil serine proteases degrade the glomerular basement membrane and lead to proteinuria. Neutrophil proteinase activity was found in the urine in only 12 of 97 patients with clinical glomerular disease; these 12 patients had rapidly progressive glomerulonephritis, severe proliferative changes, and evidence of PMN infiltration [24]. Furthermore, in other vasculitides the immunoreactive PMN elastase/α1AT complex was detected in Kawasaki's disease, and eosinophil cationic protein was found to be deposited in vascular lesions of temporal arteritis [25]. Therefore, we investigated the hypothesis that binding of cANCA to PR3 (WA) prevents the enzyme from being inactivated by its natural inhibitor by means of steric hindrance, thus leading to uncontrolled degradation of the various matrix proteins in the tissue and of the elastic fibers in vessel walls [26]. We found that IgG (anti-PR3 antibodies) isolated from the serum of several WG patients inhibited the elastinolytic activity of PR3 [27]. However, several sera did not show any inhibitory effect, indicating that some of the antibodies bind directly to the active site of the enzyme while others do not. After preincubating PR3 with the IgG preparations, we added α1AT and measured elastinolysis in suspension. In all samples elastinolysis was inhibited by more than 95 %, which was the same value obtained using α1AT together with the buffer control or the IgG preparation from a normal control. These results indicate that even those autoantibodies that do not inhibit PR3 (WA) themselves are not able to prevent inhibition by α1AT [27]. Hence, the antibody hindrance hypothesis is probably incorrect.

The theories outlined above presuppose that WA really is accessible to cANCA in vivo. We have first demonstrated in vivo that WA is translocated onto the cell membrane of PMN during relapse of the disease or under the influence of tumor necrosis factor-α (TNF-α) in vitro as established by ultrastructural localization and FACS analyses [28, 29]. In addition, several lines of evidence indicate that cANCA stimulates TNF-α primed PMN in vitro to release lysosomal proteins and toxic oxygen metabolites [30]. Since natural inhibitors in the bloodstream, such as α1AT, immediately neutralize the biologic effects of WA, the activated PMN must bind closely with the presumptive target of vasculitis, the endothelial cell. Adhesion molecules are expressed on both cell types in the presence of TNF-α (Fig. 2). Thus, cANCA in the presence of cytokines may activate neutrophils to adhere to the endothelium via adhesion molecules and to release elastinolytic PR3 [7]. Proinflammatory cytokines such as TNF-α are detectable in active WG [5, 31]. Hence, vasculitis may be induced via this two-step procedure.

In any case, as mentioned above, WG is not solely a vasculitic disease. On the contrary, it begins as a granulomatous disease (initial phase). Granuloma was the name originally given to a chronic inflammatory mass resembling a tumor. Use of the term is now restricted to histologic lesions composed largely of lymphocytes and cells of myelomonocyte lineage. Granulomas are found in patients with infectious diseases (e.g., tuberculosis, lues), immunodeficiency states (e.g., hypogammaglobulinemia), chronic granulomatous

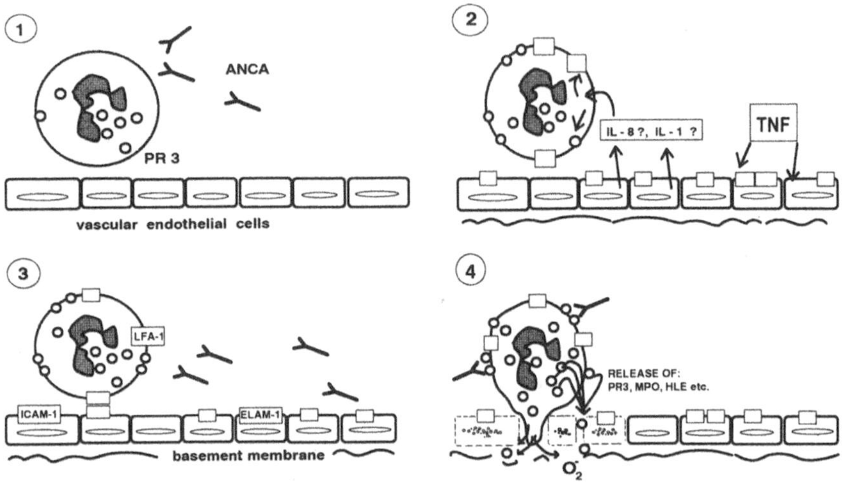

Fig. 2. Hypothetical model of ANCA-mediated PMN activation and endothelial injury. *1,* Unprimed neutrophil: PR3 mostly sequestered in azurophil granules. *2,* Priming of neutrophils by cytokines. Intracytoplasmic PR3 is translocated to the cell surface and becomes accessible to ANCA. Expression of adhesion molecules. *3,* Adhesion of neutrophils to endothelial cells. *4,* Interaction between ANCA and PR3 leads to activation of the neutrophils with degranulation, generation of O_2 radicals, and endothelial cell injury

disease, and diseases of unknown etiopathogenesis (e.g., Crohn's, Boeck's, and Wegener's diseases). In chronic granulomatous disease, neutrophils do not develop a respiratory burst after phagocytosis, and the granuloma may represent a cellular attempt to eliminate infectious agents. WG resembles chronic granulomatous disease in a few clinical aspects and in its response to treatment (e.g., with cotrimoxazole and corticosteroids). Whether exogenous agents such as cross-reacting microbial or viral antigens are involved in the local inflammatory process is unclear. In WG an association between infections, especially of the upper respiratory tract, and subsequent disease has been reported [32]. The efficacy of cotrimoxazole treatment in preventing relapses also supports the thesis that microbial factors are involved in the induction of disease activity.

If, as can be speculated, WA (PR3) is involved in defense mechanisms (e.g., against microbial infections), inhibition of WA by cANCA could result in impairment of the defense system via the following two mechanisms. (a) WA (PR3) is usually inhibited by α1AT. However, it is also known that enzyme inhibitors such as α1AT are inactivated by reactive oxygen species [33], which are released by activated neutrophils [30]. Therefore, it has been suggested that proteinase inhibitors are inactivated in the immediate vicinity of activated neutrophils, resulting in protection of the serine proteases from inhibition [34]. One could speculate that autoantibodies break through this protective shield and lead to inhibition of WA (PR3) in zones in which the enzyme is normally active. Thus granuloma formation in WG as in chronic granulomatous disease could be a compensatory mechanism for eliminating infections. However, this would not explain those cases of WG with granuloma formation in the initial phase which are ANCA negative. (b) Since WA (AGP7, p29) exhibits antimicrobial activity [14] similar to that of cathepsin G, interference of cANCA with AGP7 could result in a diminished defense. In this case, too, granuloma formation would reflect a compensation mechanism.

The disappearance of Wegener's granulomas in response to corticosteroids does not argue against this model, since in chronic granulomatous disease granulomas can also be dramatically reversed by hydrocortisone. However, this does not mean that the agents inducing the infection are combated by this treatment. Thus the granuloma can be reduced, but the disease is generally not stopped. On the other hand, granuloma formation usually suggests a state of T cell hypersensitivity. Immunohistologic studies reveal a predominance of $CD4^+$ cells in biopsies from the respiratory tract and kidneys of WG patients [35]. In the peripheral blood activated T cells (CD25 positive) are also elevated in WG and ANCA-positive vasculitides [36]. Additional indications of a T cell activation are increased levels of serum cytokines (such as TNF-α, interleukin-6, and others) during the acute disease phase and elevated soluble interleukin-2-receptor concentrations [37]. The latter have proven very useful seromarkers for the clinical activity of WG. We have demonstrated that even in complete remission they tend to be elevated in WG and enable earlier prediction of relapse than all other markers (including ANCA titer) that we have investigated so far (Fig. 3).

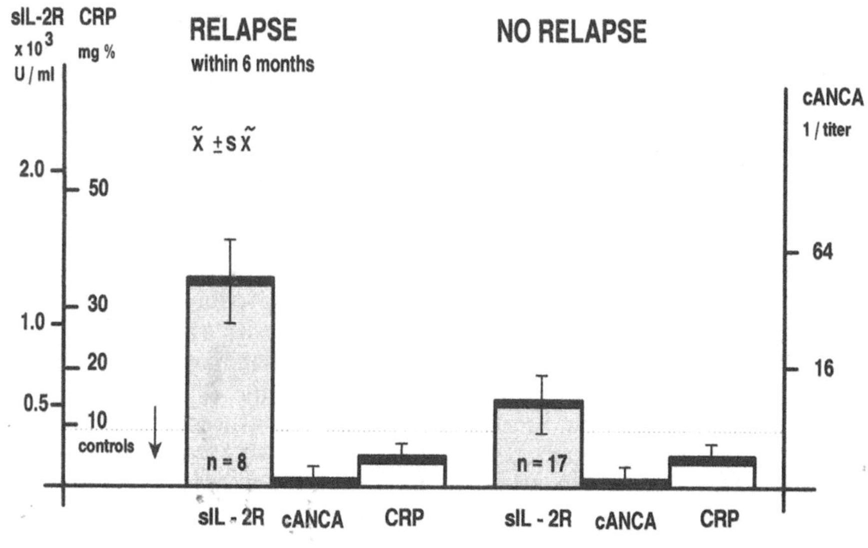

Fig. 3. Follow-up of 25 patients with generalized WG. In relapsing patients soluble interleukin-2 receptor (*sIL-2R*) levels were significantly elevated 3.5 (range 2–6) months before disease exacerbation ($p=0.05$)

The specific roles of cellular and humoral autoimmune responses in WG and ANCA-associated vasculitis remain a matter of discussion. The IgG subclass distribution of cANCA shows a high prevalence of IgG4 class antibodies [38, 39] together with increased total IgG4 and IgE levels. This contrasts with the IgG subclass distribution of, for example, antinuclear antibodies, which are mainly restricted to IgG1 and IgG3 and suggests repeated antigenic stimulation in a T cell response [40]. T cells from WG patients do respond to the cANCA target antigen (WA/PR3), reflecting an autoreactive T cell response (Mayet, University of Mainz; personal communication). Additionally, secondary responses to cross-reacting antimicrobial or antiviral structures may be involved in this process. Sequence homologies of viral and serine proteinases are thought to be a sign of a common evolutionary origin of these viral and mammalian structures [41]. The specific catalytical triad of serine proteases has been found in the core protein of Sindbis virus, a mosquito-borne alphavirus [42]. However, we found no cross-reactivity of cANCA-positive sera with Sindbis virus core protein.

pANCA and Pauci-immune Vasculitis

Besides the classic cytoplasmic staining pattern a second, perinuclear pattern can be seen in IIF on alcohol-fixed neutrophils (Fig. 1). This so-called pANCA pattern is an artifact of alcohol fixation [6] caused by the translocation of basic (positively charged) proteins to the negatively charged nucleus. If fixation is carried out with formaldehyde, which prevents the translocation of proteins, pANCA – as cANCA – exhibit a cytoplasmic staining pattern.

The most important target antigen of pANCA is myeloperoxidase, a markedly basic protein which is located within the azurophilic granules of PMN [6]. Together with H_2O_2 and halide, myeloperoxidase constitutes a potent microbicidal system within neutrophil granulocytes [43]. Myeloperoxidase is the target antigen of pANCA in about 80 % of cases [6]. However, additional target antigens such as human neutrophil elastase, cathepsin G, and lactoferrin have been described [44]. pANCA have been observed (a) in systemic vasculitides such as microscopic polyarteritis, polyarteritis nodosa, Churg-Strauß syndrome, etc. and (b) in idiopathic crescentic glomerulonephritis, thus placing these disorders within the spectrum of autoimmune diseases (Table 4). Glomerular lesions in patients with systemic and renal ANCA-associated diseases are identical, i. e., pauci-immune (no or minimal immune deposits in situ) necrotizing, and crescentic glomerulonephritis. Independent of their localization in ANCA-associated disease (e. g., kidney, lung, muscle) the vascular lesions are characterized by necrotizing inflammation and a paucity of immune deposits [45]. In most patients with pANCA-associated vasculitis (and glomerulonephritis, i. e., renal vasculitis) approximately 80 % of the pANCA are specific for myeloperoxidase (Fig. 4). The renal disease frequently presents as rapidly progressive renal failure with nephritis. One of the most life-threatening components of the systemic

Table 4. ANCA in vasculitic syndromes (from [55])

	C-ANCA	P ANCA[a]
Wegener's granulomatosis	295/383	20/383
Polyarteritis nodosa	14/49 (5/49)[b]	2/49
Churg-Strauss syndrome	4/13 (1/13)[b]	1/13
Polymyalgia rheumatica	0/62	5/62
Takayasu's arteritis	0/3	0/3
Temporal arteritis	0/24	2/24
Thrombangitis obliterans	0/6	0/6
Behçet's disease	0/21	0/21
Henoch-Schöhnlein purpura	0/18	0/18
Unclassified vasculitis	8/110	9/110
Cryoglobulinemia	0/5	0/5

[a] Hep-2 control negative
[b] PR3 ELISA

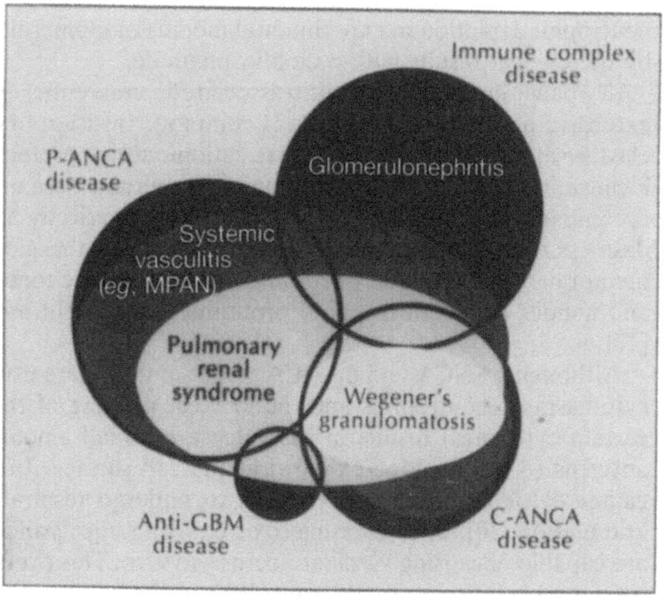

Fig. 4. Diagrammatic depiction of the interrelationships between immune pathogenic mechanisms (*four circles*) and clinicopathologic syndromes of vascular inflammation (*shaded areas*). Note that some clinicopathologic syndromes can be caused by more than one pathogenic mechanism, for example, pulmonary-renal syndrome can be caused by all four mechanisms. *C-ANCA*, cytoplasmic antineutrophil cytoplasmic autoantibody; *GBM*, glomerular basement membrane; *MPAN*, microscopic polyarteritis nodosa; *P-ANCA*, pericular antineutrophil cytoplasmic autoantibody. (From [54])

involvement is pulmonary hemorrhage caused by a necrotizing alveolar capillaritis. Although all of these symptoms can occur in WG, these vasculitides do not exhibit Wegener's granuloma. On the other hand, we found pANCA in fewer than 3% of 400 cases with biopsy-confirmed WG; cANCA and pANCA are very seldom combined in one serum.

From the immunodiagnostic point of view, pANCA and anti-myeloperoxidase antibodies are less specific for a single disease than cANCA are for WG. In addition to the group of primary vasculitis, they occur in a variety of other collagen vascular diseases.

The pathophysiology of idiopathic (primary) necrotizing vasculitides (pauci-immune vasculitis as well as the renal-restricted variant, idiopathic crescentic glomerulonephritis) is scarcely understood. This contrasts with vasculitis mediated by immune complexes, such as in collagen vascular diseases (e.g., systemic lupus erythematosus) or in allergic or infectious diseases (e.g., hepatitis-associated polyarteritis, drug-induced vasculitis). The connection between pANCA and pauci-immune vasculitis – even considering that it is not as strong as that between cANCA and WG – suggested that the in vivo reaction of these anti-lysosomal autoantibodies with their targets could be the triggering pathogenic mechanism. Neutrophils are intimately involved in the initial vascular (glomerular) injury. This is clearly indicated by the marked reduction in renal damage following neutrophil depletion in experimental models of glomerulonephritis [46] and by the clinical results with cyclophosphamide.

In pauci-immune vasculitis-associated crescentic glomerulonephritis extensive neutrophil infiltration is common. Infusion of human neutrophil elastase and cathepsin G, which are cationic serine proteases, results in their localization close to the (polyanionic) glomerular basement membrane and accompanies proteinuria [24]. Similarly, enzymatically active myeloperoxidase (perfused into rat renal arteries) binds to the glomerular basement membrane, and the subsequent infusion of nontoxic concentrations of H_2O_2 and halides results in transient proteinuria and slight proliferative changes [47].

Although cANCA and pANCA target antigens are usually located in the cytoplasm of neutrophils and monocytes, priming of these cells (e.g., by certain cytokines) results in the release of small amounts of these target antigens (e.g., myeloperoxidase) at the cell surface. In vitro, ANCA-IgG causes cytokine-primed neutrophils to undergo respiratory burst and degranulation [30], thus releasing toxic oxygen radicals and lytic enzymes that are capable of causing vascular necrosis in vivo. This oversimplified model is shown schematically for PR3/anti-PR3 in Fig. 2.

xANCA and Chronic Inflammatory Bowel Disease

In addition to the well-defined staining patterns of cANCA and pANCA a third, peculiar pattern has been described recently [48, 49]. This pattern, seen in IIF on ethanol-fixed neutrophils, appears to be a mixture of both cANCA and pANCA, with greater or lesser accentuation of cytoplasmic or perinuclear fluorescence. Some groups classify this pattern as non-p-non-cANCA while others designate it simply as pANCA. However, in addition to the peculiar staining pattern of the PMN, the correlation between xANCA and the corresponding target antigens is not nearly as clear as for pANCA or even cANCA. In our experience there is no privileged target antigen associated with xANCA. The obvious explanation that this pattern results from a mixture of autoantibodies against PR3 (WA) and myeloperoxidase in one serum proved to be incorrect. We observed xANCAs directed against human neutrophil elastase, cathepsin G, lactoferrin, myeloperoxidase, and even PR3. However, for most xANCAs we could not identify any of these target antigens. Hence, "xANCA" appears to be a "catch-all" term for peculiar staining patterns in ethanol-fixed neutrophils which are provoked not by granulocyte-specific antinuclear antibodies but by anticytoplasmic autoantibodies.

In contrast to the unproven association between xANCAs and target antigens, the correlation between xANCA and disease is much clearer. xANCAs i. e. appear to have a clearcut preference for chronic inflammatory bowel disease and related disease groups (e. g., primary sclerosing cholangitis).

Chronic inflammatory bowel disease encompasses at least two forms of intestinal inflammation: ulcerative colitis and Crohn's disease (known in its various forms as regional enteritis, Crohn's ileitis, and granulomatous colitis). In the absence of identifiable causes, Crohn's disease and ulcerative colitis are defined empirically according to their typical clinical, pathologic, radiologic, endoscopic, and laboratory features. The inflammatory process in ulcerative colitis is confined to the mucosa and superficial submucosa of the large bowel. On the macroscopic level, mucosal granularity and friability are replaced by broad areas of superficial ulceration covered with a mucopurulent exudate, leading clinically to bloody diarrhea. The histopathologic features, although nonspecific, are notable for the formation of microabscesses within crypts; the lamina propria is densely infiltrated by neutrophils and lymphocytes as well as other constituents of acute and chronic inflammation.

Although the infiltrate in acute and chronic inflammation in Crohn's disease is comparable to the infiltrate in ulcerative colitis, extension into the deeper layers of the bowel wall is a distinguishing feature of the former. The aggregation of macrophages leads to the development of noncaseating granulomata in approximately 50 % of patients, hence the term "granulomatous colitis." The diverse sites of tissue involvement and the variable degrees of inflammation give rise to a wide spectrum of clinical manifestations.

Recently, an association between ulcerative colitis and the appearance of a distinctive ANCA was reported [49, 50]. Serum from more than 70 % of patients with ulcerative colitis, but not with Crohn's disease, was found to produce the curious combined perinuclear and cytoplasmic staining pattern

Table 5. Effect of disease activity and therapy on p-ANCA reactivity of sera from three repeatedly tested patients with ulcerative colitis (from [49])

Patient no.	Age (years)	Sex	p-ANCA	Date	Treatment	Disease activity
1	46	F	+	16 Jan. 1989	No Therapy	High
			+	12 Apr. 1989	HE every 2nd day	Low
			(+)	19 June 1989	HE 2×per week	Low
			–	15 Nov. 1989	HE 1×per week	None
2	26	F	+	18 Sept. 1989	10 mg ME/day	High
			–		Subsequently, 50 mg ME pulse	
				6 Nov. 1989	20 mg ME/day	Low
3	45	F	+	8 Mar. 1989	No Therapy	High
			(+)	31 July 1989	HE 1×per day	Low
			(+)	4 Sept. 1989	HE every 2nd day	Low
			(+)	8 Nov. 1989	SASP	None

HE, 80 mg hydrocortisone enemas; ME, methylprednisolone; SASP, 3 g sulfasalazine.

called xANCA (Table 5). Later the same ANCA subtype was also observed in patients with sclerosing cholangitis [51].

Although it appears unlikely that this antibody is involved directly in the pathogenesis of ulcerative colitis, it may serve as a useful marker analogous to the anti mitochondrial antibody in primary biliary cirrhosis.

More recently, several groups of investigators have extended our knowledge of ANCA in chronic inflammatory bowel disease. In contrast to initial observations, xANCA can be found in at least 10%–20% of patients with Crohn's disease. Theoretically, one would have expected an association of ANCA rather with Crohn's disease than with ulcerative colitis, because Crohn's disease has several features in common with WG and/or vasculitis.

The granulomatous lesion in Crohn's disease resembles those in mycobacterial infections; however, as with WG, a large number of studies have failed to identify a transmitting agent. Hence, if an infectious agent is involved in the pathogenesis of Crohn's disease, alternative approaches to detection and isolation must be found. On the other hand, both cell-mediated and humoral immunity directed against epitopes common to enterobacterial antigens occur in patients with chronic inflammatory bowel disease, so that injury to the enterocyte could result from this molecular mimicry. Again, as in WG, it has been suggested that Crohn's disease is the consequence of a granulomatous angiitis which may cause multiple ischemic infarcts and lead to the remaining features of the disease [52].

Little is known about the mechanisms by which inflammatory cells are recruited to the bowel, although it is clear that neutrophils and other cellular elements are present in increased numbers in chronic inflammatory bowel disease. Preliminary observations indicate that disease activity is associated both with cANCA titer and with expression of the neutrophil-binding endothelial cell leukocyte adhesion molecule on endothelial cells of the bowel [53]. Presumably this molecule is induced by the rich mixture of interleukin-1, TNF-α, and other cytokines expressed both in tissue and the bloodstream during active inflammatory disease. Neutrophils appear to be attracted by increased concentration of the powerful chemotactic leukotrienes (e.g. B_4) as well as the formylated bacterial peptides (such as f-Met-Leu-Phe), which are known to induce degranulation of PMN. Possibly, ANCA equally activate PMN attached to the endothelial cells, thus producing the vascular damage outlined above.

Curiously, cANCA have specificity for a broad range of lysosomal proteins. This contrasts with pauci-immune vasculitis-associated pANCA (>80%: antimyeloperoxidase) and with WG-associated cANCA (>90%: anti-WA/PR3). Although the association of xANCA with chronic inflammatory disease was first described only 2 years ago, no one can expect that the immunodiagnostic data and the pathogenic role of the specific anti-lysosomal autoantibodies is complete today. On the other hand, these new autoantibodies will be able to serve as tools for clarifying the immunopathogenesis of a disease group so far only poorly understood.

References

1. Davies DJ, Moran JE, Niall JF, Ryan GB (1982) Segmental necrotising glomerulonephritis with antineutrophil antibody: possible arbovirus aetiology. Br Med J (Clin Res) 2: 606
2. Hall JB, Wadham BMcN, Wood CJ, Ashton V, Adam WR (1984) Vasculitis and glomerulonephritis; a subgroup with an antineutrophil cytoplasmic antibody. Aust NZ J Med 14: 277–278
4. van der Woude FJ, Rasmussen N, Lobatto S, Wiik A, Permin H, van Es LA, van der Giessen M, van der Hem GK, The TH (1985) Autoantibodies against neutrophils and monocytes; tool for diagnosis and marker of disease activity in Wegener's granulomatosis. Lancet I: 425–429
4. Gross WL, Lüdemann G, Kiefer G, Lehmann H (1986) Anti-cytoplasmatic antibodies in Wegener's granulomatosis (letter) Lancet I: 806
5. Nölle B, Specks U, Lüdemann J, Rohrbach MS, DeRemee RA, Gross WL (1989) Anticytoplasmatic autoantibodies: their immunodiagnostic value in Wegener's granulomatosis. Ann Intern Med 111: 28–40
6. Falk RJ, Jennette JC (1988) Anti-neutrophil cytoplasmic autoantibodies with specificity for myeloperoxidase in patients with systemic vasculitis and idiopathic and crescentic glomerulonephritis. N Engl J Med 318: 1651
7. Gross WL, Csernok E, Schmitt WH (1991) ANCA's: immunobiological aspects. Klin Wochenschr 69: 558–566
8. Wegener F (1936) Über generalisierte septische Gefäßerkrankungen. Verh Dtsch Ges Pathol 29: 202
9. Gross WL (1989) Wegener's granulomatosis. New aspect of the disease course, immundiagnostic procedures, and stage-adapted treatment. Sarcoidosis 6: 15
10. Goldschmeding R, van der Schoot DE, ten Bokkel Huinink D, Hack CE, van den Ende ME, Kallenberg CGM, von dem Borne AEGK (1989) Wegener's granulomatosis autoantibodies identify a novel diisopropylfluorophosphate-binding protein in the lysosomes of normal human neutrophils. J Clin Invest 84: 1577–1587

11. Lüdemann J, Utecht B, Gross WL (1990) Anti-neutrophil cytoplasmic antibodies in Wegener's granulomatosis recognize an elastinolytic enzyme. J Exp Med 171: 357–362
12. Kao RC, Wehner NG, Skubitz KM, Gray BH, Hoidal JR (1988) Proteinase 3: a distinct human polymorphonuclear leukocyte proteinase that produces emphysema in hamsters. J Clin Invest 82: 1963–1973
13. Baggiolini M, Bretz U, Dewald B, Feigensohn ME (1978) The polymorphonuclear leukocyte. Agents Actions. 8: 3–10
14. Gabay JE, Scott RW, Campanelli D, Griffith J, Wilde C, Marra MN, Seeger M, Nathan CF (1989) Antibiotic proteins of human polymorphonuclear leukocytes (bacteria/lysosomes/neutrophils). Proc Natl Acad Sci USA 86: 5610–5614
15. Wilde CG, Snable JL, Griffith JE, Scott RW (1990) Characterization of two azurophil granule proteases with active-site homology to neutrophil elastase. J Biol Chem 265: 2038–2041
16. Niles JR, McCluskey RT, Ahmad MF, Arnaout MA (1989) Wegener's granulomatosis autoantigen is a novel neutrophil serine proteinase. Blood 74: 1888–1893
17. Bories D, Raynal MD, Solomon DH, Darzynkiewicz Z, Cayre YE (1989) Downregulation of a serine protease, myeloblastin, causes growth arrest and differentiation of promyelocytic leukemia cells. Cell 59: 959–968
18. Campanelli DJ, Melchior M, Fu Y, Nakata M, Shuman H, Nathan C, Gabay JE (1990) Cloning of cDNA for proteinase 3: a serine protease, antibiotic, and autoantigen from human neutrophils. J Exp Med 172: 1709–1715
19. Labbaye C, Musette P, Cayre YE (1991) Wegener autoantigen and myeloblastin are encoded by a single mRNA. Proc Natl Acad Sci USA 88: 9253–9256
20. Rao NV, Wehner NG, Marshall BC, Gray WR, Gray BH, Hoidal JR (1991) Characterization of proteinase-3 (PR-3), a neutrophil serine proteinase. J Biol Chem 266: 9540–9548
21. Izaki S, Okamoto M, Hsu P-S, Epstein WL, Fukuyama K (1986) Characterization of elastase associated with granulomatous tissue remodeling. J Cell Biochem 32: 79–89
22. Braun MG, Csernok E, Gross WL, Müller-Hermelink HK (1991) Proteinase 3, the target antigen of anticytoplasmic antibodies circulating in Wegener's granulomatosis. Am J Pathol 139: 831–838
23. Katz P, Fauci AS, Yeager H, Reen BM (1981) Serum angiotensin-converting enzyme and lysozyme in granulomatous diseases of unknown cause. Ann Intern Med 94: 359–360
24. Davies M, Coles GA, Thomas GJ, Martin J, Lovett DH (1990) Proteinases and the glomerulus: their role in glomerular diseases. Klin Wochenschr 68: 1145–1149
25. Hällgren R, Gudbjörnsson B, Larsson E, Fredens K (1991) Deposition of eosinophil cationic protein in vascular lesions in temporal arteritis. Ann Rheum Dis 50: 946–949
26. van der Woude FJ, Daha MR, van Es LA (1989) The current status of neutrophil cytoplasmic antibodies. Clin Exp Immunol 78: 143–148
27. Lüdemann J, Utecht B, Gross WL (1991) Anti-cytoplasmic antibodies in Wegener's granulomatosis are directed against proteinase 3. In: Hörl WH, Schollmeyer A (eds) New aspects of human polymorphonuclear leukocytes. Plenum, New York, pp. 141–150
28. Csernok E, Lüdemann J, Gross WL, Bainton DF (1990) Ultrastructural localization of proteinase 3, the target antigen of anti-cytoplasmic antibodies circulating in Wegener's granulomatosis. Am J Pathol 137: 1113–1120
29. Csernok E, Ernst M, Schmitt WH, Bainton D, Gross WL (1991) Translocation of PR3 on the cell surface of neutrophils: association with disease activity in Wegener's granulomatosis. Arthritis Rheum 34 [Suppl 9]: 79
30. Ewert BH, Jennette JC, Falk RJ (1991) The pathogenic role of antineutrophil cytoplasmic autoantibodies. Am J Kidney Dis 18: 188–195

31. Kekow J, Szymkowiak CH, Sticherling M, Schröder JM, Christofers E, Gross WL (1992) Pro- and anti-inflammatory cytokines in primary systemic vasculitis. In: Gross WL (ed) ANCA associated vasculitides: immunodiagnostic and pathogenic value of antineutrophil cytoplasmic autoantibodies. Plenum, London (to be published)
32. DeRemee RA (1988) The treatment of Wegener's granulomatosis with trimethoprim sulfamethoxazole; illusion or vision? Arthritis Rheum 31: 1068–1072
33. Warren JS, Yabroff KR, Mandel DM, Johnson KJ, Ward PA (1990) Role of O_2^- in neutrophil recruitment into sites of dermal and pulmonary vasculitis. Free Radic Biol Med 8: 163–172
34. Weiss JS (1989) Tissue destruction by neutrophils. N Engl J Med 320: 365–379
35. Brouwer E, Cohen Tervaert JW, Weening JJ, Kallenberg CGM (1992) Kidney Int (to be published)
36. Gutfleisch J, Baumert E, Wolff-Vorbeck G, Schlesier M, Strutz HJ, Peter HH (1992) Increased expression of CD25 and adhesion molecules on peripheral blood lymphocytes of patients with Wegener's granulomatosis (WG) and ANCA positive vasculitides. In: Gross WL (ed) ANCA associated vasculitides: immunodiagnostic and pathogenic value of antineutrophil cytoplasmic autoantibodies. Plenum, London (to be published)
37. Schmitt WH, Heesen C, Csernok E, Rautmann A, Gross WL (1992) Elevated serum levels of soluble interleukin 2 receptor (sIL-2R) in Wegener's granulomatosis (WG): association with disease activity. Arthritis Rheum 35: 1088–1096
38. Bowman C, Ambrus K, Lockwood CM (1987) Restriction of human IgG-subclass expression in the population of autoantibodies to glomerular basement membrane. Clin Exp Immunol 69: 341–349
39. Nölle B, Blümke A, Lüdemann J, Rautmann A, Gross WL (1990) IgG-Subklassenverteilung bei Wegener'scher Granulomatose. Immun Infekt 18: 98–100
40. Kallenberg CGM, Cohen Tervaert JW, van der Woude FJ, Goldschmeding R, von dem Borne AEGKr, Weening JJ (1991) Autoimmunity to lysosomal enzymes: new clues to vasculitis and glomerulonephritis. Immunol Today 12: 61–64
41. Hahn CS, Strauss EG, Strauss JH (1985) Sequence analysis of three Sindbis virus mutants temperature-sensitive in the capsid protein autoprotease. Proc Natl Acad Sci USA 82: 4648–4652
42. Choi HK, Tong L, Minor W, Dumas P, Boege U, Rossmann MG, Wengler G (1991) Structure of Sindbis virus core protein reveals a chymotrypsin-like serine proteinase and the organization of the virion. Nature 354: 37–43
43. Klebanoff SJ (1975) Antimicrobial mechanisms in neutrophilic polymorphonuclear leukocytes. Semin Hematol 12: 117–142
44. Lesavre P, Noel LH, Chauveau D, Geffriaud C, Grünfeld IP (1991) Antigen specificities and clinical distribution of ANCA in kidney diseases. Klin Wochenschr 69: 552–557
45. Jennette JC, Falk RJ (1990) Antineutrophil cytoplasmic autoantibodies and associated diseases: a review. Am J Kidney Dis 15: 517–529
46. Cochrane CG, Aiken BS (1966) Polymorphonuclear leukocytes in immunologic reactions. The destruction of vascular basement membrane in vitro by neutral protease of human leukocytes. Science 16: 702
47. Johnson RJ, Guggenheim SJ, Klebanoff SJ, Ochi RF, Wass A, Baker P, Schulze M, Couser WG (1998) Morphologic correlates of glomerular oxidant injury induced by the myeloperoxidase-hydrogen peroxide-halide system of the neutrophil. Lab Invest 5: 294–301
48. Targan S, Saxon A, Landers C, Ganz T, Shanahan F (1989) Serum antineutrophil cytoplasmic autoantibodies distinguish ulcerative colitis from Crohn's disease patients. Gastroenterology 96 (2): A 505 (abstract)
49. Rump JA, Schölmerich J, Gross V, Roth M, Helfesrieder R, Rautmann A, Lüdemann J, Gross WL, Peter HH (1990) A new type of perinuclear anti-neutrophil cytoplasmic antibody (p-ANCA) in active ulcerative colitis but not in Crohn's Disease. Immunobiology 181: 406–413

50. Saxon A, Shanahan F, Landers C, Ganz T, Targan S (1990) A distinct subset of antineutrophil cytoplasmic antibodies is associated with inflammatory bowel disease. J Allergy Clin Immunol 86: 202–210
51. Snook JA, Chapmann RW, Fleming K, Jewell DP (1989) Anti-neutrophil nuclear antibody in ulcerative colitis, Crohn's disease and primary sclerosing cholangitis. Clin Exp Immunol 76: 30–33
52. Wakefield AJ, Sawyer AM, Dhillon AP (1989) Pathogenesis of Crohn's disease: multifocal gastrointestinal infarction. Lancet ii: 1057–1062
53. Podolsky DK (1991) Inflammatory bowel disease. N Engl J Med 325: 928–937
54. Jennette JC (1991) Anti neutrophil cytoplasmic autoantibody associated disease: a pathologist's perspective. Am J Kidney Dis 18: 164–170
55. Gross WL, Schmitt WH, Csernok E (1991) Antineutrophil cytoplasmic autoantibody associated diseases: a rheumatologist's perspective. Am J Kidney Dis 18: 175–179

Heat-Shock Proteins and Autoimmunity

S.H.E. Kaufmann

Introduction

The term stress has become an indispensable part of everyday vocabulary to describe the sterotype and ubiquitous response of man toward exogenous insults. More recently this term has also found its way into the vocabulary of cell biologists to describe a particular cell response. Adoption of this term by cell biologists seems appropriate because in cells a universal and ubiquitous response toward exogenous assaults can also be found (Kaufmann 1990; Young 1990). The cellular stress response is ubiquitous because it appears in every living cell of the universe and it is stereotype because in every cell the same pattern of response occurs. The cellular stress response is characterized by the increased synthesis of a certain group of proteins which, accordingly, have been termed stress proteins.

The Stress or Heat-Shock Response

In the early days of cellular stress studies, the main assault was a very simple and rather artificial one, namely incubation of cells at elevated temperature. Therefore, the reaction has been called heat-shock response and the newly synthesized polypeptides heat-shock proteins (hsp). Later, other more physiological insults were noted including anoxia, nutrient depriviation, and treatment with oxygen radicals, ethanol, heavy metal ions, or nicotin. The hsp have been grouped into distinct families according to their apparent size. Thus, hsp 90, hsp 70, hsp 60 or the small hsp have molecular masses of 90, 70, 60, and around 14 kDa, respectively. In addition, other proteins such as ubiquitin, which had already been christened, were found to belong to the hsp family. Increasing hsp synthesis under stress is not an epiphenomenon because increased hsp levels afford protection against subsequent, more serious, or even lethal injury. For example *Salmonella typhimurium* microorganisms, after being stressed by sublethal H_2O_2 concentrations, prove resistant to subsequent treatment with normally lethal concentrations of this toxic molecule (Morgan et al. 1986). Conversely, mutants of *S. typhimurium* lacking certain hsp genes are more susceptible to various insults including killing by macrophages (Fields et al. 1986).

Physiological Functions of hsp

Although hsp were first noted during stress responses, it subsequently became clear that many of them perform a pivotal role in the physiological housekeeping of cells. Thus, members of the hsp 60 and hsp 70 families interact with other polypeptides and in this way assist them in several respects without becoming part of their final functional structure. To account for these capacities, the term chaperonins was coined (Ellis and van der Vies 1991). These hsp promote the folding of nascent polypeptides; they keep nascent polypeptides in an unfolded stage; they promote protein unfolding; they arrange for protein translocation in the unfolded stage through membrane barriers; and they promote assembly of multimeric protein complexes. They fulfill all these tasks because of their particular affinity for interactive peptide regions which are hidden in the inner side of the correctly folded protein and are exposed during unfolding. At the elevated entropy of heat, proteins begin to unfold, and hsp can at least in part prevent this unfolding by virtue of the very same feature. Thus, the basic functions of hsp 70 and hsp 60 cognates under physiological and pathophysiological conditions remain virtually the same.

hsp and Immunity

Do such universal and abundant polypeptides serve as antigenic targets of the immune response? Here, the immune system faces a dilemma. On the one hand, hsp are abundant proteins of microbial infectious agents. For example, up to 10 % of all proteins of *Escherichia coli* undergoing stress are hsp (Young 1990). Since hsp of various microbial pathogens are highly similar, they could provide a general antigen for anti-infectious immunity independent of the species responsible for disease. Teleologically speaking, hsp may therefore be desirable targets for the protective host response. On the other hand, even microbial and mammalian hsp are highly similar. For example, the mycobacterial hsp 60 and its human counterpart share more than 50 % sequence homology, i.e., half of each of the two proteins are identical (Thole et al. 1987; Jindal et al. 1989). Teleologically one would argue that the immune system would be well advised to ignore antigens of such high similarity with autologous proteins to avoid autoaggression.

T cells do not recognize proteins directly but rather respond to antigenic peptides presented in the context of gene products of the major histocompatibility complex (MHC). Thus, one possible way to solve this dilemma would be focusing the immune response on those amino acid sequences that are unique for the microbial world. This, however, does not seem to be the case, and prominent T lymphocyte and B lymphocyte responses toward shared epitopes have been found to occur during infection or after immunization with microbial proteins (Mehra et al. 1986; Munk et al. 1989; Lamb et al. 1989).

Indeed, several studies have revealed that cognates of the hsp 70 and hsp 60 families are dominant antigens of various infectious agents (Kaufmann 1991). This holds true not only for patients or immune mice (Emmrich et al. 1986; Lamb et al. 1989; Kaufmann et al. 1987); even in normal healthy individuals, the frequency of hsp-specific T cells was found to be surprisingly high (Munk et al. 1988; Kabelitz et al. 1990). The demonstration of T cells with specificity for mycobacterial hsp 60 in healthy individuals without previous bacille Calmette-Guérin vaccination or any signs of *Mycobacterium tuberculosis* infection supports the notion that T cells with specificity for hsp can be induced by unrelated microbial species (Kaufmann et al. 1991). It can be envisaged that subclinical infections with opportunistic environmental microbes such as atypical mycobacteria stimulate hsp-reactive T cells which, upon infection with pathogens such as *Mycobacterium tuberculosis,* can be rapidly mobilized through a booster effect. Such T cells could provide a first line of protection and contribute to the early control of infection. Clearly, such a scenario must be considered beneficial for the host. Further in this line it has recently been shown that addition of hsp 60 or hsp 70 as carriers improves the antigenicity of subunit vaccines (Lussow et al. 1991).

hsp and Autoimmunity

T cells with specificity for regions shared by the mammalian and mycobacterial hsp 60 have been identified in normal healthy individuals. Munk et al. (1989) found that peripheral blood T cells from healthy donors, upon stimulation with mycobacterial lysates, recognize autologous targets primed with peptides corresponding to fully or almost identical regions of mycobacterial and human hsp 60. This finding indicates that T cells with specificity for autologous hsp are members of the normal T cell repertoire without detrimental consequences for the host. One might assume that under physiological conditions these T cells are not activated because autologous hsp epitopes are not presented by the MHC to the T cell system. Recently, it has become possible to isolate and identify peptides from the MHC groove which represent potential autologous T cell epitopes (Rötschke and Falk 1991). In this context it may be interesting to note that one of the first peptides isolated in this way was found to be derived from a member of the hsp 90 family (Jardetzky et al. 1991).

Moreover, it has been shown that T cells after activation with mycobacterial hsp 60 recognize and lyse stressed macrophages or Schwann's cells (Koga et al. 1989; Steinhoff et al. 1990). In these studies, class I restricted $CD8^+$ α/β T cells of naive mice were activated in vitro by high concentrations of a tryptic peptide digest of mycobacterial hsp 60. More recently, such T cells could also be activated in vivo by immunization with mycobacterial hsp 60 in ISCOM (Yamamoto et al., unpublished). Although the epitope expressed by stressed macrophages has not been identified as yet, autologous hsp 60 derived peptides appear likely candidates. In any case, these data show that T cells with specificity for mycobacterial hsp 60 indeed recognize stressed host cells. No indication for autoimmune disease, however, was found in these mice.

In summary, the findings described suggest that during microbial infection, T cells capable of recognizing shared epitopes and stressed host cells can be activated. T cells with specificity for self-hsp could be beneficial for the host since they provide a marker indicative for diseased or injured cells independent of the initial cause. In this way, cells stressed by any assault, be it an infectious, inflammatory, traumatic, or transforming process, could become recognizable for T cells of a single specificity. Thus, hsp could provide an economic marker for immune surveillance. Yet, such a scenario could become dangerous, since it could also lead to autoimmune disease.

hsp and Autoimmune Disease

Convincing evidence for hsp being central targets in autoimmune disease comes from two experimental models. Adjuvant arthritis can be induced in certain strains of rats by injection of complete Freund's adjuvant containing mycobacteria. The inflammatory process which develops in the joints has some resemblance to rheumatoid arthritis of man. Disease can be transferred by T cells which recognize mycobacterial hsp 60, and the epitope has been mapped to the amino acid sequence 180–188 (van Eden et al. 1988). This sequence shows only marginal homology with the mammalian counterpart, but the T cells cross-react with proteoglycans. Immunization with hsp 60, proper, however, does not cause arthritis in rats. Rather, pretreatment with the whole hsp polypeptide or the 180 to 188 amino acid peptide protects the animals from subsequent attempts to induce adjuvant arthritis (Van Eden et al. 1988; Feige and Cohen 1991).

In mice of the nonobese diabetic (NOD) strain a diabetic disease develops spontaneously which resembles insulin-dependent diabetes mellitus of man. T cells with specificity for mycobacterial hsp 60 can transfer disease into congenic genetically nondiabetic mice (Elias et al. 1990, 1991). The T cells recognize a shared epitope of the mycobacterial and human hsp 60 homologs. Immunization with hsp 60 in adjuvant causes disease not only in young NOD mice before onset of spontaneous diabetes but even in nondiabetic congenic animals. Yet, also in this model administration of the whole hsp 60 polypeptide or the relevant peptide causes protection against disease. Thus, the epitopes in rat adjuvant arthritis and in NOD mouse diabetes are distinct in terms of sequence as well as of conservation. Despite the central role of hsp 60 in these two forms of experimental autoimmune disease different mechanisms seem to participate. In the case of adjuvant arthritis, disease may be a matter of the mycobacterial hsp 60 only. Alternatively, cross-reactivity with unrelated tissue antigens such as proteoglycan may be considered. In the case of NOD mouse diabetes, cross-reactivity between microbial and host hsp 60 represents a possible explanation.

The findings that in both experimental models disease could be prevented by preimmunization with soluble hsp 60 may have therapeutic implications. Yet, it comes not so much to a surprise since high zone tolerance induced by immunization with soluble proteins is a well-known phenomenon in immunology (Nossal 1983).

What about man? Evidence to suggest a role for hsp 60 also exists but is far from being conclusive. In multiple sclerosis, γ/δ T cells have been found to colocalize with immature oligodendrocytes expressing high levels of hsp 60 (Selmaj et al. 1991). This finding may be interpreted to indicate that γ/δ T cells recognizing oligodendrocytes perpetuate disease by preventing remyelination. Yet, direct proof for interactions between oligodendrocytes expressing hsp 60 and γ/δ T cells remains to be shown. In patients undergoing active lupus nephritis B cell stimulation by γ/δ T cells was observed, and this response could be inhibited by antibodies with specificity for hsp 60 (Rajogoplan et al. 1990). This finding may be interpreted to say that hsp 60 is recognized directly by γ/δ T cells and serves as autoantigen in systemic lupus erythematosus. However, among the mononuclear antibodies used for blocking, one (IIIE9) is thought to be specific for *M. leprae* hsp 60 and not to be cross-reactive with mammalian hsp 60 (Dudani and Gupta 1989).

Tentatively, T cells with specificity for hsp 60 have also been implicated in human type I diabetes (Jones et al. 1990). More recently, however, the enzyme glutamic acid decarboxylase which fortuitously also has a molecular mass of 60 kDa has been more convincingly shown to be the major islet cell autoantigen in human type I diabetes (Baekeskov et al. 1990).

Strong evidence exists that reactive arthritis is caused by a variety of microbial pathogens, and indeed T cells from synovial lesions respond to lysates of these bacteria. At least some of the T cells respond to mycobacterial hsp 60, with the majority being specific for a nonconserved epitope (Res et al. 1991; Life et al. 1991). However, numerous bacterial antigens other than hsp are also recognized. Therefore, at the moment bacterial deposition in the joints and T cell stimulation by a variety of microbial antigens seems a likely explanation. In such a scenario, hsp would not represent a unique antigen. In a recent study, however, a T cell clone recognizing *Yersinia* antigens as well as mycobacterial and human hsp 60 was isolated from the synovial fluid of a reactive arthritis patient (Hermann et al. 1991). So, also here the question arises whether cross-reactive T cells with specificity for conserved regions of hsp 60 are of relevance or not.

Initial experiments provided promising results towards a role for hsp 60 specific T cells in rhematoid arthritis (Res et al. 1991; Life et al. 1991). In these studies, evidence was obtained that hsp 60 specific T cells accumulate in rheumatoid lesions. However, in subsequent analyses with numerous T cell clones contaminating *E. coli* components within the recombinant hsp 60 preparation were found to be responsible for many of the responses (Res et al. 1991). Further arguments against a role of hsp 60 in rheumatoid arthritis of adults have been raised in a recent publication (De Graeff-Meeder et al. 1991). In this study evidence was obtained that synovial fluid T cells of

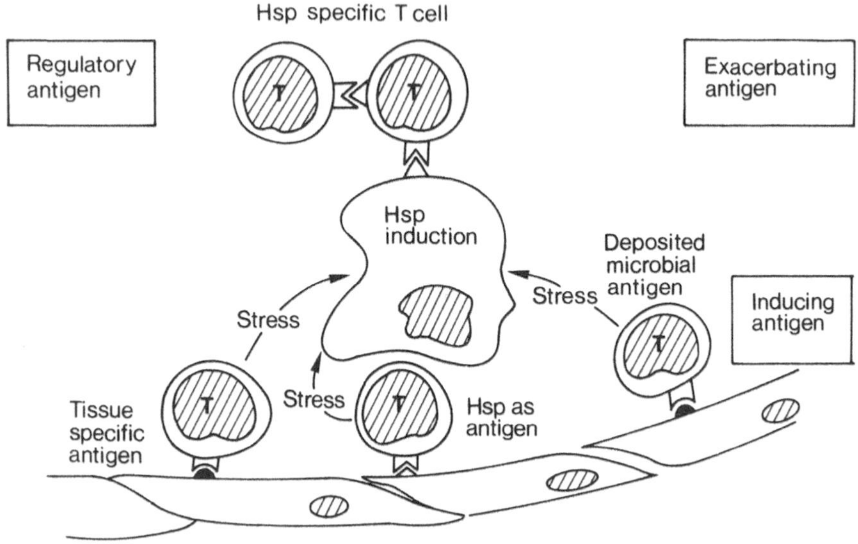

Fig. 1. Hypothetical scheme of the various possibilities by which hsp may serve as antigen in autoimmune diseases

juvenile arthritis patients show significant responses to mycobacterial and human hsp 60, implicating a conserved epitope in disease development.

Thus, the role of hsp 60 and even more so the role of shared epitopes of this protein in autoimmune diseases of man remains open. While there is sufficient evidence to justify further studies, a central and unique role of hsp 60 as initiating antigen of a variety of unrelated autoimmune diseases seems unlikely. Perhaps after initiation of disease by organ-specific antigens or by deposited microbial antigens the cells are stressed and then recognized by hsp-specific T cells. The hsp-specific T cells could then perpetuate and/or exacerbate local inflammatory responses (Fig. 1). Consistent with this assumption, increased hsp 60 expression in certain autoimmune lesions and identification of hsp-reactive α/β or γ/δ T cells has been described (Holoshitz et al. 1989; Karlsson-Parra et al. 1990; Evans et al. 1990). Autoreactive γ/δ T cells have been claimed to perform regulatory functions (Ferrick et al. 1991), and the possibility should be considered that hsp 60 reactive γ/δ T cells in autoimmune lesions may not necessarily perform effector functions but rather reflect the idle attempt of the immune system to prevent autoaggression by α/β T cells.

Acknowledgements. The author acknowledges financial support from the UNDP/World Bank/WHO Special Program for Research and Training in Tropical Diseases, German Leprosy Relief Association, EC-India Science and Technology Cooperation Program, SFB 322, Landesschwerpunkt 30. The superb help of Mrs. R. Mahmoudi is gratefully acknowledged.

References

Baekeskow S, Jan-Aanstoot H, Christgau S, Reetz A, Solimena M, Cascalho M, Folli F, Richter-Olesen H, De Camilli P (1990) Identification of the 65 K autoantigen in insulin-dependent diabetes as the GABA-synthesizing enzyme glutamic acid decarboxylase. Nature 347: 151–156

De Graeff-Meeder ER, van der Zee R, Rijkers GT, Schuurman H-J, Kuis W, Bijlsma JWJ, Zegers BMJ, van Eden W (1991) Recognition of human 60 kD heat shock protein by mononuclear cells from patients with juvenile chronic arthritis. Lancet 337: 1368–1372

Dudani AK, Gupta RS (1989) Immunological characterization of a homolog of the 65-kilodalton mycobacterial antigen. Infect Immun 57: 2786–2793

Elias D, Markovits D, Reshef T, van der Zee R, Cohen IR (1990) Induction and therapy of autoimmune diabetes in the non-obese diabetic (NOD/Lt) mouse by a 65-kDa heat shock protein. Proc Natl Acad Sci USA 87: 1576–1580

Elias D, Reshef T, Birk OS, van der Zee R, Walker MD, Cohen IR (1991) Vaccination against autoimmune mouse diabetes with a T-cell epitope of the human 65-kDa heat shock protein. Proc Natl Acad Sci USA 88: 3088–3091

Ellis RJ, van der Vies SM (1991) Molecular chaperones. Annu Rev Biochem 60: 321–347

Emmrich F, Thole J, van Embden J, Kaufmann SHE (1986) A recombinant 64 kiloDalton protein of *Mycobacterium bovis* BCG specifically stimulates human T4 clones reactive to mycobacterial antigens. J Exp Med 163: 1024–1029

Evans DJ, Norton P, Ivanyi J (1990) Distribution in tissue sections of the human GroEL stress protein homologue. APMIS 98: 437

Feige U, Cohen IR (1991) The 65-kDA heat shock protein in the pathogenesis, prevention and therapy of autoimmune arthritis and diabetes mellitus in rats and mice. Springer Semin Immunopathol 13: 99–113

Ferrick DA, Sydora B, Wallace V, Gemmell-Hori L, Kronenberg M, Mak TW (1991) Self-reactive γ/δ T lymphocytes: implications for T-cell ontogeny and reactivity. Immunol Rev 120: 51–70

Fields PI, Swanson RV, Haidaris CG, Heffron F (1986) Mutants of *Salmonella typhimurium* that cannot survive within the macrophage are avirulent. Proc Natl Acad Sci USA 83: 5189–5193

Hermann E, Lohse AW, van der Zee R, van Eden W, Mayet WJ, Probst P, Poralla T, Meyer zum Büschenfelde K-H, Fleischer B (1991) Synovial fluid-derived Yersinia-reactive Tcells responding to human 65-kDa heat-shock protein and heat-stressed antigen-presenting cells. Eur J Immunol 21: 2139–2143

Holoshitz J, Koning F, Coligan JE, De Bruyn J, Strober S (1989) Isolation of $CD4^-$ $CD8^-$ mycobacteria-reactive T lymphocyte clones from rheumatoid arthritis synovial fluid. Nature 339: 226–229

Jardetzky TS, Lane WS, Robinson RA, Madden DR, Wiley DC (1991) Identification of self peptides bound to purified HLA-B27. Nature 353: 326–328

Jindal S, Dudani AK, Singh B, Harley CB, Gupta RS (1989) Primary structure of a human mitochondrial protein homologous to the bacterial and plant chaperonins and to the 65-kilodalton mycobacterial antigen. Mol Cell Biol 9: 2279–2283

Jones DB, Hunter NR, Duff GW (1990) Heat-shock protein 65 as a ß cell antigen of insulin-dependent diabetes. Lancet 336: 583–585

Kabelitz D, Bender A, Schondelmaier S, Schoel B, Kaufmann SHE (1990) A large fraction of human peripheral blood γ/δ^+ Tcells is activated by *Mycobacterium tuberculosis* but not by its 65 kD heat shock protein. J Exp Med 171: 667–679

Karlsson-Parra A, Köderström K, Ferm M, Ivanyi J, Kiessling R, Klareskog L (1990) Presence of human 65 kD heat shock protein (hsp) in inflamed joints and subcutaneous nodules of RA patients: a clue to pathogenicity of anti-65 kD hsp immunity? Scand J Immunol 31: 283–288

Kaufmann SHE (1990) Heat shock proteins and the immune response. Immunol Today 11: 129–136

Kaufmann SHE (1991) Heat shock proteins and pathogenesis of bacterial infections. Springer Semin Immunopathol 13: 25–36

Kaufmann SHE, Väth U, Thole JER, van Embden JDA, Emmrich F (1987) Enumeration of T cells reactive with *Mycobacterium tuberculosis* organisms and specific for the recombinant mycobacterial 64 kilodalton protein. Eur J Immunol 17: 351–357

Kaufmann SHE, Schoel B, Koga T, Wand-Württenberger A, Munk ME, Steinhoff U (1991) Heat shock protein 60: implications for pathogenesis of and protection against bacterial infections. Immunol Rev 121: 67–90

Koga T, Wand-Württenberger A, DeBruyn J, Munk ME, Schoel B, Kaufmann SHE (1989) T cells against a bacterial heat shock protein recognize stressed macrophages. Science 245: 1112–1115

Lamb JR, Bal V, Mendez-Samperio P, Mehlert A, So A, Rothbard J, Jindal S, Young RA, Young DB (1989) Stress proteins may provide a link between the immune response to infection and autoimmunity. Int Immunol 1: 191–196

Life PF, Bassey EOE, Gaston HJS (1991) T-cell recognition of bacterial heat shock proteins in inflammatory arthritis. Immunol Rev 121: 113–135

Lussow AR, Barrios C, van Embden J, van der Zee R, Verdini AS, Louis JA, Lambert PH, Del Guidice G (1991) Mycobacterial heat shock proteins as carrier molecules. Eur J Immunol 21: 2297–2302

Mehra V, Sweetser D, Young RA (1986) Efficient mapping of protein antigenic determinants. Proc Natl Acad Sci USA 83: 7013–7017

Morgan RW, Christman MF, Jacobson FS, Storz G, Ames BN (1986) Hydrogen peroxide-inducible proteins in *Salmonella typhimurium* overlap with heat shock and other stress proteins. Proc Natl Acad Sci USA 83: 8059–8063

Munk ME, Schoel B, Kaufmann SHE (1988) T cell responses of normal individuals towards recombinant protein antigens of *Mycobacterium tuberculosis*. Eur J Immunol 18: 1835–1838

Munk ME, Schoel B, Modrow S, Karr RW, Young RA, Kaufmann SHE (1989) Cytolytic T lymphocytes from healthy individuals with specificity to self epitopes shared by the mycobacterial and human 65 kDa heat shock protein. J Immunol 143: 2844–2849

Nossal GJV (1983) Cellular mechanisms of immunologic tolerance. Annu Rev Immunol 1: 33–62

Rajagopalan S, Zordan T, Tsokos GC, Datta SK (1990) Pathogenic anti-DNA autoantibody-inducing T helper cell lines from patients with active lupus nephritis: isolation of $CD4^{-}8^{-}$ T helper cell lines that express the γ/δ T cell antigen receptor. Proc Natl Acad Sci USA 87: 7020–7024

Res P, Thole J, de Vries R (1991) Heat-shock proteins and autoimmunity in humans. Springer Semin Immunopathol 13: 81–98

Rötzschke O, Falk K (1991) Naturally occurring peptide antigens derived from the MHC class-I-restricted processing pathway. Immunol Today 12: 447–455

Selmaj K, Brosnan CF, Raine CS (1991) Colocalization of lymphocytes bearing γ/δ T-cell receptor and heat shock protein $hsp65^{+}$ oligodendrocytes in multiple sclerosis. Proc Natl Acad Sci USA 88: 6452–6456

Steinhoff U, Schoel B, Kaufmann SHE (1990) Lysis of interferon-γ activated Schwann cells by crossreactive CD8 α/β T cells with specificity to the mycobacterial 65 kDa heat shock protein. International Immunol 2: 279–284

Thole JER, Kevlen WJ, Kolk AHJ, Groothuis DG, Berwald LC, Tiesjema RH, van Embden JDA (1987) Characterization, sequence determination, and immunogenicity of a 64-kilodalton protein of *Mycobacterium bovis* BCG expressed in *Escherichia coli* K-12. Infect Immun 50: 800–806

Van Eden W, Thole JE, van der Zee R, Noordzij A, van Embden JD, Hensen EJ, Cohen IR (1988) Cloning of the mycobacterial epitope recognized by T lymphocytes in adjuvant arthritis. Nature 331: 171–173

Young RA (1990) Stress proteins and immunology. Annu Rev Immunol 8: 401–420

Cytochrome P450 Enzymes as Autoantigens in Autoimmune Hepatitis

M. P. Manns

Introduction

Autoantibodies against several subcellular components of liver tissue are associated with inflammatory liver diseases [1]. While antimitochondrial antibodies are associated with primary biliary cirrhosis (PBC), antinuclear antibodies, liver-kidney-microsomal (LKM) antibodies, and antibodies against soluble liver antigen characterize three different subgroups of idiopathic autoimmune chronic active hepatitis (CAH) (Table 1) [2]. The etiology of these serologically distinct subgroups of CAH is unknown. A loss of tolerance against liver tissue is regarded as the main pathogenetic mechanism. In contrast to virus-induced liver diseases, these autoimmune variants of CAH respond well to immunosuppressive treatment. Furthermore, these disease associated autoantibodies may give further insights into pathogenesis and may provide clues to their etiology. In recent years the identification and characterization of hepatocellular autoantigens has made significant progress related to the development of new techniques, including molecular cloning.

Three members of the cytochrome P450 family of proteins have been identified as human autoantigens. They are specifically recognized by LKM antibodies detectable in sera from patients with either drug-induced or idiopathic autoimmune hepatitis. Cytochrome P450 proteins belong to a family of mono-oxygenases which metabolize drugs, hormones, and carcinogens. In this chapter the present knowledge on cytochrome P450s as human autoantigens, their corresponding autoantibodies, and the clinical relevance of these findings are reviewed.

Cytochrome P450 IID6 (LKM-1 Antigen)

LKM-1 autoantibodies characterize autoimmune hepatitis type II (Table 1) [2, 3] and do not occur in PBC [4]. LKM-1 antibodies react with cytochrome P450 IID6 (previously termed DB1; Table 2). This has been shown after screening a human liver cDNA expression library with human autoantibodies [5] and by biochemical studies demonstrating that these sera specifically inhibit P450-IID6-mediated drug metabolism in isolated human liver microsomes [6]. P450 IID6 is known to metabolize more than 25 commonly used

Table 1. Heterogeneity of hepatitis B surface antigen negative chronic hepatitis

	ANA	LKM-1	SLA	SMA	AMA	Anti-HCV	Anti-GOR	Therapy
Chronic hepatitis C	–	–	–	–	–	+	+	Interferon
Autoimmune hepatitis								
Type 1	+	–	–	+	–	–	–	Immunosuppression
Type 2 a	–	+	–	–	–	–	–	Immunosuppression
Type 2 b	–	+	–	–	–	+	+	?
Type 3	–	–	+	+/–	+/–	–	–	Immunosuppression
Type 4	–	–	–	+	–	–	–	Immunosuppression
Primary billiary cirrhosis	–	–	–	–	+	–	–	UDCA, etc.

ANA, Antinuclear antibodies; *LKM-1,* liver-kidney-microsomal antibodies against cytochrome P450 IID6; *SLA,* antibodies against soluble liver antigens; *SMA,* smooth muscle antibodies; *AMA,* antimitochondrial antibodies; *HCV,* hepatitis C virus; *UDCA,* ursodesoxycholic acid.

drugs, among them β-blockers, antiarrhythmic drugs, and tricyclic antidepressants. Due to a genetic polymorphism, 5%–10% of whites do not express P450 IID6 protein in their livers; these individuals are poor metabolizers [7]. Patients with LKM-1 antibody-positive CAH express functionally intact protein in their livers, i.e., they are extensive metabolizers, although LKM-1 autoantibodies inhibit the function of this P450 enzyme in vitro [8]. This means that these autoantibodies do not sufficiently penetrate the intact liver cell membrane to inhibit the function of these enzymes located in the smooth endoplasmic reticulum. Recently, P450 IID6 was shown to be expressed on the surface of human hepatocytes [9]. Furthermore, we localized the immunodominant epitope to a linear sequence of P450 IID6. The smallest segment recognized by LKM-1 autoantibodies encodes for eight amino acids; six of these eight amino acids share complete sequence homology with the immediate early protein (IE 175) of herpes simplex virus type I [10]. At present, the relevance of this molecular mimicry is under investigation. Of 189 liver tissue-derived T cell clones from four patients with LKM-1 antibody-positive CAH, five specifically responded to human recombinant cytochrome P450 IID6 [11].

Sera from 90% of patients with LKM antibodies as determined by fluorescence react with recombinant cytochrome P450 IID6 (LKM-1 antigen) in western blots [12]. Clinically, patients with LKM-1 antibody-positive CAH have a young age at onset, female predominance, low IgA levels, frequent association with extrahepatic autoimmune syndromes, and a good response to immunosuppressive therapy.

Cytochrome P450 IIC9 (LKM-2 Antigen)

Autoantibodies reacting with a different microsomal antigen were identified by immunofluorescence and termed LKM-2 [13]. They react with cytochrome P450 IIC9, responsible for the metabolism of ticrynafen and mephenytoin (Table 2) [14, 15]. LKM-2 antibodies have been described only in France. Their occurrence is linked to hepatitis caused by the diuretic drug tienilic acid (ticrynafen). This drug is distributed only in France and the United States. LKM-2 antibodies, as LKM-1 antibodies, inhibit the function of their P450 enzyme in vitro. Cytochrome P450 IIC9 is also genetically polymorphic.

Table 2. Microsomal autoantigens in liver diseases

Mol.wt. (kD χ)	Nomenclature	Biochemical definition	Disease association
50	LKM-1	P450 IID6	Autoimmune CAH
50	LKM-2	P450 IIC9	Drug-induced hepatitis (tienilic acid)
?	LKM-3	?	Chronic hepatitis D
50	LM	P450 IA2	Autoimmune CAH, dihydralazine hepatitis
55	–	?	Autoimmune CAH
64	–	?	Autoimmune CAH

Cytochrome P450 IA2

Of the sera from patients with idiopathic autoimmune type CAH that react with a 50-kDa microsomal protein 10% do not recognize recombinant P450 IID6 (LKM-1 antigen) [12]. One of these rare microsomal autoantigens has been identified as cytochrome P450 IA2 [16]. P450 IA2 is a dioxin-inducible protein responsible for the metabolism of phenacetin in man [17]. It is liver specific. Autoantibodies against this protein are also inhibitory, as shown by their inhibition of ethoxyresorufin oxidation in human liver microsomes [16]. These antibodies were found in an 8-year-old boy suffering from CAH, alopecia, nail dystrophy and vitiligo [18]. The disease responded well to immunosuppressive treatment, leading to normalization of liver enzymes and liver histology 1 year after start of treatment. Independently, a French group of investigators described anti-P450 IA2 antibodies in dihydralazine-induced hepatitis [19].

Discussion

The identification of different members of the cytochrome P450 family of proteins as human autoantigens has various implications for hepatology, pharmacology and autoimmunity. Molecular cloning of these P450s provides us with recombinant autoantigens that can be used as specific and sensitive diagnostic reagents improving the diagnosis of autoimmune hepatitis. This may help to better separate individuals that profit from immunosuppressive drug therapy from those who profit from interferons, which are nowadays given in virus-induced liver diseases [20, 21].

Interestingly, all microsomal proteins identified as human autoantigens in inflammatory liver diseases are drug-metabolizing enzymes (Table 2). Their corresponding autoantibodies inhibit enzyme function in vitro, and the autoepitopes are highly conserved regions of the molecules. Furthermore, these immunologically distinct proteins are closely located together in the endoplasmatic reticulum. While different mitochrondrial enzymes (i.e., subunits of pyruvate dehydrogenase complex) are recognized by autoantibodies in PBC [22, 23], nuclear enzymes involved in messenger RNA processing have been indentified as autoantigens in systemic rheumatological disorders [24]. Almost all of these autoantibodies seem to be inhibitory. The precise identification of autoepitopes may further elucidate the topology of these enzymes. Further studies will have to evaluate the T cell response against these P450 autoantigens. This may help to clarify the role of these antigens in the pathogenesis of autoimmune liver diseases. In this context, it is of particular interest that the P450 enzymes identified as human autoantigens (P450, IID6, IIC9, and 1A2) are genetically polymorphic. The prevalence of LKM antibody-positive liver disease is low, comparable to other autoimmune disorders. The rarity of these autoimmune diseases may be related to a genetic background based on both a genetic polymorphism of the major histocompatibility complex and the target antigen itself.

The relationship between autoimmunity to cytochrome P450 proteins and possible etiological agents of autoimmune liver diseases has become of particular interest. While the relationship between LKM-2 antibodies and cytochrome P450 IIC9 has become a model for an immune-mediated drug-induced liver disease [14] P450 IA2 seems to be a target for drug induced (dihydralazine) and idiopathic autoimmune hepatitis [16, 19]. LKM-3 antibodies in chronic hepatitis D may also recognize a P450 protein. However, the antigen must still be identified at its molecular level. A very interesting relationship exists between hepatitis C virus (HCV) and LKM-1 antibody associated liver disease. Although anti-HCV antibodies were detected frequently by first-generation tests in all kinds of autoimmune diseases, specificity for anti-HCV was confirmed by second-generation enzyme-linked immunosorbent assays and HCV-RNA polymerase chain reaction only for a proportion of patients with LKM-1 antibody-associated autoimmune hepatitis type II. The association between HCV infection and LKM-1 antibody-associated liver disease is less than 10 % in the United Kingdom, more than 80 % in Italy [25], 40 % in the Federal Republik of Germany [26], and 48 % in France [27]. Our patients with HCV-associated autoimmune hepatitis type II are positive for HCV antibodies and anti-GOR. Anti-GOR is a HCV-specific autoantibody [28]. These anti-HCV-positive patients are older, have a less female predominance, lower disease activity, and respond less favorably to corticosteroids. HCV seems to induce autoimmunity to GOR regulary while HCV-infected patients very rarely may develop autoimmunity to cytochrome P450 proteins. Interestingly, the anti-HCV-negative population of autoimmune hepatitis type II is clinically different from anti-HCV-positive patients. This is particularly evident concerning the response to corticosteroids. Herpes simplex virus type I is a candidate for triggering anti-HCV-negative autoimmune hepatitis type II since the immunodominant B cell epitope of P450 IID6 exhibits sequence homology with the IE 175 protein of herpes simplex virus 1 [10]. Patients with anti-HCV-negative but not anti-HCV-positive autoimmune hepatitis type II exhibit an immunogenetic background compatible with an autoimmune disorder, i.e., increase in HLA antigens B8 and DR3 and null alleles of complement factor C4A, which is regarded as an HLA class III antigen (Manns et al., unpublished data).

References

1. Manns M (1989) Autoantibodies and antigens in liver diseases – updated. J Hepatol 9: 272–280
2. Manns M, Gerken G, Kyriatsoulis A et al. (1987) Characterization of a new subgroup of autoimmune chronic active hepatitis by autoantibodies against a soluble liver antigen. Lancet I: 292–294
3. Homberg JC, Abuaf N, Bernard O et al. (1987) Chronic active hepatitis associated with anti-liver/kidney microsome autoantibody type I: a second type of "autoimmune hepatitis". Hepatology 1: 1333–1339
4. Manns M, Meyer zum Büschenfelde K-H, Slusarczyk J, Dienes H-P (1984) Detection of liver-kidney microsomal autoantibodies by radioimmunoassay and their relation to anti-mitochondrial antibodies in inflammatory liver diseases. Clin Exp Immunol 57: 600–608
5. Manns M, Johnson EF, Griffin KJ et al. (1989) The major target antigen of liver and kidney microsomal autoantibodies in idiopathic autoimmune hepatitis is cytochrome P450 db1. J Clin Invest 83: 1066–1072
6. Zanger UM, Hauri HP, Loeper J et al. (1988) Antibodies against human cytochrome P450 db 1 in autoimmune hepatitis type II. Proc Natl Acad Sci USA 27: 8256–8260
7. Gonzales FJ, Skoda RC, Kimura S et al. (1988) Characterization of the common genetic defect in humans deficient in debrisoquine metabolism. Nature 331: 442

8. Manns M, Zanger U, Gerken G et al. (1990) Patients with type II autoimmune hepatitis express functionally inact cytochrome P450 db1 that is inhibited by LKM-1 autoantibodies in vitro but not in vivo. Hepatology 12: 127–132
9. Loeper J, Descatorie V, Maurice M et al. (1990) Presence of cytochrome P450 on human hepatocyte plasma membrane. Recognition by several autoantibodies. Hepatology 12: 909
10. Manns M, Griffin KJ, Sullivan KF et al. (1990) Molecular mimicry between intermediated early protein (IE1 75) of herpes simplex virus type I in cytochrome P450 db1 (IID6), a major autoantigen in autoimmune hepatitis. Hepatology 12: 907
11. Löhr H, Manns M, Trautwein C et al. (1991) Clonal analysis of liver infiltrating T cells in patients with chronic active hepatitis (AI-CAH). Clin Exp Immunol 84: 297–302
12. Manns M, Johnson EF, Griffin KJ et al. (1989) Human recombinant LKM (P450 db1) antigen as diagnostic reagent for autoimmune hepatitis. Hepatology 10: 637
13. Homberg J-C, André C, Abuaf N (1984) A new anti-liver-kidney microsome antibody (anti-LKM-2) in tienilic acid-induced hepatitis. Clin Exp Immunol 55: 561–570
14. Beaune PH, Dansette PM, Mansuy D et al. (1987) Human anti-endoplasmic reticulum autoantibodies appearing in a drug induced hepatitis directed against a human liver cytochrome P450 that hydroxylates the drug. Proc Natl Acad Sci USA 84: 551–555
15. Meier UT, Meyer UA (1987) Genetic polymorphism of human cytochrome P450 (S)-mephenytoin 4-hydrolase. Studies with human autoantibodies suggest a functionally altered cytochrome P450 isoenzyme as course of the genetic deficiency. Biochemistry 26: 8466–8474
16. Manns MP, Griffin KJ, Quattrochi LC et al. (1990) Identification of cytochrome P450 IA2 as a human autoantigen. Arch Biochem Biophys 280: 229–232
17. Quattrochi LC, Pendurthi UR, Okino ST et al. (1986) Human cytochrome P450 4 mRNA and gene: part of a multigene family that contains Alu sequences in its mRNA. Proc Natl Acad Sci USA 83: 6731–6735
18. Sacher M, Blümel P, Thaler H, Manns M (1990) Chronic active hepatitis associated with vitiligo, nail dystrophy, alopecia and a new variant of LKM antibodies. J Hepatol 10: 364–369
19. Bourdi M, Larrey D, Nataf J et al. (1990) Anti-liver endoplasmic reticulum autoantibodies are directed against human cytochrome P450 IA2. J Clin Invest 85: 1967–1973
20. Vento S, di Perri G, Luzzati R et al. (1990) Type 2 autoimmune hepatitis and hepatitis C virus infection. Lancet 335: 921–922
21. Ruiz-Moreno M, Rua JA, Carreno V et al. (1991) Autoimmune chronic active hepatitis type 2 manifested during interferon therapy in children. J Hepatol 12: 265–266
22. Mackay IR, Gershwin ME (1989) Molecular basis of mitochondrial autoreactivity in primary bilary cirrhosis. Immunol Today 10: 315–318
23. Fussey SPM, Guest JR, James OFW et al. (1988) Identification and analysis of the major M2 autoantigens in primary biliary cirrhosis. Proc Natl Acad Sci USA 85: 8654
24. Tan EM, Feltkamp TEW, Alarcon-Segovia D et al. (1988) Reference reagents for antinuclear antibodies. Arthritis Rheum 31: 1331
25. Lenzi M, Johnson PJ, McFarlane IG et al. (1991) Antibodies to hepatitis C virus in autoimmune liver disease: evidence for geographical heterogenity. Lancet 338: 1370–1378
26. Manns M, Michel G, Ritter A et al. (1991) Anti-GOR reflects hepatitis C virus (HCV) specific autoimmunity. J Hepatol 13 [Suppl 2]: 49
27. Lunel F, Maisoneuvre P, Marcellin P et al. (1991) Relationship between anti-HCV antibodies measured by a quantitative riba assay and response to interferon in patients with chronic non A non B hepatitis. J Hepatol 13 [Suppl 2]: 47
28. Michel G, Ritter A, Gerken G et al. (1992) Anti GOR and hepatitis C virus in autoimmune liver disease. Lancet 339: 267–269

Myelin-Specific Autoimmune T Cells in the Pathogenesis of Multiple Sclerosis: Their Characteristics and Possible Approaches to Immunospecific Therapy

H. Wekerle

Introduction

Multiple sclerosis (MS) is one of the numerous human inflammatory diseases with suspected, though not formally confirmed autoimmune pathogenesis. It is clear that MS is not caused by humoral autoantibodies, which definitely have a central effector function in diseases such as myasthenia gravis and pemphigoid. It appears rather that the immunopathological changes typically seen in the myelinated parts of the central nervous system (CNS) are caused by cellular rather than by humoral autoimmune mechanisms. There are diverse lines of evidence suggesting that autoaggressive T cells cause MS by attacking the body's own myelinated tissues. These include the association of disease susceptibility with certain haplotypes of the major histocompatibility complex (MHC), in particular with its class II genes. Second, the histological changes in the MS lesion are highly suggestive of a T cell mediated inflammatory reaction (see below). These changes share essential features with experimental autoimmune encephalomyelitis (EAE), a myelin-specific autoimmune disease inducible in animals by immunization against myelin components.

This chapter summarizes the current information on myelin-specific T cells in the human immune system. In particular, possibilities of novel, T cell specific immunotherapies of MS and other putatively autoimmune diseases are examined.

Myelin Basic Protein Specific, Autoaggressive T Cells in Experimental Autoimmune Encephalomyelitis

EAE is an inducible, myelin-specific autoimmune disease which is commonly considered as a valid model for the initial stages of the autoimmune pathogenesis of MS (Lassmann 1983; Raine 1984; Wekerle et al. 1986). EAE lesions are characterized by several pathological changes. These include (a) mononuclear infiltrates, concentrated mainly around postcapillary microvessels of the CNS white matter; the cells contained within these infiltrates are predominantly lymphocytes (mainly CD4 but also some CD8 T cells and a few B cells); (b) disturbance of the endothelial blood-brain barrier, with marked edema formation and fibrin deposits; and (c) activation of local glia. Many astrocytes are activated, showing gliotic changes such as enhanced expression of cytoskeletal glial fibrillary acidic protein. In addition, there are numerous activated microglia cells, which express MHC class I and class II antigens and hence closely resemble infiltrating blood-derived macrophages.

It should be stressed, however, that demyelination, i.e., large-scale destruction of myelin and oligodendrocytes, is rarely seen in the most common EAE variants. Primary demyelination is neither prominent in EAE actively induced in Lewis rats by immunization with myelin basic protein (MBP) nor in EAE transferred with MBP-specific T cell lines (Lassmann 1983). However, large-scale demyelination can be seen produced in these systems by cotransferring of humoral antibodies directed to myelin surface molecules (Linington et al. 1988).

Paterson (1960) was the discoverer of encephalitogenic T cells. He was the first to note that EAE can be transferred to naive host animals by lymphocytes but not by autoantibodies reacting against MBP. Formal confirmation for the pathogenic role of MBP-specific autoimmune T cells was provided by Ben-Nun et al. (1981), who succeeded in isolating MBP-monospecific clonable T cells lines from MBP primed Lewis rats and showed that these cells are able to transfer lethal EAE to completely normal, syngeneic recipient rats. The first encephalitogenic T cell line, Z1a, has been kept in permanant culture for more than 12 years, and at least some sublines still exhibit unchanged antigen specificity and autoaggressive potential. More recently, Schluesener and Wekerle (1985) showed that encephalitogenic MBP-specific T cell lines can be isolated not only from in vivo primed but even from unprimed, completely naive Lewis rats. MBP-specific T cell lines from unprimed rats shared their major characteristics with T cell lines isolated from immunized donor animals (Fig. 1).

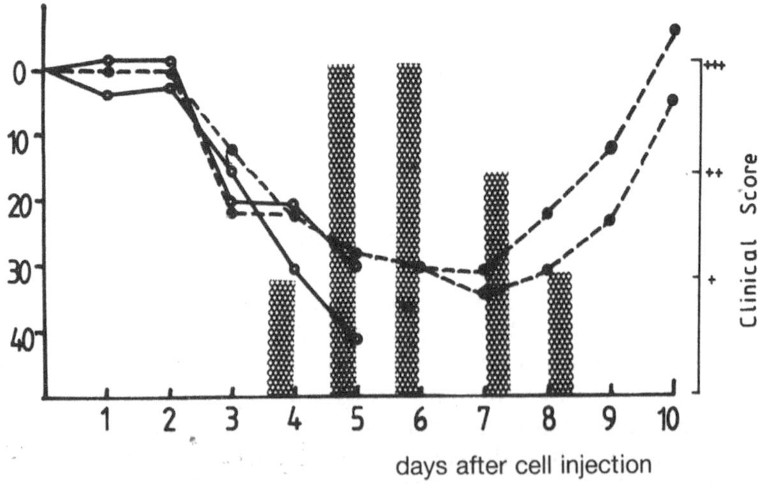

Fig. 1. Encephalitogenic activity of MBP-specific T cells in the Lewis rat. Time course of weight loss *(curves)* versus clinical signs *(bars)* in recipient rats receiving 3×10^6 *(open circles)* and 2×10^6 *(full circles)*. (From Sun et al. 1988)

These findings have important implications. It should be noted that the encephalitogenic T cell lines were isolated from peripheral immune organs. They were established by activating and propagating immunologically mature T cells. Since mature, immunocompetent T cells keep their antigen receptors unaltered by somatic mutation (Davis and Bjorkman 1988), one may conclude that T cells with autoimmune response potential are continuously present within the rat donors' immune systems. These findings clearly refute traditional theories of self tolerance which were based exclusively on the deletion of self-reactive lymphocytes from the immune repertoire.

Encephalitogenic T cells isolated from rodents exhibit some highly unusual functional characteristics. All encephalitogenic T cells described so far are members of the $CD4^+$ subset (Pettinelli and McFarlin 1981; Ben-Nun and Cohen 1982; Holda and Swanborg 1982) and consequently recognize "their" autoantigenic epitope in the molecular context of MHC class II molecules (Ben-Nun et al. 1983; Fontana et al. 1984). The encephalitogenic T cell response both in the Lewis rat (Hashim 1977; Kibler et al. 1977; Holoshitz et al. 1983) and in the PL/J mouse (Zamvil et al. 1987) is strictly focused on discrete, individual peptide segments of the MBP molecule, namely sequence 68–88 in the Lewis rat, and 1–11 in the PL/J mouse (Fritz and McFarlin 1989). Equally unexpected is the highly restricted repertoire of T cell receptor variable genes used by encephalitogenic T cells. In the PL/J mouse (Acha-Orbea et al. 1988; Urban et al. 1988) and, curiously, also in the Lewis rat (Burns et al. 1989; Chluba et al. 1989), almost all encephalitogenic T cells use the Vβ8.2 gene, often in combination with Vα2. Finally, it is of note that encephalitogenic T cells, while expressing the CD4 "helper" phenotype, are very efficient killer cells (Sun and Wekerle 1986; Fallis and McFarlin 1989). The association between the cytotoxic and autoaggressive potential of myelin-specific T cell lines is extremely close. All encephalitogenic T cells described so far are effective killer cells in culture (Wekerle et al. 1989). Although not formally confirmed, this suggests that cytotoxic mechanisms similar to those demonstrable in vitro are also involved in mediating tissue damage.

Myelin Basic Protein Specific T Cells in Multiple Sclerosis

Experimental research into cellular autoimmunity is considerably complicated by several factors. First, the human MHC is more complex than its rodent counterparts; second, humans are as a rule outbred and heterozygous. To accumulate valid data on the recognition properties of human myelin-specific, autoimmune T cells, a technique is required that allows the establishment of *multiple* T cell lines (or clones) from *all* MS patients (and if any possible healthy donors as well).

A culture system fulfilling these conditions has recently been developed by Pette et al. (1990 a). This selection method ("split-well culture") is based on the primary culture of peripheral blood T lymphocytes distributed into multiple wells of microtiter plates at low cell numbers. Upon confrontation with MBP (or other myelin autoantigens) some of these microcultures start to be activated and to enter cell division. In a second step the proliferating cultures are transferred to two adjacent wells of another plate. One of the twin wells is cultured with and the other one without MBP. Only those wells are selected for further expansion which specifically respond to MBP. This method, which is now used by many laboratories interested in MS and other autoimmune disorders, is extremely efficient. It allows, as required, to derive abundant numbers of T cell lines not only from any MS patient but also from healthy volunteers. Furthermore, due to the low T cell numbers seeded initially, many although not all of the lines derived by this method are truly monoclonal, as documented by retrospective analysis of the T cell receptor genes used (Fig. 2).

Detailed analyses of large numbers of human MBP-specific T cells carried out by several groups have yielded convergent results. It now appears that the human anti-MBP T cell response significantly differs from the reaction seen in rodents. In contrast to rodent anti-MPB T cells, there is not a particular MBP epitope dominating the human T cell response, either in the general population or in humans with particular MHC haplotypes. Although certain MBP sequences (positions 80–105 and 139–153) may be more antigenic than others, any other segment of the molecule may qualify as a human T cell epitope (Martin et al. 1990; Ota et al. 1990; Pette et al. 1990 b). A striking diversity of MBP epitopes recognized by human T cells is by no means limited to polymorphic populations but is demonstrable in individual human donors as well (Richert et al. 1989 a; Ota et al. 1990; Pette et al. 1990 a).

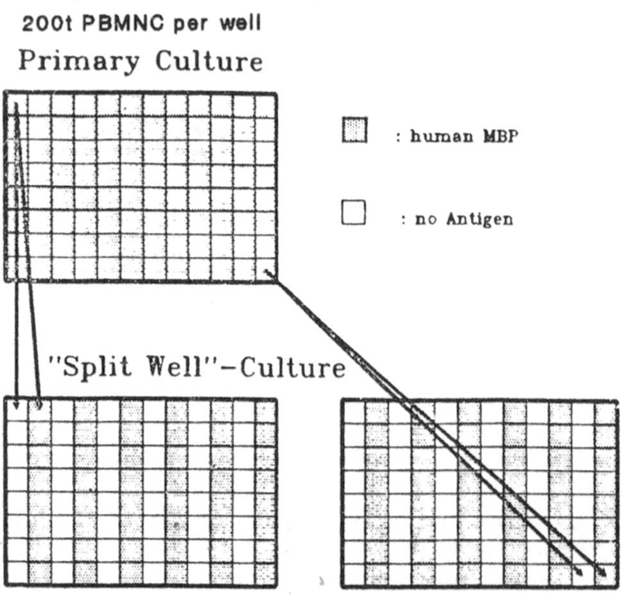

Fig. 2. Primary selection of MBP-specific T cell lines from human peripheral blood ("Split well" culture system)

General identification of human T cell epitopes on MBP has been carried out using series of overlapping synthetic peptides spanning the entire length of the MBP molecule as antigen and autologous peripheral blood monocytes as antigen-presenting cells (APC). The administration of APC transfected with individual MHC class II products established additionally that any individual class II molecule is able to present several distinct MBP epitopes to appropriate T cells. The DR2a molecule has been investigated most thoroughly, both since it is a product of an MHC haplotype associated with increased MS risk in white populations (Compston 1986), and because of the availability of transfectant APC (Wilkinson et al. 1988). Studies using DR2 gene transfected L cells showed first that the majority of the majority of MBP-specific T cells from DR2-positive donors are restricted by the DR2a (DRA/DRB5*0101) while a significant minority recognize its epitope in the context of DR2b (DRA/DRB5*1501; Pette et al. 1990 b; Jaraquemada et al. 1990). Second, these studies made it clear that each of the two nonallelic class II molecules are able to present a minimum of five (DR2a) or two (DR2b) different MBP peptide sequences (Pette et al. 1990 b). Conversely, individual MBP peptides may be presented to T cells by a variety of MHC class II molecules from distinct haplotypes (Martin et al. 1991).

MBP-specific T cell lines can be isolated from normal donors almost as easily as from MS patients (Burns et al. 1983; Tournier-Lasserve et al. 1988; Chou et al. 1989, 1991; Martin et al. 1990; Ota et al. 1990; Pette et al. 1990 b). Although some groups initially noted some skewed epitope recognition profiles in MS versus normal donor derived T cell panels (Ota et al. 1990; Chou et al. 1989), at present no significant MS-specific T cell repertoire has been identified (Fig. 3).

There is no direct evidence that the MBP-specific T cells isolated from MS patients are indeed involved in the donor's pathogenesis, and one may even question more the pathogenic potential of the T cells derived from normal donors. It should be noted, however, that studies in rat EAE argue strongly in favor of the autoaggressive capacity of the human autoreactive T cells. Schluesener and Wekerle (1985) isolated MBP-specific T cell lines from completely normal, not preimmunized Lewis rats. These T cells were lethally encephalitogenic, as shown in transfer experiments. This was the first demonstration of potentially autoaggressive T cell clones in a healthy mammalian immune system; the extrapolation to the human T cell repertoire seems especially legitimate as rat and human MBP-specific T cells share important common functional properties. In the Lewis rat all encephalitogenic T cells are cytotoxic to MBP-presenting APC (Sun and Wekerle 1986; Wekerle et al. 1989). At least some of the human MBP-specific T cells are cytotoxic as well (Weber and Buurman 1988; Richert et al. 1989 b; Martin et al. 1990) and thus in principle qualify as pathogenic effectors.

Taken together the accumulated data presently indicate that, in contrast to the encephalitogenic T cell response in the Lewis rat and the PL/J mouse, human MBP-specific T cells recognize a very broad spectrum of MBP peptide epitopes. MBP-specific T cells are present both in the immune system of MS

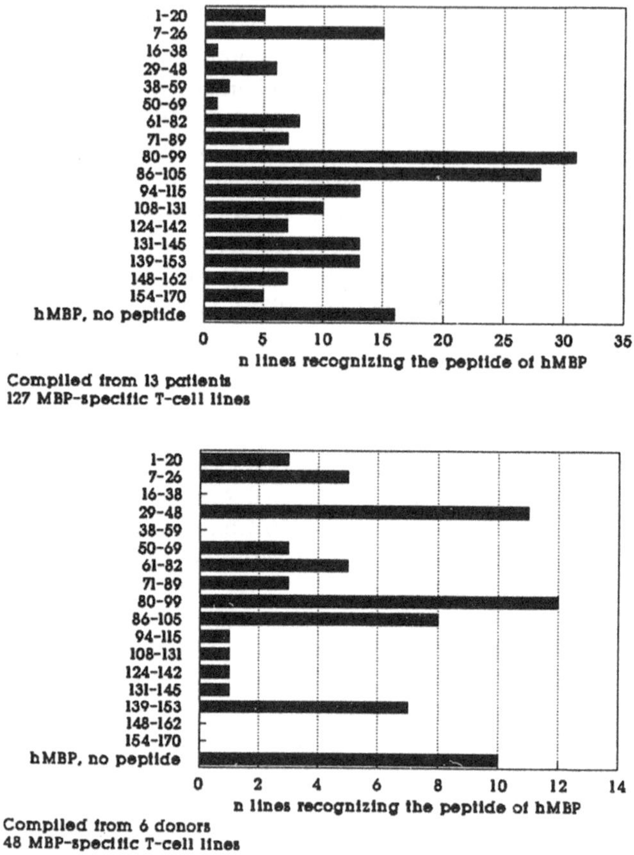

Fig. 3. MBP epitope recognition by T cell lines from MS patients and healthy donors. *Ordinate,* synthetic MBP peptides (amino acid positions) used for epitope typing; *abscissa,* number of T cells responding to individual peptides

patients and in healthy individuals. Furthermore, no MS specific epitope has been identified.

A comparably complex situation emerges with regard to the use of T cell receptor (TcR) genes in human MBP specific T cells. Early reports showing restricted gene use in MS patients have been cautioned by more recent studies. Oksenberg et al. (1990) amplified the TcR-specific message from RNA derived from MS rain material and found the use of limited Vα gene repertoires. More recent studies have demonstrated that limited TcRV gene expression may possibly be seen in long-standing, "burnt-out" plaques but not in fully developed active infiltrates (Wucherpfennig et al. 1992).

Examination of the TcR genes used by MBP-specific T cell lines has provided an equally complex picture. Some preliminary studies seemed to indicate a limited TcRV gene use (Wucherpfennig et al. 1990; Chou et al. 1991). More recently most groups have found evidence for a multiplicity of V genes to be used even by very similar T cell clones (Martin et al. 1991; Richert et al. 1991; Wucherpfennig et al. 1991; Giegerich et al. 1992). This has been confirmed in a large series of primarily cloned T cell lines using Vβ-specific monoclonal antibodies and cytofluorometry (Meinl et al. 1991).

T cell lines recognizing similar MBP epitopes in identical MHC class II context exhibit diverse TcRV gene usage (Giegerich et al. 1992; Martin et al. 1992), and T cell clones expressing the same Vβ genes may recognize disparate MBP epitopes (Kotzin et al. 1991; Meinl et al. 1991), Finally, as is the case with MBP peptide epitopes, there is no significant difference between TcR of T cell clones from normal or MS donors (Meinl et al. 1991; Giegerich et al. 1992).

Idiotypic Therapy?

The limited repertoire of TcRV genes used by encephalitogenic T cells from the Lewis rat and the PL/J mouse, in context with the inducibility of counterregulatory T cells by vaccination regimens, led two groups to manipulate Lewis rat EAE by immunization with synthetic peptides representing TcR sequences commonly used by MBP-specific T cells (Howell et al. 1989; Vandenbark et al. 1989). The results reported were extremely encouraging. They suggested that vaccination with synthetic peptides indeed protects inbred rat from later induction of myelin-directed autoimmune disease by activate immunization or by passive transfer. The mechanisms underlying EAE protection were not fully clarified. Both induction of TcR specific antibodies (Offner et al. 1991) and downregulatory "anti-idiotypic" T cells (Vandenbark et al. 1989) were discussed as possible regulatory circuits.

We examined the possible adaptability of TcR peptide vaccination in a human in vitro model. As paradigm we selected the T cell clone HW.BP3, isolated from a healthy donor, which recognizes MBP sequence 139–153 in the context of the DR2a molecule (Pette et al. 1990b) and the TcR genes which had been cloned and sequenced (Giegerich et al. 1992). Following the strategy successfully applied in the Lewis rat, we selected potential T cell epitope sequences from the TcR β chain of clone HW.BP3 and synthesized peptides located on the Vβ and the VDJ junctional regions. In a second step T cell lines were selected from the donor's peripheral blood lymphocytes responding to either TcR (HW.BP3) peptide. Indeed, a panel of "anti-idiotypic," peptide-specific T cell lines were isolated. They all expressed the $CD4^+$ $CD8^-$ membrane phenotype and recognized their target peptides in context of DR molecules. All the T line selected were efficiently cytotoxic against any APC presenting the peptides in proper MHC class II context. Confrontation of the TcR (HW.BP3) specific T cell lines with the MBP-reactive target cell line HW.BP3 led to ambiguous results. First, HW.BP3 cells, which upon activation expressed ample amounts of DR molecules, efficiently presented exogenous peptide antigen to the complementary autologous T cell lines. This was assessed by induction of proliferation, by cytotoxic assays, and by determination of interleukin-2 release. No activation of the TcR-specific T cell lines, however, was seen in the *absence* of exogenous peptides. In other words, the MBP-specific T cell clone HW.BP3 was unable to process and present in recognizable form its *endogenous* TcR proteins to the TcR peptide specific T cells.

The data so far represent the first formal confirmation of the existence of TcR-specific T cells within the same immune system. They fail, however, to demonstrate positive or negative mutual regulation between both populations in vitro. However, this does by no means exclude the possible presence of such interactions in vivo. It should be noted that there are examples of T cells ignoring autoantigens in vitro although reactions in vivo have been demonstrated by the same cells in EAE (Mannie et al. 1985) and in experimental autoimmune uveoretinitis (Kotake et al. 1990; Fling et al. 1991).

Conclusion

Work originally intended to elucidate T cell mechanisms in MS has led to radically new concepts in at least two areas of immunology. First, it has become clear that the CNS is by no means absolutely secluded from the mechanisms of immune surveillance. It became clear that activated but not resting T cells have the capacity to pass through the endothelial blood-brain barrier and thus may reach CNS parenchymal cells, some of which can be induced to express MHC antigens.

Second, analyses of myelin-specific T cells provided the first evidence for the existence of potentially autoaggressive T cell clones in the *healthy* immune repertoire. Myelin-specific T cells are readily demonstrable in the immune system of healthy humans as well as in rats. In the rat it has been shown that these T cells may mediate lethal EAE, provided they have been activated before transfer. One may thus conclude that myelin-specific autoimmune disease is caused by accidental activation of potentially autoimmune T cells preformed in the immune system. Alternatively, protection from autoimmunity may be guaranteed by downregulatory mechanisms keeping the autoimmune T cell clones in an nonpathogenic, resting state.

At least in the rat new therapeutic strategies have been reported which specifically suppress myelin specific T cell clones in vivo. Direct adaptation of these approaches to treat human disease is, however, still complicated by several factors. First, clinical immunology deals with outbred, heterozygous populations. Identification of MHC products directly involved in pathogenic T cell responses will be a prerequisite for specific immunotherapies. Second, although MBP may well have a role in the autoimmune pathogenesis of *some* MS patients, it is not probable that this myelin protein is responsible for *all* pathogenic T cell responses. Other myelin determinants or even CNS autoantigens unrelated to myelin may have roles, which must be specified in each individual patient. Third, in deplorable contrast to the Lewis rat, the human T cell response to myelin autoantigens is extremely complex. So far no one TcR variable gene has been identified which is associated with an MS-related autoimmune response.

Notwithstanding these problems, the fact that T cells specific for TcR sequences from autologous MBP-specific T cells have been isolated from the human immune system provides hope that T cell directed immunotherapy may not remain a fantasy.

Acknowledgements. I am grateful to the many colleagues in Würzburg and Munich who provided the experimental basis for this synopsis.

References

Acha-Orbea H, Mitchell DJ, Timmermann L, Wraith DC, Tausch GS, Waldor MK, Zamvil SS, McDevitt HO, Steinmann L (1988) Limited heterogeneity of T cell receptors from T lymphocytes mediating autoimmune encephalomyelitis allows specific immune intervention. Cell 54: 263–273

Ben-Nun A, Cohen IR (1982) Experimental autoimmune encephalomyelitis (EAE) mediated by T cell lines: process of selection of lines and characterization of the cells. J Immunol 129: 303–308

Ben-Nun A, Wekerle H, Cohen IR (1981) The rapid isolation of clonable antigen-specific T lymphocytes capable of mediating autoimmune encephalomyelitis. Eur J Immunol 11: 195–199

Ben-Nun A, Lando Z, Dorf ME, Burakoff SJ (1983) Analysis of cross-reactive antigen-specific T cell clones. Specific recognition of two major histocompatibility complex (MHC) and two non-MHC antigens by a single clone. J Exp Med 147: 2147–2153

Burns J, Rosenzweig A, Zweiman B, Lisak RP (1983) Isolation of myelin basic protein-reactive T cell lines from normal human blood. Cell Immunol 81: 435–440

Burns FR, Li X, Shen H, Offner H, Chou YK, Vandenbark AA, Heber-Katz E (1989) Both rat and mouse T cell receptors specific for the encephalitogenic determinant of myelin basic protein use similar Vα and Vβ chain genes even though the major histocompatibility complex and encephalitogenic determinants being recognized are different. J Exp Med 169: 27–40

Chluba J, Steeg C, Becker A, Wekerle H, Epplen JT (1989) T cell receptor β chain usage in myelin basic protein-specific rat T lymphocytes. Eur J Immunol 19: 279–284

Chou YK, Vainiene M, Whitham RH, Bourdette DN, Chou C-HJ, Hashim G, Offner H, Vandenbark AA (1989) Response of human T lymphocyte lines to myelin basic protein: association of dominant epitopes with HLA class II restriction molecules. J Neurosci Res 23: 207–216

Chou YK, Henderikx P, Vainiene M, Whitham R, Bourdette D, Chou CH-J, Hashim G, Offner H, Vandenbark AA (1991) Specificity of human T clones reactive to immunodominant epitopes of myelin basic protein. J Neurosci Res 28: 280–290

Compston DAS (1986) Genetic factors in the etiology of multiple sclerosis. In: McDonald WI, Silberberg DH (eds) Multiple sclerosis. Butterworths, London, pp 56–73

Davis MM, Bjorkman PJ (1988) T-cell antigen receptor genes and T-cell recognition. Nature 334: 395–402

Fallis RJ, McFarlin DE (1989) Chronic relapsing experimental allergic encephalomyelitis: cytotoxicity effected by a class II-restricted T cell line specific for an encephalitogenic epitope. J Immunol 143: 2160–2165

Fling SP, Donoso LA, Gregerson DS (1991). In vitro unresponsiveness to autologous sequences of the immunopathogenic autoantigen, S-antigen. J Immunol 147: 483–489
Fontana A, Fierz W, Wekerle H (1984) Astrocytes present myelin basic protein to encephalitogenic T cell lines. Nature 307: 273–275
Fritz RB, McFarlin DE (1989) Encephalitogenic epitopes of myelin basic protein. In: Sercarz E (ed) Antigenic determinants and immune regulation. Karger, Basel, pp 101–125
Giegerich G, Pette M, Meinl E, Epplen JT, Wekerle H, Hinkkanen A (1992). Diversity of T cell receptor α and β chain genes expressed by human T cells specific for similar myelin basic protein peptide/major histocompatibility complexes. Eur J Immunol 22: 753–758
Hashim GA (1977) Experimental allergic encephalomyelitis in Lewis rats: chemical synthesis of disease-inducing determinant. Science 196: 1219–1221
Holda JH, Swanborg RH (1982) Autoimmune effector cells. II. Transfer of experimental allergic encephalomyelitis with a subset of T lymphocytes. Eur J Immunol 12: 453–455
Holoshitz J, Frenkel A, Ben-Nun A, Cohen IR (1983) Autoimmune encephalomyelitis (EAE) mediated or prevented by T lymphocyte lines directed against diverse antigenic determinants of myelin basic protein. Vaccination is determinant specific. J Immunol 131: 2810–2813
Howell MD, Winters ST, Olee T, Powell HC, Carlo DJ, Brostoff SW (1989). Vaccination against experimental allergic encephalomyelitis with T cell receptor peptides. Science 246: 668–671
Jaraquemada D, Martin R, Rosen-Bronson S, Flerlage M, McFarland HF, Long EO (1990) HLA-DR2a is the dominant restriction molecule for the cytotoxic T cell response to myelin basic protein in DR2Dw2 individuals. J Immunol 145: 2880–2885
Kibler RF, Fritz RB, Chou FC-H, Chou C-HJ, Peacocke NY, Brown NM, McFarlin DE (1977) Immune response of Lewis rats to peptide C1 (residues 68–88) of guinea pig and rat myelin basic proteins. J Exp Med 146: 1323–1331
Kotake S, Wiggert B, Zhang X-Y, Redmond TM, Chader GJ, Gery I (1990) Stimulation in vitro of lymphocytes for induction of uveoretinitis without any significant proliferation. J Immunol 145: 534–539
Kotzin BL, Karuturi S, Chou YK, Lafferty J, Forrester JM, Better M, Nedwin GE, Offner H, Vandenbark AA (1991) Preferential T-cell receptor β-chain variable gene use in myelin basic protein-reactive T-cell clones from patients with multiple sclerosis. Proc Natl Acad Sci USA 88: 9161–9165
Lassmann H (1983) Comparative neuropathology of chronic experimental allergic encephalomyelitis and multiple sclerosis. Springer, Berlin Heidelberg New York
Linington C, Bradl M, Lassmann H, Brunner C, Vass K (1988) Augmentation of demyelination in rat acute allergic encephalomyelitis by circulating mouse monoclonal antibodies directed against a myelin/oligodendrocyte glycoprotein. Am J Pathol 130: 443–454
Mannie MD, Paterson PY, U'Pritchard DC, Flouret G (1985) Induction of experimental allergic encephalomyelitis (EAE) in the Lewis rat with purified synthetic peptides: delineation of antigen determinants for encephalitogenicity, in vitro activation of cellular transfer, and proliferation of lymphocytes. Proc Natl Acad Sci USA 82: 5515–5519
Martin R, Jaraquemada D, Flerlage M, Richert JR, Whitaker J, Long EO, McFarlin DE, McFarland HF (1990) Fine specificity and HLA restriction of myelin basic protein-specific cytotoxic T cell lines from multiple sclerosis patients and healthy individuals. J Immunol 145: 540–548
Martin R, Howell MD, Jaraquemada D, Flerlage M, Richert J, Brostoff S, Long EO, McFarlin DE, McFarland HF (1991) A myelin basic protein peptide is recognized by cytotoxic T cells in the context of four HLA-DR types associated with multiple sclerosis. J Exp Med 173: 19–24
Martin R, Utz U, Coligan JE, Richert JR, Flerlage M, Robinson E, Stone R, Biddison WE, McFarlin DE, McFarland HF (1992) Diversity in fine specificity and T cell receptor usage

of the human $CD4^+$ cytotoxic T cell response specific for the immunodominant myelin basic protein peptide 87–106. J Immunol 148: 1359–1366

Meinl E, Saruhan G, Weber F, Schönbeck S, Goebels N, Bröhm M, Hohlfeld R, Wekerle H (1991) Multiple sclerosis: heterogeneity of T cell-receptors used by human T lymphocytes specific for myelin basic protein. Neurology 43 [Suppl 1]: 257 (abstract)

Offner H, Hashim GA, Vandenbark AA (1991) T cell receptor peptide therapy triggers autoregulation of experimental encephalomyelitis. Science 251: 430–432

Oksenberg JR, Stuart S, Begovich AB, Bell RB, Erlich HA, Steinman L, Bernard CCA (1990) Limited heterogeneity of rearranged T-cell receptor Vα transcripts in brains of multiple sclerosis patients. Nature 345: 344–346

Ota K, Matsui M, Milford EL, Mackin GA, Weiner HL, Hafler DA (1990) T-cell recognition of an immunodominant myelin basic protein epitope in multiple sclerosis. Nature 346: 183–187

Paterson PY (1960) Transfer of allergic encephalomyelitis in rats by means of lymph node cells. J Exp Med 111: 119–135

Pette M, Fujita K, Kitze B, Whitaker JN, Albert E, Kappos L, Wekerle H (1990 a) Myelin basic protein-specific T lymphocyte lines from MS patients and healthy individuals. Neurology 40: 1770–1776

Pette M, Fujita K, Wilkinson D, Altmann DM, Trowsdale J, Giegerich G, Hinkkanen A, Epplen JT, Kappos L, Wekerle H (1990 b) Myelin autoreactivity in multiple sclerosis: recognition of myelin basic protein in the context of HLA-DR2 products by T lymphocytes of multiple sclerosis patients and healthy donors. Proc Natl Acad Sci USA 87: 7968–7972

Pettinelli CB, McFarlin DE (1981) Adoptive transfer of experimental allergic encephalomyelitis in SJL/J mice after in vitro activation of lymph node cells with myelin basic protein: requirement for Lyt-1+2- T lymphocytes. J Immunol 127: 1420–1423

Raine CS (1984) Analysis of autoimmune demyelination: its impact upon multiple sclerosis. Lab Invest 50: 608–635

Richert JR, Robinson ED, Deibler GE, Martenson RE, Dragovic LJ, Kies MW (1989 a) Evidence for multiple human T cell recognition sites on myelin basic protein. J Neuroimmunol 23: 55–66

Richert JR, Robinson ED, Deibler GE, Martenson RE, Dragovic LJ, Kies MW (1989 b) Human cytotoxic T-cell recognition of a synthetic peptide of myelin basic protein. Ann Neurol 26: 342–346

Richert JR, Robinson ED, Johnson AH, Bergman CA, Dragovic LJ, Reinsmoen NL, Hurley CK (1991) Heterogeneity of the T cell receptor β gene rearrangements generated in myelin basic protein-specific T cell clones isolated from a patient with multiple sclerosis. Ann Neurol 29: 299–306

Schluesener HJ, Wekerle H (1985) Autoaggressive T lymphocyte lines recognizing the encephalitogenic region of myelin basic protein: in vitro selection from unprimed rat T lymphocyte populations. J Immunol 135: 3128–3133

Sun D, Wekerle H (1986) Ia-restricted encephalitogenic T lymphocytes mediating EAE lyse autoantigen-presenting astrocytes. Nature 320: 70–72

Tournier-Lasserve E, Hashim G, Bach MA (1988) Human T-cell response to myelin basic protein in multiple sclerosis patients and healthy subjects. J Neurosci Res 19: 149–156

Urban JL, Kumar V, Kono DH, Gomez C, Horvath SJ, Clayton J, Ando DG, Sercarz EE, Hood L (1988) Restricted use of T cell receptor V genes in murine autoimmune encephalomyelitis raises possibilities for antibody therapy. Cell 54: 577–592

Vandenbark AA, Hashim G, Offner H (1989) Immunization with a synthetic T-cell receptor V-region peptide protects against experimental autoimmune encephalomyelitis. Nature 341: 541–544

Weber WEJ, Buurman WA (1988) In vitro functional blocking of myelin basic protein-specific cytolytic human T lymphocyte clones by immunosuppressive drugs and monoclonal antibodies. J Neuroimmunol 22: 1–10

Wekerle H, Linington C, Lassmann H, Meyermann R (1986) Cellular immune reactivity within the CNS. Trends Neurosci 9: 271–277

Wekerle H, Pette M, Fujita K, Nomura K, Meyermann R (1989) Autoimmunity in the nervous system: functional properties of an encephalitogenic protein. Prog Immunol 7: 813–820

Wilkinson D, De Vries RRP, Madrigal JA, Lock CB, Morgenstern JP, Trowsdale J, Altmann DM (1988) Analysis of HLA-DR glycoproteins by DNA-mediated gene transfer. Definition of DR2β gene products and antigen presentation to T cell clones from leprosy patients. J Exp Med 167: 1442–1458

Wucherpfennig KW, Ota K, Endo N, Seidman JG, Rosenzweig A, Weiner HL, Hafler DA (1990) Shared human T cell receptor Vβ usage to immunodominant regions of myelin basic protein. Science 248: 1016–1019

Wucherpfennig KW, Weiner HL, Hafler DA (1991) T-cell recognition of myelin basic protein. Immunol Today 12: 277–282

Wucherpfennig KW, Newcombe J, Li H, Keddy C, Cuzner ML, Hafler DA (1992) T cell receptor Vα-Vβ repertoire and cytokine gene expression in active multiple sclerosis lesions. J Exp Med 175: 993–1002

Zamvil SS, Mitchell DJ, Moore AC, Schwarz AJ, Stiefel W, Nelson PA, Rothbard JB, Steinman L (1987) T cell reactivity for class II (I-A) and the encephalitogenic N-terminal epitope of the autoantigen myelin basic protein. J Immunol 139: 1075–1079

Adverse Immune Reactions to Drugs (Gold, Procainamide) and Environmental Chemicals (Mercury, Platinum): The Role of Phagocytic Cells in Generating Immunogenic Metabolites

M. Kubicka-Muranyi, C. Goebel, P. Griem, H.-C. Schuppe, J. Uetrecht, and *E. Gleichmann*

Introduction

Adverse Immune Reactions to Chemicals of Low Molecular Weight

Adverse immune reactions to drugs, sometimes termed drug hypersensitivity reactions, account for a considerable proportion of all adverse drug reactions [32]. These reactions pose a difficult problem for the development of new drugs because they are not detected in standard toxicology assays. Consequently, many drugs have had to be removed from the market shortly after they were introduced because of what was considered to be an unacceptable risk of adverse immune reactions [4, 42]. The term adverse immune reaction to drugs is used when the following criteria are fulfilled:

a) a certain percentage, usually a small one, of the persons treated with the drug develop a reaction;
b) the reaction does not resemble the pharmacologic actions of the drug;
c) reactions occur only after an induction period of at least 4–7 days after primary exposure to the drug but ensue promptly after reexposure;
d) reactions occur with very small doses of the drug; and
e) signs and symptoms consist of those characteristic of immunopathologic reactions, including both allergic and autoimmune reactions.

Although the term adverse immune reaction implies involvement of the immune system, for many drugs this has not been formally demonstrated. Compared with drugs, however, even less is known about the occurrence of adverse immune reactions to environmental chemicals. As far as pathogenesis is concerned, it is a reasonable hypothesis that the same principles apply to both types of chemical exposure.

In the present paper we review experimental work from our laboratories concerning the pathogenesis of adverse immune reactions to low molecular weight chemicals and their metabolites. The compounds to be discussed in detail are *gold salts* and *procainamide (PA)*, both of which are drugs, and *salts of mercury* and *platinum*, both of which occur at the workplace and in the environment.

M. M. Eibl, C. Huber, H. H. Decker, U. Wahn (Eds.)
Symposium in Immunology I
Symposium in Immunology II

Concept for the Pathogenesis of Adverse Immune Reactions to Chemicals

The clinical characteristics of adverse immune reactions to drugs can vary considerably among different drugs and also for the same drug in different individuals. In many cases reactions are confined to specific organs, such as the skin, liver, or bone marrow. However, *systemic reactions* are also frequent in which there is fever, skin rash, and lymphadenopathy along with involvement of internal organs. The adverse immune reactions to gold (Table 1) and PA are examples of such generalized immunopathological effects. The clinical picture of generalized adverse immune reactions to drugs is strikingly similar to that of a systemic graft-versus-host (GVH) reaction, and it has been proposed that GVH-like mechanisms underly the pathogenesis of many adverse immune reactions to drugs [24, 25, 31]. In the GVH reaction the pivotal reactions are by grafted T lymphocytes that react to incompatible tissue antigens of the host. Depending on the donor T cell subset(s) predominating in the reaction and the cytokines produced by them, the more distal effector mechanisms and the immunopathologic picture of the GVH reaction can vary considerably [25, 31]. The concept of GVH-like reactions to drugs or chemicals postulates that the etiologic agent involved, i.e., the drug or chemical, alters either MHC (major histocompatibility complex) molecules or MHC-embedded self peptides. In either case autologous T cells would react to the MHC-peptide complex in a GVH-like fashion.

Although the hypothesis of GVH-like T cell reactions to drugs was proposed more than 15 years ago [24], the experiments designed to support this concept have been progressing slowly. This is due mainly to the difficulty in measuring T cell reactions to drugs in vitro. Presumably, two intrinsic

Table 1. Adverse immunological side effects of *gold (I)* drugs, such as Na_2AuTM, and their genetical association

	Man	Mouse
Dermatitis	+	
Stomatitis	+	
Alveolitis	+	
Eosinophilia	+	
Spleen and lymph node enlargement		+
IC glomerulonephritis	+	+
IgG ↑, IgE ↑	+	+
ANA	+	+
Thrombopenia	+	
Granulocytopenia	+	
IgG ↓, IgA ↓	+	
Aplastic anemia	+	
MHC	+	+
Slow sulfoxidation status	+	

properties of drugs are responsible for this. Firstly, it is now clear that T cells only recognize short peptides, including self peptides, presented to them by MHC molecules [10]. Most drugs, however, are nonproteins and in all likelihood cannot themselves be directly embedded into the MHC groove. To sensitize T cells, nonprotein compounds must somehow alter the physiologic cleavage of self peptides and/or their mode of presentation by MHC molecules. Hence, the use of terms such as T cell reactions to drug X or metabolite Y are actually incorrect, although for the sake of brevity we use them in this paper. Secondly, most drugs, including most of those known to cause adverse immune reactions, are designed not to undergo direct protein binding. Before being capable of altering the presentation of self peptides in one way or another, most drugs of low molecular weight must probably be metabolized into reactive intermediates.

The Popliteal Lymph Node Assay in Rodents: A Test System for Detecting T Cell Sensitization to Chemicals and Their Metabolites

Two experimental systems in rodents have proven particularly useful in elucidating T cell reactions to chemicals respectively their metabolites in vivo. The first is the *direct popliteal lymph node assay (PLNA)*, which was introduced into immunotoxicology by H. Gleichmann [29, 30] to demonstrate primary immune reactions to diphenylhydantoin. The second, the *adoptive transfer PLNA*, is an extension of the former; it was developed by H. Gleichmann and coworkers for measuring secondary T cell reactions to the diabetogen streptozotocin [45] and is described in detail in the context of experiments performed with gold (see below). In the report of an International Workshop on Immunotoxicology [3], both the direct PLNA and the adoptive transfer PLNA were recommended as predictive test systems for detecting the sensitizing potential of drugs and chemicals during the preclinical and premarketing phase of toxicity testing.

By now the *direct PLNA* has been used by several groups of investigators [26, 43, 44, 76, 85]. In this assay the test compound is injected subcutaneously without adjuvant into one hind foot pad of a mouse or rat. A primary immune response, if present, is detected 1 week later by an increase in either weight, cell number, cell proliferation, or a change in cell composition of the draining PLN when compared to the values obtained from the contralateral PLN (for review see [26]). Secondary immune responses can be detected after the primary PLN reaction reverted to normal. A small dose of the test compound is then injected into the same foot pad, and the secondary PLN reaction is measured 1 week later [38, 75, 76]. Alternatively, secondary immune responses can be detected by the adoptive transfer PLNA [see "Biooxidation of Gold (I) to Gold (III)"]. A problem with the direct PLNA is, however, that it gives *false-negative* reactions to gold, hydralazin, and PA, all of which are notorious for frequently causing adverse immune reactions in humans [23, 43,

44, 75]. To overcome this problem the testing of *metabolites* in both the direct PLNA and the adoptive transfer PLNA can be employed (see "Immune Reactions to Gold Salts Induced in Experimental Animals").

The Potential of Phagocytic Cells to Generate Immunogenic Drug Metabolites

Usually the generation of reactive drug metabolites is discussed in the context of liver mono-oxygenases. However, it is doubtful whether *liver* enzymes play the major role in generating the reactive intermediate metabolites assumed to cause systemic adverse immune reactions of the *generalized type*, i.e., outside of the liver. Probably, many intermediates are far too reactive and have too short a biological half-life to escape the organ in which they are produced. Therefore, one of us [89, 92] has proposed that in the case of extrahepatic immune reactions to drugs the reactive intermediate metabolites suspected of eliciting the adverse immune reactions are generated extrahepatically. As ubiquitous cells which might generate reactive intermediate metabolites attention has focused on neutrophils, monocytes, and macrophages [88, 89]. These cells not only phagocytose foreign matter but are also equipped with various oxidizing enzymes that physiologically serve to kill infectious agents but may as well oxidize chemicals. For instance, during the respiratory burst of activated neutrophils and monocytes the enzyme myeloperoxidase (MPO) converts hydrogen peroxide (H_2O_2) and chloride ion (Cl^-) to *hypochlorous acid (HOCl,* or *bleach)*, a powerful oxidant. In vitro, HOCl has proven capable of generating reactive intermediates from a great variety of different drugs and chemicals [89]. The generation by activated leukocytes of reactive intermediates has been formally demonstrated for several drugs, including PA [89, 91]. Monocytes and macrophages also act as antigen-presenting cells in that they cleave proteins, including self proteins, into short peptides and via their MHC molecules present them to T cells along with accessory signals [47, 72, 87]. In the present paper, we review recent data obtained with gold and PA that are first to show *T cell reactions* to reactive intermediate metabolites generated by phagocytic cells or, more exactly, to undefined self proteins/peptides presumably altered by metabolites.

Adverse Immune Reactions to Gold Drugs

Observations in Humans Treated with Gold

All antirheumatic gold drugs, such as gold (I) disodium thiomalate [GST, $Na_2Au(I)TM$], contain gold in the gold (I) oxidation state. The mechanism of action of gold drugs is unknown, but they are effective in the treatment of rheumatoid arthritis. With respect to both their therapeutic and their adverse effects gold drugs have been termed slow acting because there is a lag period of several weeks to months before they become effective [11, 48]. Eventually adverse immune reactions necessitate discontinuation of gold therapy in up to one-third of patients [9, 33, 49]. As reviewed elsewhere [75], the types of immunopathologic alteration developing under gold therapy resemble those seen during the GVH reaction; these are summarized in Table 1. The pathogenic mechanisms, however, that trigger these reactions are poorly understood.

Immune Reactions to Gold Salts Induced in Experimental Animals

At least some of the immunopathologic side effects seen in man also develop in susceptible mouse strains treated with weekly intramuscular injections of GST (Table 1). Equimolar injections of the carrier disodium thiomalate (ST, Na_2TM), by contrast fail to induce any of these abnormalities [64, 67, 75]. As in humans, genes linked to the MHC as well as non-MHC genes are involved in the immunologic susceptibility of mice to GST [67]. Strain-dependent susceptibility to treatment with a gold (I) drug has also been demonstrated in rats. Brown Norway rats developed an increased IgE level, proteinuria, and autoantibodies to the glomerular basement membrane, whereas Lewis rats failed to do so [86].

Both the GVH-like picture of the immunopathologic reactions to gold (I) drugs and their association with the MHC suggest that *T cells* play a central role in their pathogenesis [25]. When this hypothesis was tested in susceptible mouse strains [75], a perplexing result was obtained. The gold (I) drug GST, although a potent inducer of adverse immune reactions upon weekly intramuscular injections, failed to elicit T cell reactions in the direct PLNA. By contrast, equimolar amounts of gold (III) salts readily induced a T cell dependent PLN reaction.

Biooxidation of Gold (I) to Gold (III)

To explain this discrepancy the hypothesis has been proposed that in vivo the gold (I) of GST, a slow-acting drug, is gradually oxidized to gold (III), and that it is the latter which elicits T cell sensitization and thus initiates the GVH-like side effects. This was experimentally tested by Schuhmann et al. [75] using the adoptive transfer PLNA. The results of this experiment demonstrated that, indeed, weekly intramuscular injections of gold (I), given in the form of GST, sensitized T cells neither to gold (I) nor to ST but to gold (III) even though the latter had never been administered to the T cell donors.

In the *adoptive transfer PLNA* [26, 45, 46, 75] the test compound, such as GST, is first administered to donor animals according to a schedule that is relevant to human use of this compound. (In humans, GST is given by repeated intramuscular injections.) Subsequently, T cells of the donor animals are injected subcutaneously into one hind foot pad of a syngeneic recipient animal. The recipient serves merely as an indicator of reactivity of the transferred T cells because, in addition to the donor T cells, the test compound or one of its metabolites is injected into the same foot pad. As in the direct PLNA, lymph node weight, cell number, or cell proliferation is measured 6 days later. By means of this assay system it can be asked whether T cells of the donor animals have been sensitized to the test compound or a metabolite. If in their new environment the donor T cells reencounter the antigen to which they have been sensitized, they mount a secondary immune response. The latter manifests itself by quantitative and qualitative changes of lymphoid cells in the draining PLN of the recipient. The dose of test antigen used in the adoptive transfer PLNA is always below the minimal dose required for inducing a primary PLN response. Thus, a primary PLN response of the recipient animal is avoided, but anamnestic responses of the donor T cells transferred can be detected.

On the basis of their findings Schuhmann et al. [75] concluded that the adverse immune effects of gold (I) salts are in fact caused by gold (III) which must be generated in vivo through oxidation of gold (I). In both animals and humans, gold is known to be accumulated and stored in the lysosomes of monocytes and macrophages [7, 22, 41]. Here, gold (I) might be oxidized to gold (III) by reactive oxygen species, such as HOCl (Fig. 1). In fact, in a cell-free system in vitro, which contained the HOCl-generating factors H_2O_2, Cl^-, and MPO, gold (III) was generated from GST [5]. Furthermore, gold (III), other than gold (I) [40], can irreversibly oxidize proteins [78, 97] and thus may be considered a reactive intermediate metabolite. Altered self protein(s), in turn, if presented by MHC molecules on the surface of macrophages, could elicit GVH-like reactions by T cells. In the presence of protein, gold (III) exists only for a few minutes [39, 78] because immediately after its generation gold (III) oxidizes proteins and is thus itself reduced again.

In the study of Schuhmann et al. [75] sensitized T cells were used as a probe to detect alterations induced by gold (III), a short-lived reactive intermediate metabolite that in biological samples is not or is only with difficulty detectable by physicochemical methods. Because T cells are known not to react to free metal ions, such as gold (III), but react to MHC-embedded peptides [72], the observed T cell reactions cannot have been directed to gold (III) itself, but to self protein(s)/peptide(s) altered by this highly reactive heavy metal ion. In other words, the observed T cell reactions presumably were not directed to the metabolite but to its footprints left on self protein(s)/peptide(s) or on MHC molecules themselves.

More recently the group at Düsseldorf was able to provide further experimental evidence for the concept (Fig. 1) that biooxidation of gold (I) to gold (III) takes place in phagocytic cells, such as monocytes and macrophages. T cells of mice were primed to gold (III) either by weekly intramuscular injections of gold (I) in the form of GST, or by three

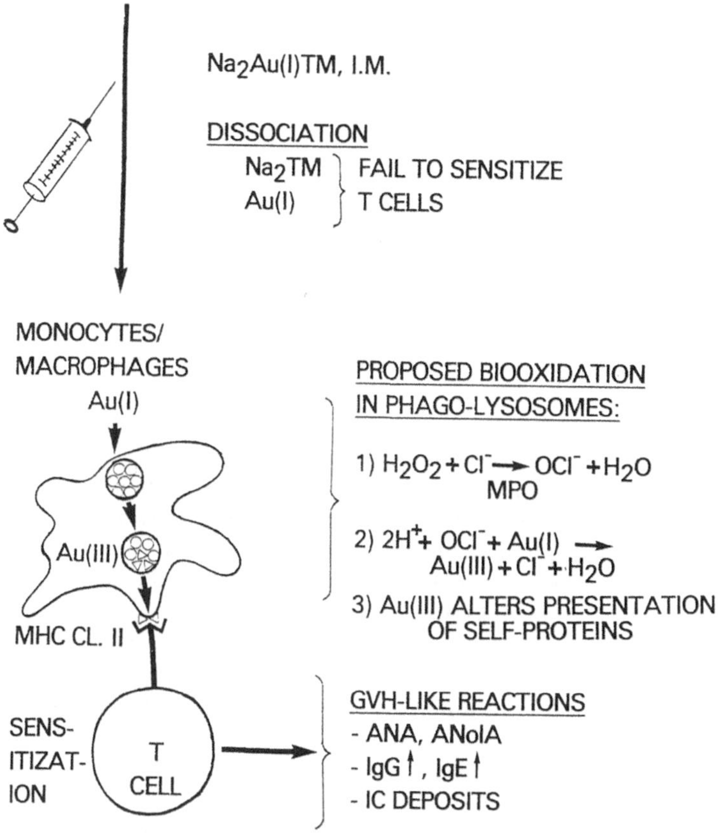

Fig. 1. Concept of adverse immune reactions to gold (I) drugs. Oxidation of gold (I) could take place either inside the phago-lysosomes (as shown in the figure) or outside on the cell surface after myeloperoxidase (*MPO*) has been secreted by activated monocytes or neutrophils. In the latter case, direct oxidation of cell surface proteins, such as MHC molecules, could take place as a consequence of generation of gold (III)

subcutaneous injections of $HAu(III)Cl_4$. Then, using the adoptive transfer PLNA the transferred T cells of these animals were found to react in an anamnestic fashion not only to gold (III) salt but also to homogenized macrophages pretreated with GST, i.e., gold (I). The macrophages used were either cells of a syngeneic macrophage cell line that had been incubated with GST in vitro or peritoneal cells obtained from donors that had received weekly intramuscular injections of GST for 12 weeks (C. Goebel and M. Kubicka-Muranyi, unpublished results).

In *humans* who had been treated with gold (I) drugs for rheumatoid arthritis and had subsequently developed dermatitis, anamnestic T cell responses to gold (III) were also observed ([27, 69, 94] and T. Tonn, unpublished results). Verwilghen et al. [94] found that when peripheral blood lymphocytes of 17 patients with acute gold dermatitis were tested in the lymphocyte transformation test in vitro, the cells of 13 of them reacted to gold (III) but not to GST or other heavy metal salts.

While the results of Verwilghen et al. [94] clearly reflect the differential immunogenicity of gold (I) and gold (III) salts and thus confirm in humans the findings obtained in mice [75], the picture is not quite as clearcut in all investigations. In a few patients a positive reaction to both gold (III) and gold (I) was observed (T. Tonn, unpublished results). Here, it can be argued that the putative reaction to gold (I) was in fact directed towards gold (III) that was generated by monocytes through oxidation of gold (I) during the 1-week culture period. This explanation, however, can only be applied with difficulty to the findings of Romagnoli et al. [69]. They found that two T cell clones obtained from the same patient reacted to both gold (I) and gold (III) even when the antigen-presenting cells (Epstein-Barr virus transformed autologous B cells) were glutaraldehyde fixed. It is generally agreed that glutaraldehyde fixation inactivates enzyme activities in cells [10, 79]; if true, this would also pertain to the enzymes involved in the oxidation of gold (I) to gold (III). A possible explanation for the inability of the two T cell clones to distinguish between gold (I) and gold (III) could be that the gold (I) salt induces a conformational change of MHC class II molecules [80]. Conceivably, the two T cell clones studied by Romagnoli et al. [69] were specific for class II molecules thus changed. Because gold (III) is rapidly reduced to gold (I) by protein, it may have caused identical reactions as gold (I) in this particular case.

Possible Pharmacological Implications of the Biooxidation of Gold (I) to Gold (III)

Generation of the highly reactive intermediate gold (III) could also be relevant with respect to the unknown pharmacological mechanism of action of gold (I) drugs. Three anti-inflammatory mechanisms of gold (III) may be envisaged (Fig. 2). Firstly, the generation in phagocytic cells of gold (III) from gold (I) scavenges reactive oxygen species. Secondly, as already mentioned, gold (III) is a highly reactive chemical that irreversibly cross-links and thus denatures proteins [97]. The candidate proteins to be denatured by gold (III) are those nearest to the site of oxidation of gold (I) to gold (III). Presumably these are the proteins located in the phago-lysosomes of phagocytic cells [27, 28], such as lysosomal enzymes, which are known to enhance inflammation when released from cells. Thirdly, gold (III) may interfere with those lysosomal enzymes involved in antigen-processing or may directly alter MHC molecules. Both mechanisms could result in reduced production or presentation of arthritogenic (self) peptides. These anti-inflammatory effects of gold should be enhanced and prolonged by the fact that gold (III) is very short-lived in the presence of protein because, when oxidizing proteins, gold (III) is rereduced to gold (I) [39, 78]. In fact, as

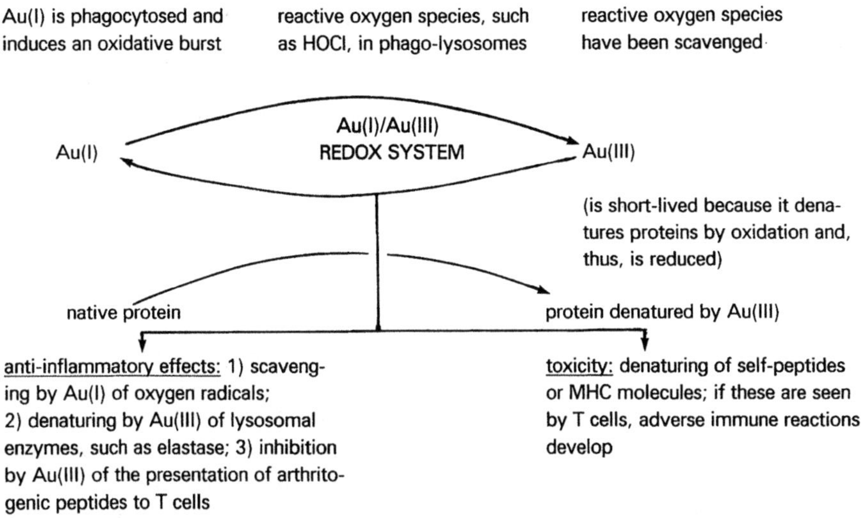

Fig. 2. Proposed mechanism of action of gold (I) drugs in phagocytic cells

pointed out by C. F. Shaw III (personal communication, 1991), on the basis of the findings of Schuhmann et al. [75] gold therapy may introduce a gold (I)/gold (III) *redox system* into phagocytic cells. If this view is correct, the three anti-inflammatory actions of gold (I)/gold (III) described above would be effective over a prolonged period of time.

The arguments for phagocytic cells as potential sites for the generation of reactive drug metabolites [89] are summarized above. Regarding the actual immunogenicity of drug metabolites thus generated, the findings with gold (I)/gold (III) described above were the first to give experimental support to this important concept. Gold (III), however, is a somewhat unusual intermediate whose generation in the body has been demonstrated only in the indirect fashion outlined above. In contrast, the production by phagocytes of reactive metabolites of PA [73, 88, 89] is generally accepted. Therefore, we recently started to perform similar experiments with PA and its reactive metabolites using the same experimental approach as with gold (I)/gold (III). These experiments are described below ("Murine T Cell Reactions to Reactive Intermediate Metabolite of Procainamide").

Adverse Immune Reactions to Procainamide

Observations in Humans Treated with Procainamide

During therapy with the antiarrhythmic drug PA, a common adverse side effect is a generalized autoimmune disease resembling systemic lupus erythematosus (SLE). The incidence of antinuclear autoantibodies (ANA) associated with long-term use of PA is close to 90%, and that of clinically manifest lupus approaches 30% [73, 89]. The clinical signs and symptoms of PA-induced SLE, given in the order of decreasing prevalence, include the following: arthralgia, lung involvement, fever, weight loss and fatigue, myalgia, splenomegaly, arthritis, and pericarditis [73].

Metabolism of Procainamide

The structure of PA and its metabolites are shown in Figure 3. PA is an arylamine, a class of compound that is notorious for eliciting adverse immune reactions leading to allergy and/or autoimmunity. Arylamines can be metabolized by two different pathways, both of which involve alteration of the amino (arylamine) group [73, 89]. The predominant metabolic pathway consists of acetylation of the amino group via *N*-acetyltransferase. Acetyltransferase activity is found mainly in the liver, and in both humans and mice its level is genetically controlled [73, 84, 98]. Rapid acetylation is an autosomal dominant trait giving rise to the fast acetylator phenotype. Slow acetylators are homozygous for a recessive gene controlling hepatic acetyltransferase activity and have approximately twofold higher blood levels of the unacetylated drug at equivalent therapeutic doses.

The second metabolic pathway of PA, which consists of *N*-hydroxylation of the arylamine group, is utilized preferentially by slow acetylators. It is assumed that the products of this pathway, hydroxylamine-PA (HAPA), nitroso-PA, and perhaps *N*-chloro-PA (Fig. 3), are responsible for PA-induced SLE [73, 89]. This view is based on three different lines of indirect evidence. Firstly, ANA appear more quickly in slow acetylators, and the slow acetylator phenotype predominates in symptomatic patients during the first 6 months of the therapy [73]. Secondly, the reactive metabolites formed by activated neutrophils or monocytes [90] as well as the synthetic *N*-chloro-PA [91] did bind covalently to cells and soluble protein, whereas PA and *N*-acetyl-PA showed only weak or insignificant covalent binding to hepatic protein [20] or nonactivated leukocytes [90]. Thirdly, *N*-acetyl-PA used as a drug is not associated with lupus even in patients who have had PA-induced SLE [73, 89]. In short, there is suggestive evidence that *N*-acetylation of the arylamine group prevents autoimmunization, whereas *N*-hydroxylation favors it. In view of the concept that immunogenic drug metabolites may be generated by extrahepatic phagocytic cells (see "The Potential of Phagocytic Cells to Generate Immunogenic Drug Metabolites"), important findings were that in vitro the reactive intermediate metabolites of PA could be generated by incubating PA either directly with the MPO/H_2O_2/Cl^- system or with activated leukocytes [90–92].

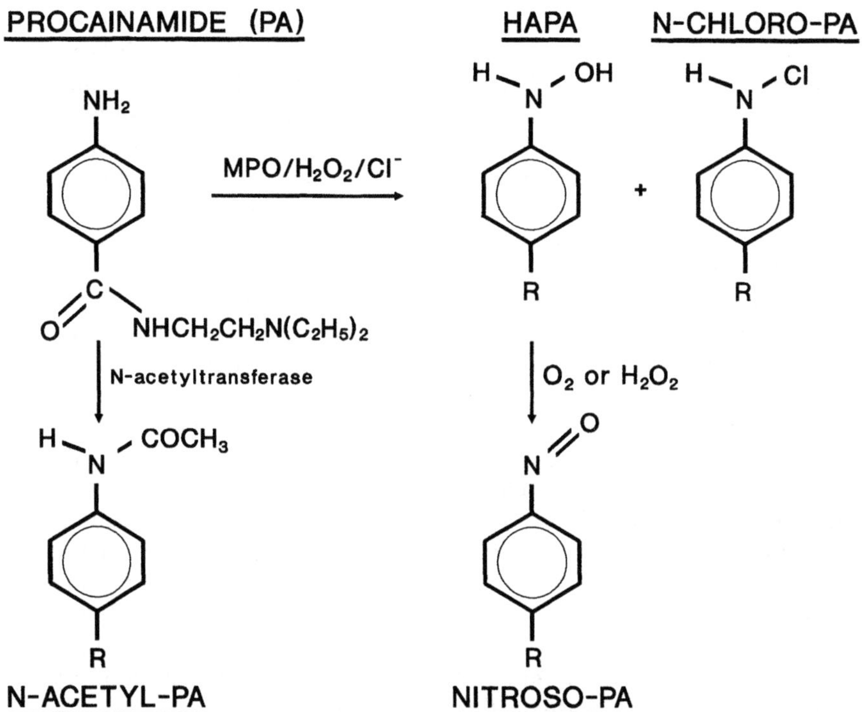

Fig. 3. Pathways of detoxication and bioactivation of procainamide (PA). The *N*-acetyl-PA formed by the action of *N*-acetyltransferase is a stable derivative of PA that cannot react with protein and is thus eliminated from the body. In contrast, the PA metabolites generated by the $MPO/H_2O_2/Cl^-$ system are very reactive and short-lived. The nitrogen carries a partially positive charge and can therefore bind covalently to nucleophilic groups such as thiol and amino groups of protein. It should be noted that *N*-hydroxylation of PA can also be performed by hepatic mixed-function mono-oxygenases (not depicted here; see [45])

Murine T Cell Reactions to Reactive Intermediate Metabolites of Procainamide

To address the question of whether the metabolites generated by *N*-hydroxylation of PA are indeed capable of eliciting specific T cell reactions, direct PLNA were performed in mice. The metabolites were prepared by treating PA with hypochlorous acid (HOCl) and were shown to consist of HAPA and small amounts of other metabolites, such as nitroso-PA and *N*-chloro-PA (J. Uetrecht, unpublished findings). In confirming previous results [23, 43, 44], injection of PA (1.6 mg/mouse) into C57BL/6 mice completely failed to induce a reaction in the direct PLNA. In contrast, the same amount of reactive PA metabolite(s) induced a vigorous PLN reaction, and there was an excellent dose-effect relationship in the range of 0.2–1.6

mg/mouse. Using the adoptive transfer PLNA, the T cells of C57BL/6 mice that had received three injections of the reactive metabolite were shown to be sensitized to these metabolites (R. Goebels and M. Kubicka-Muranyi, unpublished results). It should be mentioned here that the false-negative direct PLN reactions could also be overcome by incubating the drug with activated liver microsomes as a source of oxidizing enzymes prior to its injection [44].

Chronic treatment with the *original compound PA*, combined with stimulation of phagocytic cells by phorbol myristate acetate (PMA), also sensitized splenic T cells to the reactive metabolite(s). C57BL/6 mice, which are fast acetylators, received weekly three subcutaneous injections of PA (4 mg/mouse) and a one intraperitoneal injection of PMA (600 ng/mouse). When tested in the adoptive transfer PLNA, after 4 months of treatment their splenic T cells were found to respond to the reactive metabolite(s) but continued to ignore the original compound PA. Finally, the same result was obtained when A/J mice, which are *slow acetylators*, were treated with PA without additional injections of PMA (M. Kubicka-Muranyi et al., submitted for publication). Hence, these findings are analogous to those obtained with GST [75] (see "Immune Reactions to Gold Salts Induced in Experimental Animals") and once again underline the utility of the adoptive transfer PLNA. More importantly, they provide direct experimental support for the concept [73, 89] that the compounds derived by *N*-hydroxylation of PA are generated in vivo and sensitize T lymphocytes.

Immunopathologic Alterations Induced by Mercury Compounds

Observations in Humans Exposed to Mercury

Several case reports suggest that human exposure to mercurials may induce a nephrotic syndrome due to immune glomerulonephritis [21], and a case of systemic autoimmune disease following occupational exposure to Hg has been described [68]. When patients with amalgam fillings and chronic oral inflammation were tested for contact hypersensitivity to Hg salts, 62% of these patients but only 3% of controls were found to be positive [19].

Chemical Nature of Mercurials and Their Disposition in the Body

The chemical nature of the Hg compounds involved in the case reports mentioned above has not been identified in all cases. It is known, however, that in animals and man Hg can undergo a variety of chemical reactions [51, 59]. On the one hand, metallic Hg, Hg (0), may be oxidized to ionic Hg by catalases and peroxidases, while on the other hand ionic Hg may be reduced to Hg (0) by superoxide anion (O_2^-) [34, 50, 51]. Conversion of organic Hg to inorganic Hg and vice versa also occurs [83]. Consistent with this metabolism of Hg in the body, different Hg compounds have proven capable of inducing identical or similar immunopathologic alterations in rats and mice [13, 14, 21]. The only requirement for induction of these alterations was that genetically susceptible strains were used [15, 52, 67]. As with gold, a substantial fraction of Hg is accumulated and stored in the lysosomes of phagocytic cells [8, 18]. Moreover, in susceptible strains of mouse and rat the immunopathologic alterations induced by salts of the two heavy metals are almost identical [31]. In contrast to gold, however, the immunopathologic alterations in animals exposed to $HgCl_2$ develop much more rapidly than those seen after exposure to the slow-acting drug GST, i.e., gold (I) [12, 17, 35, 52, 58, 64, 75, 86]. This may be explained by the view that in the case of gold (I) salts an oxidation of gold (I) to gold (III) is required to precede, whereas in the case of Hg (II) no further oxidation of the heavy metal is needed for the alteration of proteins and hence for T cell reactions and the development of immunopathologic alterations.

Animal Experiments with Mercurials

To investigate the immunopathologic effects of mercurials in detail, experimental models were established in rabbits, rats, and mice (for review see [2, 16, 21, 31]). In susceptible mouse strains, a treatment consisting of repeated subcutaneous $HgCl_2$ injections, which are hardly toxic by conventional criteria of toxicity [82], suffices to induce a systemic autoimmune disease. The hallmark of this disease is a massive *T cell dependent B cell stimulation* which results in an increase in total serum IgE and IgG, especially IgG1, formation of high titers of antinucleolar autoantibodies (ANolA) and eventually immune glomerulonephritis.

Susceptible mouse strains, such as A.SW and B10.S, express the H-2^s haplotype; strains that carry the H-2^d haplotype, such as B10.D2/n, are largely resistant to these immunostimulatory effects of $HgCl_2$ [36, 37, 52, 58, 64, 66, 67].

Treatment of H-2^s mice with neutralizing antibodies against murine interleukin-4 (IL-4) completely abrogated the $HgCl_2$-induced rise in total serum IgE (160-fold) and partly prevented the rise in IgG1, but failed to prevent the rise in IgG2A [58]. ANolA of the IgG1 subclass [58], and the $HgCl_2$-induced increase in expression of class II MHC molecules on B cell [95] likewise proved to be IL-4 dependent. For the following reasons it is likely that the IgE increase and autoimmune disorder inducible by $HgCl_2$ are at least partially due to an increased IL-4 production by $CD4^+$ T cells. Firstly, mice and rats that were depleted of T cells by monoclonal antibody against $CD4^+$ or were congenitally athymic failed to develop the autoimmune disease upon $HgCl_2$ treatment [62, 74]. Secondly, the autoimmune disease and increased IgE production could be transferred to syngeneic recipients using $CD4^+$ T cells from $HgCl_2$-treated donors [63]. Thirdly, $HgCl_2$ treatment induced a strong increase in IL-4 messenger RNA (mRNA) of purified $CD4^+$ T cells obtained from susceptible H-2^s mice, whereas the increase in resistant H-2^d mice was very weak [95]. These findings suggest that H-2^s mice preferentially respond to $HgCl_2$ by their Th2 cells [95], because Th2 cells, unlike Th1 cells, produce IL-4 and thus stimulate B cells [53].

Although H-2^d strains fail to respond to $HgCl_2$ with the strong B-cell stimulation seen in H-2^s mice, they are by no means immunologic nonresponders to $HgCl_2$. Upon repeated injections of $HgCl_2$ the percentage of splenic $CD4^+$ T cells expressing the activation marker $CD45RB^{low}$ is as high in H-2^d mice as in H-2^s mice [95]. Following epicutaneous $HgCl_2$ administration, the T cells obtained from the draining lymph nodes of H-2^d mice produce significantly more interferon-γ than those of H-2^s mice (C. Stringer and M. Doth, unpublished results).

What is the exact stimulus that activates T cells in $HgCl_2$-treated animals? Using the adoptive transfer PLNA, Kubicka-Muranyi et al. [46] demonstrated that the T cells of $HgCl_2$-treated H-2^s mice respond in an anamnestic fashion to an injection of either $HgCl_2$ or proteins obtained from macrophages and spleen cells of $HgCl_2$-treated syngeneic animals. Comparable observations, which likewise point to anamnestic reactions of Hg-specific T cells, were made in Brown Norway rats [96]. However, the precise antigens involved in the reactions of Hg-specific T cells have not yet been identified. Because Hg (II) has a high affinity to protein thiol groups, T cell reactions specific for Hg may be directed to one or more of the following Hg-induced alterations of proteins: (a) Hg (II) bound to MHC class II molecules, (b) Hg (II) bound to MHC-embedded self peptides, or (c) an altered set of presented self peptides that is generated because Hg (II) inhibits single proteases in the processing pathway or binds to the self proteins being processed.

It should be noted, however, that autoreactive $CD4^+$ T cells reacting to MHC class II molecules on normal syngeneic cells have also been described [46, 61, 63, 71], and it has been shown that lines of such autoreactive T cells can induce autoantibody formation and IgE production upon transfer to syngeneic Brown Norway rats not treated with $HgCl_2$ (L. Pelletier and P. Druet, personal communication 1992). Further experiments are needed to decide whether activation of such autoreactive T cells or of Hg-specific T cells is the primary event that triggers the immunopathologic alterations seen in the $HgCl_2$ model, and what the exact contributions of Th1 and Th2 cells are.

Hypersensitivity Reactions to Platinum Salts

Observations in Humans Exposed to Platinum

The signs and symptoms of Pt-induced allergy consist of rhinitis, conjunctivitis, asthma, and occasionally urticaria or contact dermatitis. With latency periods of a few weeks to several years, the incidence of Pt refinery workers with hypersensitivity reactions was as high as 73% some 40 years ago (for review see [70]). Despite of a threshold limit value of 2μg Pt/m^3 ambient air at the work place, up to 50% of exposed workers still develop immediate-type hypersensitivity to Pt salts. Current knowledge seems to indicate that the immunotoxicologic relevance of Pt is confined mainly to complex halide salts, such as $[Pt(IV)Cl_6]^{2-}$ and $[Pt(II)Cl_4]^{2-}$, whereas metallic Pt and Pt oxides are thought to be nonallergenic [70].

Until recently, exposure to Pt compounds was restricted to occupational settings, primarily in mining areas, Pt metal refineries, and catalyst factories. However, the introduction of Pt-containing catalytic converters in automobiles gave rise to concern that the emission of yet undefined Pt compounds could constitute a new environmental pollutant. At present, there is no evidence that the amount or quality of Pt compounds released into the environment from automobile catalysts contribute to the rate of immediate-type allergies in industrialized countries. However, a sufficient data base for drawing definitive conclusions is not available. The amount and quality of Pt compounds emitted need to be exactly characterized, and the same is true for the chemical fate of Pt in the environment and in living organisms [70]. With regard to sensitization, the possible role of complex formation and redox reactions of Pt in vivo is completely unknown. Comparable with the biooxidation of gold and mercury [see "Biooxidation of Gold (I) to Gold (III)" and "Chemical Nature of Mercurials and Their Disposition in the Body"), in vivo generation of reactive Pt compounds must be considered for adequate risk assessment.

Animal Experiments with Platinum Salts

Although some effects inducible by Pt compounds have been studied in experimental animals, the mechanism of sensitization is still unclear. Upon high-dose primary exposure to halide salts of Pt, elevated plasma histamine levels were detected in guinea pigs and rats [60] and bronchial hyperreactivity found in cynomolgus monkeys [6]. In rats, tetra- and hexachloroplatinates acted synergistically with classical adjuvants in enhancing both total IgE production and a specific IgE response against unrelated proteins [54, 55]. Attempts to demonstrate Pt-specific IgE remained inconclusive. Cellular events, such as T cell sensitization, have not yet been investigated. However, adequate risk assessment concerning human exposure to Pt requires improved understanding of structure-function relationships of different Pt compounds with respect to their sensitizing potential.

Recently, such experiments have been initiated using the direct PLNA in mice [76]. It was found that a single subcutaneous injection of hexachloroplatinates without adjuvants induced a vigorous primary immune reaction in the draining PLN. This reaction required the presence of T lymphocytes because athymic mice failed to respond. Dose-response curves were established showing peak reactions around day 6 after a single injection of 90–180 nmol $Na_2[PtCl_6]$ or $(NH_4)_2[PtCl_6]$ per animal. Genetic differences between various inbred mouse strains were detected, and structure-function relationships were established [76]. Following chronic low-dose treatment of susceptible mice with $Na_2[PtCl_6]$, persistent Pt-specific immunity could be demonstrated by means of the adoptive transfer PLNA [77]. Interestingly, animals exposed via the nasal route (comparable with inhalative exposure) were sensitized at least as successfully as mice injected subcutaneously or intraperitoneally. Uptake of Pt into peritoneal macrophages was shown in animals treated intraperitoneally (H. C. Schuppe et al., unpublished results). Both Pt-exposed macrophages and Pt-specific T lymphocytes may be used to study the possibility of in vivo generation of immunogenic Pt compounds (see above) following exposure to primarily nonallergenic Pt compounds.

Conclusions and Prospects

An understanding of the pathogenesis of adverse immune reactions to low molecular weight chemicals requires expertise in both immunology and toxicology – in other words, an *immunotoxicological* approach. The results with gold and PA reviewed above provide experimental support for the concept [89] that in many adverse immune reactions to drugs specific T cell reactions are elicited not by the original compound but by reactive intermediate metabolites produced in phagocytic cells. It is therefore hardly surprising that GST and PA give false-negative results in the direct PLNA. Intrinsic features of the direct PLNA – such as (a) the single injection of the test compound, (b) the short anatomical distance from the site of injection to the site of the response in the draining PLN, and (c) the short period of time between injection of the test compound and examination of the PLN – apparently fail to provide sufficient opportunity for the generation of and subsequent T cell sensitization to these metabolites.

Concerning test systems, the adoptive transfer PLNA in mice proved to be of great value in demonstrating specific T cell reactions to low molecular weight chemicals or their metabolites. With respect to measuring T cell reactions in vitro, we have had little success up to now ([56]; M. Kubicka-Muranyi and P. Griem, unpublished results). Nevertheless, for a thorough understanding of the complex chain of events termed adverse immune reactions to drugs it is necessary to establish T cell clones specific to drug metabolites or the altered self proteins/peptides involved.

Detection of the reactive intermediate gold (III) by means of sensitized T cells [27, 75, 94] provides a novel approach. By contrast, when gold (III) is to be detected by means of physicochemical techniques in biological material, it is extremely difficult, if not impossible, to distinguish between the different oxidation states of this heavy metal.

The experiments designed to unravel the mechanism of adverse immune reactions to the antirheumatic drug GST have also provided new and intriguing insights into the possible *pharmacological* action of gold (I) drugs.

These slow-acting drugs can be considered as "prodrugs" that are targeted to the phago-lysosomes of monocytes and macrophages. Here, they might introduce a long-lived and biologically very effective gold (I)/gold (III) redox system. Gold (III), a reactive intermediate metabolite of gold (I), could account for both the beneficial and the adverse side effects of gold therapy (Fig. 2).

Gold (I) salts are the prototype of so-called disease-modifying antirheumatic drugs. Generally speaking, it is surprising how little is known about the mechanisms underlying the pharmacological action of these agents [65]. Could some of these agents act in a similar way as proposed for gold (I) salts? Two candidates in this respect are *chloroquine* and *dapsone*, both of which are used as antirheumatic drugs. Chloroquine is a known lysosomotropic agent that raises the acid pH in lysosomes; this quality is used in experiments designed to prevent enzymatic cleavage of proteins into (immunogenic) peptides [1, 57]. Dapsone has an antileukotactic effect and has been shown to inactivate MPO [81]. As with PA, the metabolism of dapsone by activated neutrophils likewise leads to the formation of the hydroxylamine and nitro metabolites [93]. Before developing batteries of new antirheumatic drugs whose mechanisms of action are not properly understood, from a scientific point of view it is preferable to unravel the mechanism of action of existing drugs with proven therapeutic value.

Acknowledgements. We would like to thank Rainer Goebels, Torsten Tonn, Clive Stringer, and Margit Doth, Düsseldorf, for permission to quote their unpublished results. We are grateful to Charlotte Esser, Christina Stein, Margit Doth, and Joachim Kremer for critical reading of the manuscript and to Barbara Lohmar for expert secretarial work.

References

1. Adorini L, Appella E, Doria G, Cardinaux F, Nagy ZA (1989) Competition for antigen presentation in living cells involves exchange of peptides bound by class II MHC molecules. Nature 342: 800–803
2. Albini B, Blurich I, Andres GA (1983) Mercuric chloride-induced immunologically mediated diseases in experimental animals. In: Porter GA (ed) Nephrotoxic mechanisms of drugs and environmental toxins. Plenum Medical, London, pp 413–424
3. Anonymous (1990) Report of an International Workshop held in Hannover on 6th–10th November 1989. In: Dayan AD, Hertel RF, Heseltine E, Kazantzis G, Smith EM, Van der Venne MT (eds) Immunotoxicity of metals and immunotoxicology. IPCS Joint symposia, no 15. Plenum, New York, pp 3–15
4. Bakke OM, Wardell WM, Lasagna L (1984) Drug discontinuations in the United Kingdom and the United States, 1964–1983; issues of safety. Clin Pharmacol Ther 35: 559–567
5. Beverly B, Couri D (1987) Role of myeloperoxidase (MPO) in aurothiomalate metabolism. Fed Proc 46: 854
6. Biagini RE, Moorman WJ, Smith RJ, Lewis TR, Bernstein IL (1983) Pulmonary hyperreactivity in cynomolgus monkeys (Macaca fascicularis) from nose-only inhalation exposure to disodium hexachloroplatinate Na_2PtCl_6. Toxicol Appl Pharmacol 69: 377–384

7. Brown DH, Smith WE (1980) The chemistry of the gold drugs used in the treatment of rheumatoid arthritis. Chem Soc Rev 2: 217–241
8. Christensen M, Mogensen SC, Rungby J (1988) Toxicity and ultrastructural localization of mercuric chloride in cultered murine macrophages. Arch Toxicol 62: 440–446
9. Davis P (1979) Undesirable effects of gold salts. J Rheumatol 6 [Suppl 5]: 18–23
10. Delovitch TL, Semple JW, Philips ML (1988) Influence of antigen processing on immune responsiveness. Immunol Today 9: 216–219
11. Dillard CJ, Tappel AL (1986) Are some major in vivo effects of gold related to microenvironments of decreased selenium? Med Hypotheses 20: 407–420
12. Druet P, Pelletier L (1991) Chemical-induced autoimmunity. Eur Cytokine Net, special issue for the CIT, pp 43–49
13. Druet P, Druet E, Potdevin F, Sapin C (1978) Immune type glomerulonephritis induced by $HgCl_2$ in BN rat by mercuric chloride. Ann Immunol 12: 777–792
14. Druet P, Teychenne P, Mandet C, Bascou C, Druet E (1981) Immune-type glomerulonephritis induced in the Brown-Norway rat with mercury-containing pharmaceutical products. Nephron 28: 145–148
15. Druet P, Sapin C, Druet E, Hirsch F (1983) Genetic control of mercury-induced immune response in the rat. In: Porter GA (ed) Nephrotoxic mechanisms of drugs and environmental toxins. Plenum Medical, London, p 425–435
16. Druet P, Hirsch F, Pelletier L, Druet E, Baran D, Sapin C (1987) Mechanisms of chemical-induced glomerulonephritis. In: Fowler BA (ed) Mechanisms of cell injury: implications for human health. Wiley, New York (copyright by Dr S Bernhard, Dahlem Konferenzen), pp 153–173
17. Druet P, Pelletier L, Rossert J, Druet E, Hirsch F, Sapin C (1989) Autoimmune reactions induced by metals. In: Kammüller ME, Bloksma N, Seinen W (eds) Autoimmunity and toxicology. Elsevier (Biomedical Divison), Amsterdam, pp 347–361
18. Eley BM (1990) A study of mercury redistribution, excretion and renal pathology in guinea pigs implanted with powdered dental amalgam for between 2 and 4 years. J Exp Pathol 71: 375–393
19. Finne K, Goeransson K, Winkler L (1982) Oral lichen planus and contact allergy to mercury. Int J Oral Surg 11: 236–239
20. Freeman RW, Uetrecht JP, Woosley RL, Oates JA, Harbison RD (1981) Covalent binding of procainamide in vitro and in vivo to hepatic protein in mice. Drug Metab Dispos 9: 188–193
21. Friberg L, Eneström S (1990) Inorganic mercury. In: Dayan AD, Hertel RF, Heseltine E, Kazantzis G, Smith EM, Van der Venne MT (eds) Immunotoxicity of metals and immunotoxicology, vol 15. Plenum, New York, pp 163–173
22. Ghadially FN (1979) The aurosome. J Rheumatol 6: 45–50
23. Gleichmann E, Gleichmann H (1989) Der popliteale Lymphknoten (PLK)-Test bei Nagern, ein einfacher Funktionstest zur Entdeckung sensibilisierender Chemikalien. In: Grosdanoff P, Kraupp O, Schulte-Hermann R, Schütz W (eds) Toxikologische und klinisch-pharmakologische Prüfungen. De Gruyter, Berlin, pp 259–280
24. Gleichmann E, Gleichmann H, Wilke W (1976) Autoimmunization and lymphomagenesis in parent-F1 combinations differing at the major histocompatibility complex: model for spontaneous disease caused by altered self-antigens? Transplant Rev 31: 157–224
25. Gleichmann E, Pals ST, Rolink AG, Radaszkiewicz T, Gleichmann H (1984) Graft-versus-host reactions: clues to the etiopathology of a spectrum of immunological diseases. Immunol Today 5: 324–332
26. Gleichmann E, Kind P, Schuppe H-C, Merk H (1990) Tests for predicting sensitization to chemicals and their metabolites, with special reference to heavy metals. In: Dayan AD, Hertel RF, Heseltine E, Kazantzis G, Smith EM, Van der Venne MT (eds) Immunotoxicity of metals and immunotoxicology, vol 15. Plenum, New York, pp 139–152

27. Gleichmann E, Kubicka-Muranyi M, Kind P, Goldermann R, Goerz G, Merk H, Rau R (1991) Insights into the mechanism of gold action provided by immunotoxicology: biooxidation of gold (I) to gold (III) detected by sensitized T cells. Rheumatol Int 11: 219–220
28. Gleichmann E, Kubicka-Muranyi M, Griem P, Goebel C (1992) An Au (I)Au (III) redox system underlies the anti-inflammatory effect of gold (I) drugs, such as sodium aurothiomalate. A hypothesis. Br J Rheumatol 31: 45
29. Gleichmann H (1981) Studies on the mechanism of drug sensitization: T-cell-dependent popliteal lymph node reaction to diphenylhydantoin. Clin Immunol Immunopathol 18: 203–211
30. Gleichmann H, Pals ST, Radaszkiewicz T (1983) The T cell-dependent B cell proliferation and activation induced by administration of the drug diphenylhydantoin (DPH) to mice. Hematol Oncol 1: 165–176
31. Goldman M, Druet P, Gleichmann E (1991) A role for Th2 cells in systemic autoimmunity: insights from allogeneic diseases and chemically induced autoimmunity. Immunol Today 12: 223–227
32. Goldstein RA, Patterson R (1984) Summary. J Allergy Clin Immunol 74: 643–644
33. Gran JT, Husby G, Thorsby E (1983) HLA DR antigens and gold toxicity. Ann Rheum Dis 42: 63–71
34. Halbach S, Ballatori N, Clarkson TW (1988) Mercury vapor uptake and hydrogen peroxide detoxification in human and mouse red blood cells. Toxicol Appl Pharmacol 96: 517–524
35. Hirsch F, Condere J, Sapin C, Fournie G, Druet P (1982) Polyclonal effect of $HgCl_2$ in the rat, its possible role in an experimental autoimmune disease. Eur J Immunol 2: 620–625
36. Hultman P, Eneström S (1988) Mercury induced antinuclear antibodies in mice: characterization and correlation with renal immune complex deposit. Clin Exp Immunol 71: 269–274
37. Hultman P, Eneström S (1989) Mercury induced B cell activation and antinuclear antibodies in mice. J Clin Lab Immunol 28: 143–150
38. Hurtenbach U, Nagata N, Gleichmann E (1987) Immunity to D-penicillamine: genetic, cellular, and chemical requirements for induction of popliteal lymph node enlargement in the mouse. J Immunol 139: 411–416
39. Isab AA, Sadler PJ (1977) Reactions of gold (III) ions with ribonuclease A and methionine derivates in aqueous solution. Biochim Biophys Acta 492: 322–330
40. Issa FA, Kradolfer T, Geier G (1991) Extremely rapid Au(I)-transfer reactions between S-donor ligands. J Inorg Biochem 43:617
41. Jakobson E, Andreasen A, Graudal H, Danscher G (1989) Autometallographic demonstration of gold uptake in cultured synovial fluid cells from patients with rheumatoid arthritis. Scand J Rheumatol 18: 161–164
42. Kammüller ME, Seinen W (1988) Structural requirements for hydantoins and 2-thiohydantoins to induce lymphoproliferative popliteal lymph node reactions in the mouse. Int J Immunpharmacol 10: 997–1010
43. Kammüller ME, Thomas CC, De Bakker JM, Bloksma N, Seinen W (1989) The politeal lymph node assay in mice to screen for the immune disregulation potential of chemicals. A preliminary study. Int J Immunopharmacol 11: 293–300
44. Katsutani N, Shionoya H (1992) Popliteal lymph node enlargement induced by procainamide. J Immunopharmacol 14: 681–686
45. Klinkhammer C, Popowa P, Gleichmann H (1988) Specific immunity to the diabetogen streptozotocin: cellular requirements for induction of lymphoproliferation. Diabetes 37: 74–80
46. Kubicka-Muranyi M, Behmer O, Uhrberg M, Klonowski H, Bister J, Gleichmann E (1993) Murine systemic autoimmune disease induced by mercuric chloride ($HgCl_2$): Hg-specific helper T cells react to antigen stored in macrophages. Int J Immunopharmacol (in press)

47. Lanzavecchia A (1990) Receptor-mediated antigen uptake and its effect on antigen presentation to class II-restricted T lymphocytes. Annu Rev Immunol 8: 773–793
48. Lipsky PE (1984) Remittive therapy in rheumatoid arthritis: clinical uses and mechanisms of action. Agents Actions 14: 181–204
49. Lockie LM, Smith DM (1985) Forty-seven years experience with gold therapy in 1019 rheumatoid arthritis patients. Sem Arthritis Rheum 14: 238–246
50. Magos L, Halbach S, Clarkson TW (1978) Role of catalase in the oxidation of mercury vapor. Biochem Pharmacol 27: 1373–1377
51. Meguro T, Ishii K, Ogata M (1990) Exhaled metalic mercury in acatalasemic, hypocatalasemic and normal mice injected with mercury (II) chloride. Acta Med Okayama 44: 251–256
52. Mirtcheva J, Pfeiffer C, De Bruijn JA, Jacquesmart F, Gleichmann E (1989) Immunological alterations inducible by mercuric compounds. III. H-2A acts as an immune response and H-2E as an immune "suppression" locus for $HgCl_2$-induced antinucleolar autoantibodies. Eur J Immunol 19: 2257–2261
53. Mosmann TR, Coffmann RL (1989) TH1 and TH2 cells: different patterns of lymphokine secretion lead to different functional properties. Annu Rev Immunol 7: 145–173
54. Murdoch RD, Pepys J (1984) Immunological responses to complex salts of platinum. II. Enhanced IgE antibody responses to ovalbumin with concurrent administration of platinum salts in the rat. Clin Exp Immunol 58: 478–485
55. Murdoch RD, Pepys J (1986) Enhancement of antibody production by mercury and platinum group metal halide salts. Kinetics of total and ovalbumin-specific IgE synthesis. Int Arch Allergy Appl Immunol 80: 405–411
56. Nagata N, Hurtenbach U, Gleichmann E (1986) Specific sensitization of Lyt-1+2- T cells to spleen cells modified by the drug D-penicillamine or a stereoisomer. J Immunol 136: 136–142
57. Nuchtern IG, Biddison WE, Klausner RD (1990) Class II molecules can use the endogenous pathway of antigen presentation. Nature 343: 74–76
58. Ochel M, Vohr H-W, Pfeiffer C, Gleichmann E (1991) IL-4 is required for the IgE and IgG1 increase and IgG1 autoantibody formation in mice treated with mercuric chloride. J Immunol 146: 3006–3011
59. Ogata M, Ikeda M, Sugata Y (1979) In vitro mercury uptake by human acatalasemia erythrocytes, lungs and liver homogenates. Ind Health 34: 218–222
60. Parrot JL, Hebert R, Saindelle A, Ruff F (1969) Platinum and platinoses. Allergy and histamine release due to some platinum salts. Arch Environ Health 19: 685–691
61. Pelletier L, Pasquier R, Hirsch F, Sapin C, Druet P (1986) Autoreactive T cells in mercury-induced autoimmune disease. In vitro demonstration. J Immunol 137: 2548–2554
62. Pelletier L, Pasquier R, Rossert J, Druet P (1987) $HgCl_2$ induces non-specific immunosuppression in Lewis rats. Eur J Immunol 17: 49–54
63. Pelletier L, Pasquier R, Rossert J, Vial MC, Mandet C, Druet P (1988) Autoreactive T cells in mercury-induced autoimmunity. Ability to induce the autoimmune disease. J Immunol 140: 750–754
64. Pietsch P, Vohr H-W, Degitz K, Gleichmann E (1989) Immunological alterations inducible by mercuric compounds. II. $HgCl_2$ and gold sodium thiomalate enhance serum IgE and IgG concentrations in susceptible mouse strains. Int Arch Allergy Appl Immunol 90: 47–53
65. Pullar T (1990) Disease modifying drugs for rheumatoid arthritis: yesterday's treatment today or today's treatment tomorrow? Br J Clin Pharmacol 30: 501–510
66. Reuter R, Tessars G, Vohr H-W, Gleichmann E, Lührmann R (1989) Mercuric chloride induces autoantibodies against U3 small nuclear ribonucleoprotein in susceptible mice. Proc Natl Acad Sci USA 86: 237–241
67. Robinson GCJ, Balazs T, Egorov IG (1986) Mercuric chloride-, gold sodium thiomalate-, and D-penicillamine-induced antinuclear antibodies in mice. Toxicol Appl Pharmacol 86: 159–169

68. Röger JD, Zillekens D, Hartmann AA, Burg G, Gleichmann E (1992) Systemic autoimmune disease in a patient with long-standing exposure to mercury. Eur J Dermatol 2: 168–170
69. Romagnoli P, Spinas GA, Sinigaglia F (1992) Gold-specific T cells in rheumatoid arthritis patients treated with gold. J Clin Invest 89: 254–258
70. Rosner G, Merget R (1990) Allergenic potential of platinum compounds. In: Dayan AD, Hertel RF, Heseltine E, Kazantzis G, Smith EM, Van der Venne MT (eds) Immunotoxicity of metals and immunotoxicology. Plenum, New York, pp 93–104
71. Rossert J, Pelletier L, Pasquier R, Druet P (1988) Autoreactive T cells in mercury-induced autoimmunity. Demonstration by limiting dilution analysis. Eur J Immunol 18: 1764–1766
72. Rothbard JB, Gefter ML (1991) Interactions between immunogenic peptides and MHC proteins. Annu Rev Immunol 9: 527–561
73. Rubin RL (1989) Autoimmune reactions induced by procainamide and hydralazine. In: Kammüller ME, Bloksma N, Seinen W (eds) Autoimmunity and toxicology. Elsevier Science (Biomedial Division), Amsterdam, pp 119–150
74. Saegusa J, Yamamoto S, Iwai H, Ueda K (1990) Antinucleolar autoantibody induced in mice by mercuric chloride. Ind Health 28: 21–30
75. Schuhmann D, Kubicka-Muranyi M, Mirtcheva J, Günther J, Kind P, Gleichmann E (1990) Adverse immune reactions to gold: chronic treatment with an Au (I) drug sensitizes mouse T cells not to Au (I), but to Au (III) and induces autoantibody formation. J Immunol 145: 2132–2139
76. Schuppe H-C, Haas-Raida D, Kulig J, Bömer U, Gleichmann E, Kind P (1992a) T-cell-dependent popliteal lymph node reactions to platinum compounds in mice. Int Arch Allergy Immunol 97: 308–314
77. Schuppe H-C, Lerchenmüller C, Kulig J, Gleichmann E, Kind P (1992b) Specific immunity to platinum compounds in mice. Abstract no 28. In: Abstracts of the 8th Internat Congr Immunol, Budapest, 23–28 Aug. Springer, Budapest, p 619
78. Shaw III CF (1979) The mammilian biochemistry of gold in inorganic perspective of chrysotherapy. Inorg Perspect Biol Med 2: 287–355
79. Shimonkevitz R, Kappler J, Marrack P, Grey H (1983) Antigen recognition by H-2 restricted T cells. I. Cell-free antigen processing. J Exp Med 158: 303–316
80. Sinigaglia F, Takacs B, Romagnoli P (1992) Immunologically relevant interactions between metals and peptide-MHC complex. Abstract no 29. In: Abstracts of the 8th Internat Congr Immunol, Budapest, 23–28 Aug. Springer, Budapest, p 619
81. Stendahl O, Molin L, Dahlgren C (1978) The inhibition of polymorphonuclear leukocyte cytotoxicity by dapsone. J Clin Invest 78: 214–220
82. Stiller-Winkler R, Radaszkiewicz T, Gleichmann E (1988) Immunopathological signs in mice treated with mercury compounds I. Identification by the popliteal lymph node assay of responder and nonresponder strains. Int J Immunopharmacol 4: 475–484
83. Suda I, Totoki S, Takahashi H (1991) Degradation of methyl and ethyl mercury into inorganic mercury by oxygen free radical-producing system: involvement of hydroxyl radical. Arch Toxicol 65: 129–134
84. Tannen RH, Weber WW (1980) Antinuclear antibodies related to acetylator phenotype in mice. J Pharmacol Exp Ther 213: 485–490
85. Thomas C, Groten J, Kammüller ME, De Bakker JM, Seinen W, Bloksma N (1989) Popliteal lymph node reactions in mice induced by the drug zimeldine. Int J Immunopharmacol 11: 698–702
86. Tournade H, Guery J-C, Pasquier R, Nochy D, Hinglais N, Guilbert B, Druet P, Pelletier L (1991) Experimental gold-induced autoimmunity. Nephrol Dial Transplant 6: 621–630
87. Townsend A, Bodmer H (1989) Antigen recognition by class I-restricted T lymphocytes. Annu Rev Immunol 7: 601–624
88. Uetrecht JP (1988) Mechanism of drug-induced lupus. Chem Res Toxicol 1: 133–143

89. Uetrecht JP (1992) The role of leucocyte generated reactive metabolites in the pathogenesis of idiosyneratic drug reactions. Drug Metabolism Rev 24: 299–366
90. Uetrecht JP, Sokoluk B (1992) Comparative metabolism and covalent binding of procainamide by human leukocytes. Drug Metab Dispos 20: 120–123
91. Uetrecht JP, Zahid N (1991) N-chlorination and oxidation of procainamide by myeloperoxidase: toxicoligical implications. Chem Res Toxicol 4: 218–222
92. Uetrecht JP, Zahid N, Rubin R (1988a) Metabolism of procainamide to a hydroxylamine by human neutrophils and mononuclear leukocytes. Chem Res Toxicol 1: 74–78
93. Uetrecht JP, Zahid N, Shear NH, Biggar WD (1988b) Metabolism of dapsone to a hydroxylamine by human neutrophils and mononuclear cells. J Pharmacol Exp Ther 245: 274–279
94. Verwilghen J, Kingsley GH, Gambling L, Panayi GS (1992) Activation of gold specific T lymphocytes in rheumatoid arthritis patients receiving gold. Arthritis Rheum (in press)
95. Vliet van E, Uhrberg M, Stein C, Gleichmann E (1993) MHC control of IL-4-dependent enhancement of B cell la-expression and Ig class switch in mice treated with mercuric chloride. (Submitted for publication)
96. Warfvinge G, Larsson Ä (1990) Spontaneous lymphocytic infiltrates of oral mucosa in $HgCl_2$ induced autoimmuneity of BN rats: phenotypic characteristics and contact hypersensitivity to Hg. Reg Immunol 3: 83–96
97. Witkiewicz PL, Shaw CF III (1981) Oxidative cleavage of peptide and protein disulphide bonds by gold (III): a mechanism for gold toxicity. JCS Chem Comm 523: 1111–1114
98. Woosley RL, Drayer DE, Reidenberg MM, Nies AS, Carr K, Oates JA (1978) Effect of acetylator phenotype on the rate at which procainamide induces antinuclear antibodies and the lupus syndrome. N Engl J Med 298: 1157–1159

New Therapeutic Trends in Autoimmunity

Current Principles and Perspectives in the Treatment of Autoimmune Disease

H. H. Peter

Autoimmune diseases are thought to result from a dysregulation of the immune system leading to loss of self-tolerance and autoaggression via antigen-specific T and B cell responses. Whether or not these responses are directed against true autoantigens or cross-reacting epitopes of microbial origin remains a matter of intense debate and research (Schwimmbeck et al. 1987; Steglitz et al. 1989; Hermann 1991; Smiley and Hoffmann 1991; Kaufmann 1990). Nevertheless, an ever-increasing number of high-titer autoantibodies of the IgG and IgA isotypes are being reported (Brostoff et al. 1991; Pisetzky 1991). Most of these autoantibodies are associated with distinct clinicopathologic conditions. Thus, various types of antinuclear antibodies (ANA) are specific markers of certain collagen vascular diseases, antimitochondrial antibodies (ANA) are associated with autoimmune liver disease and antineutrophil cytoplasmic autoantibodies (ANA) with necrotizing granulomatous vasculitis or crescentic glomerulonephritis (Jennette and Falk 1992).

The ultimate goal of any treatment of autoimmune disease remains the reinstitution of tolerance. Not all the various immunologic interventions

Table 1. Immunologic interventions and their effectiveness in clinical autoimmune diseases

Type of intervention	Example	Effectiveness in autoimmune disease
Immunoprophylaxis	Antigen avoidance	No evidence
Specific vaccination	Active immunity	No evidence
Immunosuppression	Steroids, AZA, MTX, CyA, CYC, TLI, anti-CD4	+++
Immunosubstitution	ivIgG, cytokines (e.g. IFN-8)	+
Immune reconstitution	BMT	No evidence
Immunostimulation	BRM	No evidence
Immune elimination	Plasma/leukapheresis photopheresis	+ +

AZA, Azathioprine; MTX, methotrexate; CyA, cyclosporin A; CYC, cyclophosphamide; TLI, total lymphoid irradiation; ivIgG, intravenous immunoglobulins; BMT, bone marrow transplantation; BRM, biologic response modifiers.

M. M. Eibl, C. Huber, H. H. Decker, U. Wahn (Eds.)
Symposium in Immunology I
Symposium in Immunology II

Table 2. Immunosuppressive drugs and range of dosage

Group	Drug	Dosage range
Steroids	Prednisone	0.25–1.0 mg/kg per day
Antimetabolites	Azathioprine, methotrexate	2–4 mg/kg per day 7.5–15 mg per week
Antimalarials	Chloroquine, hydroxychloroquine	1–2 × 250 mg per day 2 × 200 mg per day
Alkylants	Cyclophosphamide, chlorambucil	2–3 mg/kg per day 0.05–0.1 mg/kg per day
Gold salts	Auranofin, Na-aurothiomalate	6 mg per day, orally 50 mg per week, i.m.[§]
Chelating agent	d-Penicillamine	300–600 mg per day orally
Immunophilin ligands	Cyclosporin A, FK 506	5 mg/kg per day
Androgens	Danazol	2–4 × 200 mg per day
Sulfones	Dapsone	200–300 mg per day

[§] When effective cumulative dose (approxinately 1000 mg Aurothiomalate) is reached dose reduction to 50 mg every 2–4 weeks.

conceivable in experimental immunology for achieving this goal have been found suitable in clinical autoimmunity (Table 1). Thus, there is as yet no way to immunize against autoimmune disease, nor has bone marrow transplantation reached the level of sophistication and effectiveness to make it an acceptable treatment of clinical autoimmune disease. The various forms of drug-mediated immunosuppression (Klippel 1987; McCune and Friedman 1992) remain the keystone of current treatment principles in autoimmune disease (Table 2). Depletion of lymphoid tissue by anti-T cell globulin (Balaban et al. 1991), total nodal irradiation (Strober et al. 1988), plasma-

Table 3. Treatment of autoimmune diseases: current principles and research perspectives

Current principles	Research perspectives
Immunosuppressive drugs	Specific elimination of pathogenic T cells by "humanized" monoclonals against CD4, TcR, VLA, CD8, ICAM-1
Ionizing radiation UV light	Vaccination or blockade with relevant peptides
Plasmapheresis	Extracorporal manipulation of immune competent cells
Leukapheresis Photopheresis	Targeting of drugs to critical molecules, cells, sites
Thoracic duct drainage Diets	Inhibition of autoantigen expression (e.g., with anti-sense oligonucleotides or somatic gene targeting)

and leukapheresis (Kalden 1985), photopheresis (Rook et al. 1992), and attempts to modulate the immune system by intravenous gammaglobulins (Morell and Nydegger 1986; Dwyer 1992) cytokines (Hofschneider et al. 1992) and specific diets (Kjeldsen-Kragh et al. 1991) complete the available immunosuppressive armamentarium (Table 1 and 3). Research perspectives in this field are ample and extend from treatment with "humanized" monoclonal anti-T cell antibodies (e.g., anti-CD4; Reiter et al. 1991) to T cell blockade with peptides (Wrouth et al. 1989) or inhibition of autoantigen expression in target tissues (Table 3; Skeith and Davies 1992; Trentham 1992).

A hallmark in the treatment of rheumatoid arthritis and systemic lupus erythematosus has been the introduction of corticosteroids (Dubois 1956). The various anti-inflammatory and immunosuppressive effects of steroids accounting for their clinical benefit can be summarized as follows:

Anti-inflammatory

Reduction of:
- Vascular permeability
- Leukocyte adherence to endothelial cells
- Phagocytosis and bactericidal activity of granulocytes and macrophages
- Interleukin-1 synthesis

Inhibition of:
- Arachodonic acid metabolism via macrocortin-mediated blockade of phospholipase A_2
- Macrophage response to interferon-γ

Immunosuppressive

Inhibition of:
- Interleukin-1 action on T and B cells
- Antigen processing in antigen-presenting cells
- T cell proliferation
- Interleukin-2 and interferon-γ production
- Delayed-type hypersensitivity

Induction of:
- Lympho- and monocytopenia
- Increased catabolism of proteins, including immunoglobulins and cytokines

Among the effects of prednisone, one is rarely mentioned: the rapid and impressive disappearance of polyclonal B cell lymphocytosis in peripheral blood, explaining in part the inhibition of autoantibody production (Fig. 1). Corticosteroids cause a wide spectrum of side effects:

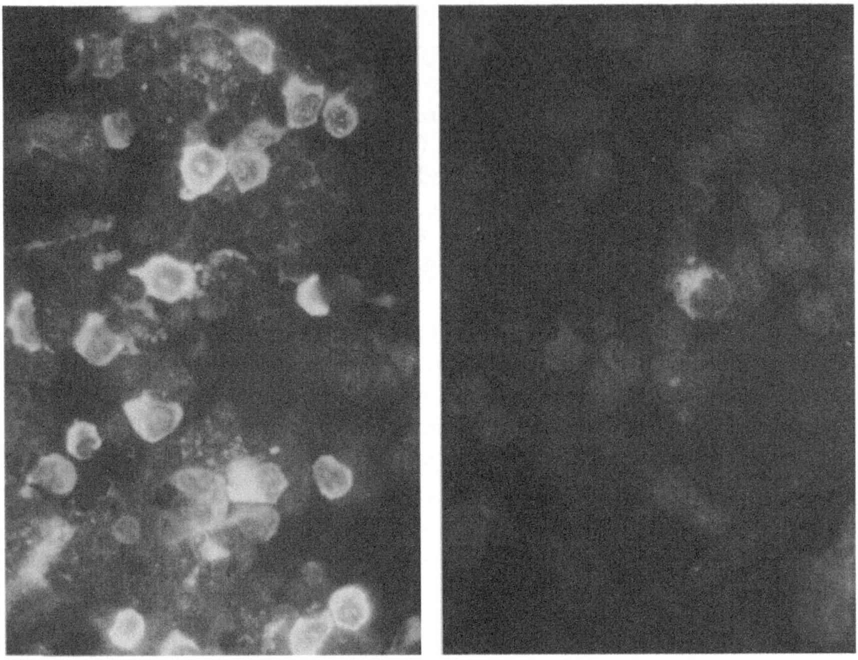

a b

Fig. 1a, b. Mononuclear cell fraction of peripheral blood from a 30-year-old patient with active systemic lupus erythrematosus. **a** Prior prednisone treatment; note the massive increase in cytoplasmic Ig positive B lymphocytes and plasma cells. **b** One week after prednisone treatment (1 mg/kg per day) the B cell lymphocytosis has disappeared

Steroid action	*Resulting pathology*
Increase of:	
Gluconeogenesis	Hyperglycemia, diabetes
Protein catabolism	Myopathy, skin atrophy
Lipid metabolism	Steroid-induced Cushing's disease
Na^{+} retention	Hypertension, glaucoma,
Neuropsychological activity	Pseudotumor cerebri, Steroid psychosis
Inhibition of:	
Osteoblasts and calcium resorption	Osteoporosis Bone necrosis
Specific and nonspecific immune system	Viral, bacterial, and fungal infections
Antithrombotic principles	Thrombophilia

Therefore, when patients are treated for prolonged periods (e.g., for systemic lupus erythrematosus) with doses exceeding 7.5 mg prednisone equivalent per day, the following guidelines for the use of steroids should carefully be followed:

- Use derivatives with low mineralocorticoid side effects (e.g., prednisone, prednisolone, fluocortolon).
- Avoid steroids with long biological half-life.
- Use lowest effective dose for shortest period necessary.
- Prefer topical steroids for dermatologic indications.
- Use "alternate-day" modus.
- Caveats:
  Avoid steroids in bacterial infections such as sepsis, pneumonia, meningitis, pancreatitis, endocarditis, tuberculosis.
  Steroids increase peptic ulcer risks in hypoalbuminemia
  Steroids may cause bony infarction.
- Initial prednisone dosage schedules in systemic lupus erythrematosus:
  Without visceral disease: 0.25–0.5 mg/kg per day.
  With visceral disease: 0.5–1.0 mg/kg per day.
  "Lupus crisis:" 250–500 mg methylprednisolone intravenously followed by 100 mg every 8 h; alternatively a 500- to 1000-mg pulse daily for 3 days.

To avoid or minimize the steroid side effects disease-modifying antirheumatic drugs (DMARDs) with steroid-sparing potential should to be combined regularly with long-term prednisone treatment. This group of drugs comprises antimalarials (chloroquine, hydroxychloroquine), antimetabolites (azathioprine, methotrexate), alkylating agents (cyclophosphamide, chlorambucil), immunophilin ligands (cyclosporin A, FK 506), gold salts, chelating agents (d-penicillamin), androgens (danazol), and sulfone derivatives (dapsone) (Table 2). There are certain, although not undisputed, rules as to which drug should be the first-line DMARD in rheumatoid arthritis (Zeidler and Raspe 1990; Wilske and Healey 1989).

In our hospital we start systemic immunosuppressive treatment with antimalarials or salazosulfapyridine; in the case of treatment failure we switch to gold salts or d-penicillamin, continue with antimetabolites or cyclosporin A, and finally turn to alkylating agents and/or leukaphoresis:

1. Salazosulfapyridine, hydroxy-/chloroquine
2. Au-thiomalate (intramuscularly), auranofin, d-penicillamine
3. Azathioprine, methotrexate, cyclosporin A
4. Cyclophosphamide, chlorambucil
5. Plasma-/leukapheresis, total nodal irradiation

In contrast to this schedule, some centers consider methotrexate as today's first-line DMARD, which should be used in early rheumatoid arthritis

(Jeurissen et al. 1991). Further studies are needed to confirm this approach (Brooks 1992). It is noteworthy, however, that there are also principles for a local immunosuppressive therapy of oligo- and/or monarthritis (Zeidler and Raspe 1990). Our concept of a stepwise increase in local aggressiveness in the treatment of rheumatoid arthritis is shown as follows:

1. Cryotherapy
2. Local, intra-articular steroids
3. Radiosynoviorthese, chemical synovectomy
4. Synovectomy
5. Functional surgery, joint replacement

Whenever possible we prefer local therapy to avoid the considerable side effects of the various systemic immunosuppressive treatments.

In summary, the current status of immunosuppressive therapy in autoimmune diseases is unsatisfactory because of its empirical approach, its unselective, systemic mode of action, the prolonged treatment periods required, and its many side effects. The current status of and future hopes for immunosuppressive therapy in autoimmune diseases can be summarized as follows:

Current status	*Future hopes*
Empirical approach	Smart approach
Unselective	Selective
Unspecific	Specific
Systemic > local	Local > systemic
Long treatment periods	Short treatment periods
Many side effects	Little or no side effects
Costly	Inexpensive
Little understanding of:	To be able to:
– Autoimmune pathogenesis	– Understand and prevent
– Genes controlling it	– Identify persons at risk
– Treatments improving it disease	– Interfere early with disease

This therapeutic dilemma has its origin in our ignorance regarding autoimmune pathogenesis and genes controlling it. Future hopes envisage a smart, knowlegable approach to therapy of autoimmune diseases based on a profound understanding of the autoimmune pathogenesis, ways to identify the people at risk and means to interfere with early disease manifestations.

References

Balaban EP, Zashin SJ, Geppert TD, Lipsky PE (1991) Treatment of systemic sclerosis with antithymocyte globulin. Arthritis Rheum 34: 244–245

Brooks P (1992) Current issues of methotrexate and cyclosporine. Curr Opin Rheumatol 4: 309–313

Brostoff J, Scadding GK, Male D, Roitt IM (1991) Clinical immunology. Gower Medical, London

Dubois EL (1956) Prednisone and prednisolone in the treatment of systemic lupus erythematosus. JAMA 161: 427–433

Dwyer JM (1992) Manipulation of the immune system with immune globulin. N Engl J Med 326: 107–116

Jeurissen MEC, Toderbooms AM, van de Putte LBA et al. (1991) Methotrexate versus azathioprine in the treatment of rheumatoid arthritis. Arthritis Rheum 34: 961–972

Jennette JC, Falk RJ (1992) Disease associations and pathogenic role of antineutrophil cytoplasmic autoantibodies in vasculitis. Curr Opin Rheumatol 4: 9–15

Hermann E, Lohse AW, Van der Zee R, Van Eden E, Mayet WJ, Probst P, Poralla T, Meyer zum Büschenfelde KH, Fleischer B (1991) Synovial fluid-derived Yersinia-reactive T cells responding to human 65-kDa heat-shock protein and heat-stressed antigen-presenting cells. Eur J Immunol 21: 2139–2143

Hofschneider PH, Lemmel EM, Gans W et al. (1992) Double blind controlled phase III multicenter clinical trial with interferon gamma in rheumatoid arthritis. Rheumatol Int. 12: 175–185

Kalden JR (1985) Plasmapheresis. In: Gupta S, Talal N (eds) Immunology of rheumatic diseases. Plenum Medical, New York, pp 741–765

Kaufmann SHE (1990) Heat shock proteins: a link between rheumatoid arthritis and infection? Curr Opin Rheumatol 2: 430–432

Kjeldsen-Kragh J, Haugen m, Borchgrevink CF, Labrum E, Eek M, Mowinkel P, Hovi K, Forre O (1991) Controlled trial of fasting and one-year vegetarian diet in rheumatoid arthritis. Lancet 338: 900–902

Klippel JH (1987) Immunosuppressive therapy. In: Lahita RG (ed) Systemic lupus erythematosus. Wiley, New York, pp 923–945

McCune WJ, Friedman AW (1992) Immunosuppressive drug therapy for rheumatic disease. Curr Opin Rheumatol 4: 314–321

Morell A, Nydegger KE (eds) (1986) Clinical use of intravenous immunoglobulins. Academic, London

Pisetzky DS (1991) Autoantibodies and their idiotypes. Curr Opin Rheumatol 3: 731–737

Reiter C, Kakavand B, Rieber EP, Schattenkirchner M, Riethmüller G, Krüger K (1991) Treatment of rheumatoid arthritis with monoclonal anti CD4 antibody M-T151. Arthritis Rheum 34: 525–536

Rook AH, Freundlich B, Jegasothy BV et al. (1992) Treatment of systemic sclerosis with extracorporeal photochemotherapy – results of a multicenter trial. Arch Dermatol 128: 337–346

Schwimmbeck PL, Yu DT, Oldstone MB (1987) Antibodies to HLA-B27 in the sera of HLA-B27$^+$ patients with ankylosing spondylitis and Reiter's syndrome: molecular mimicry with Klebsiella pneumoniae as potential mechanism of autoimmune disease. J Exp Med 171: 1635–1647

Skeith KJ, Davies P (1992) New horizons in the medical treatment of rheumatoid arthritis. Curr Opin Rheumatol 4: 365–371

Smiley JD, Hoffmann WL (1991) The role of infections in rheumatic diseases: molecular mimicry between bacterial and human stress proteins. Am J Med Sci 301: 138–149

Steglitz H, Fosmire S, Lipsky P (1989) Identification of a 2-MD from Shigella flexneri plasmid associated with reactive arthritis. Arthritis Rheum 32: 937–946

Strober SM, Farinas EH, Fieldeh et al. (1988) Treatment of lupus nephritis with total lymphoid irradiation: observations during a 12–79 month follow-up. Arthritis Rheum 31: 850–858

Trentham DE (1992) Novel immunomodulating and immunotherapies and novel therapies and strategies for inflammatory arthropathy. Curr Opin Rheumatol 4: 322–324

Wilske KR, Healey LA (1989) Remodelling the pyramid: a concept whose time has come. J Rheumatol 16: 557–565

Wrouth DC, Smilek DE, Mitchell DJ, Steinman L, McDevitt HO (1989) Antigen recognition in autoimmune encephalomyelitis and the potential for peptide-mediated immunotherapy. Cell 59: 247–255

Zeidler H, Raspe HH (1990a) Systemische Pharmakotherapie. In: Zeidler H (ed) Rheumatologie. IMG, vol 6. Urban and Schwarzenberg Munich, pp 314–327

Zeidler H, Raspe HH (1990b) Lokale Therapie. In: Zeidler H (ed) Rheumatologie. IMG, vol 6. Urban and Schwarzenberg, Munich, pp 328–334

Immunological Intervention with Chimeric CD4 Monoclonal Antibodies

G. Riethmüller, C. Reiter, and *E. P. Rieber*

Introduction

The idea of turning the weaponry of the immune system against itself is attributed to Eli Metchnikoff, who used a rabbit antiserum against primitive phagocytes for modulating their function. Today, the great efforts of international leukocyte differentiation workshops charting the unknown territory of the human immune system on the molecular level with the help of the murine immune system have provided hundreds of murine monoclonal antibodies recognizing defined targets on the formerly white map of the human lymphoid cell surface. Rather unexpectedly, monoclonal antibodies have also turned out to be the key to the genes encoding many of the lymphocyte surface molecules which are critical not only for initiation of an adaptive immune response but also for maintenance of memory and induction of tolerance. Some of these molecules are also used for navigational purposes by the mobile lymphocytes and are needed for their functioning as effector cells at appropriate targets.

It is obvious that these surface molecules pose as ideal targets for therapeutic approaches with reagents as versatile as antibodies. Their innate versatility allows one to attack individual epitopes on these surface molecules and to select defined pairs of antibodies to optimize their immune modulating capacity. Thus not only the selective elimination of lymphocyte subpopulations but also more subtle manipulations such as induction of anergy or apoptosis and initiation of specialized functions may now become amenable to a therapeutic approach with monoclonal antibodies. Furthermore, as knowledge of the natural ligands of many surface molecules progresses, the antigen-binding domains of an antibody may now be replaced by the binding domains of the natural ligand, and fusion molecules of Ig and ligand can be obtained that may serve as elegant inhibitors of receptor-ligand interactions.

In view of the large number of potential target molecules the question becomes important as to which particular target to choose. Because of the high costs of developing and producting recombinant antibodies cost/benefit analyses concerning the field of indication and the potential market size have a great influence on the process of decision making.

In contrast to the old anti-lymphocyte or anti-thymocyte globulins, which always exhibited pan-T-lymphocyte reactivity, monoclonal antibodies can now be chosen which aim at only one of the numerous lymphocyte subpopulations. Among many possible targets the CD4 molecule on T helper lymphocyte stands out as a prime candidate since it is a distinct feature of cells inducing and maintaining an immune response. Moreover, the CD4 molecule itself as a coreceptor of the antigen receptor on T lymphocytes is intimately involved in recognition of antigen presented by class II MHC molecules. Indeed, in experimental autoimmune diseases of mice and monkeys, treatment with CD4 monoclonal antibodies has proven effective in almost every system tested (Waldmann 1989). Even in advanced stages of experimental encephalomyelitis in rhesus monkeys, a notoriously severe autoimmune disease, infusions of CD4 antibody halt or even reverse the otherwise lethal course (van Lambalgen and Jonker 1987). Another remarkable demonstration of the efficacy of CD4 antibodies has been the prevention and treatment of genetically determined lupus nephritis in mice (Wofsy and Seaman 1985). One of the main advantages of the CD4 target may be reduced to its unique role as a coreceptor with the T cell receptor (TCR) antigen receptor on T cells. When stimulated on its own and not in association with the TCR-CD3 complex, CD4 appears to transmit a negative signal into the cell's interior, leading under certain circumstances to apoptosis. Thus CD4 antibody does not induce a massive cytokine release syndrome in vivo, which complicates current CD3 antibody therapy.

The experience of two phase I trials in rheumatoid arthritis with murine CD4 antibodies has shown that in chronic diseases in which multiple courses of antibody treatment are needed a less immunogenic CD4 antibody is greatly desired. To reduce the immunogenicity of the murine antibody a chimerization with human immunoglobulin was performed by which the Fc fragment, the most immunogenic portion of a xenogeneic immunoglobulin, is replaced by the human IgG_1 constant regions of L and H chains (Looney et al. 1992). Previously, the particular immunogenicity of the Fc portion had been established in mice by experiments showing that the Fc part of immunoglobulin functions as a carrier providing "helper" determinants for the increased induction of Fv or Fab specific antibodies.

For chimerization a rather broad panel of more than 110 different CD4 antibodies was available. Therefore in a first selection step antibodies were screened for the following criteria: specifictiy to the two terminal domains of the CD4 molecules, affinity in the order of $10^9\,M^{-1}$, blocking activity on T cell clones in antigen-dependent stimulatory tests, and lack or deficiency in antigen-modulating activity. Of the candidate group of about 20 CD4 antibodies cM-T412 was chosen because it fulfilled these criteria in an almost optimal manner (Riethmüller et al. 1992).

First Clinical Experience with CD4 Antibodies

In view of the broad spectrum of experimental autoimmune diseases responding to CD4 antibody therapy the attempt was warranted to apply one of our CD4 antibodies to autoimmune disorders of man. Herzog et al. (1989) tested a murine CD4 antibody from our laboratory in a small group of patients with rheumatoid arthritis and observed promising results. A similar effect was observed in another group of rheumatoid arthritis patients receiving a double dose of the same antibody (Reiter et al. 1991).

In this open trial a better defined group of ten patients with active rheumatoid arthritis was treated with a daily dose of 20 mg MT151 – twice as much as in the previous trial – for 7 days. Six of the ten treated patients showed a good clinical response. Clinical improvement was greatest 2 weeks after the therapy and lasted from 4 weeks to 6 months, while, as in the first study, effects on laboratory parameters were minimal. There was an indication of a decline in C-reactive protein serum levels in patients showing a distinct clinical response. Interestingly, immediately after infusion soluble CD4 molecules were detected in serum, and complement components such as C5 were found on CD4 antibody coated circulating CD4 T cells. An inhibitory effect on antigen- or mitogen-driven proliferation was most pronounced 2–4 h after injection, which was also reversible after 24 h (Herzog et al. 1989; Walker et al. 1989).

Four of the initially responding patients were treated a second time after a 6-month interval, with responses lasting from 3 to 3 months in three of them. In one of the latter patients a mild anaphylactic reaction was observed. This patient was later shown to have developed IgE antibodies against mouse IgG. Thus far this patient has remained the only patient with an anayphylactic complication. The presence of human anti-mouse IgG antibodies in all of the treated patients was taken as evidence that the clinical observed improvement was not bought by the high price of a severe immunosuppression since a primary immune response against the foreign protein determinants of murine immunoglobulin could still be induced. This notion is supported by the finding that none of the patients reported increased episodes of viral or bacterial infection.

It was gratifying to note in a third independent study with a different murine antibody using a similar regimen of 0.3 mg/kg daily for 7 days, a response rate similar to the two previous trials was observed in ten patients with active rheumatoid arthritis (Horneff et al. 1991).

With the experience on murine CD4 antibodies in rheumatoid arthritis a larger trial with chimeric CD4 antibody (cM-T412) was initiated. An earlier phase I trial had shown that up to 100 mg cM-T412 was well tolerated as a short-term intravenous infusion without major side effects. At two different centers – Munich and Leiden – 32 patients with active rheumatoid arthritis were treated in an open study with chimeric CD4 monoclonal antibodies (cM-T412). For 7 consecutive days the patients received either 10 mg ($n=15$), 50 mg ($n=13$), or 100 mg ($n=4$) cM-T412 intravenously. The patients treated with 50 mg cM-T412 daily showed a significant improvement in the Ritchie pain index, number of swollen joints, morning stiffness, grip strength, and the patient's assessment of disease activity. The clinical effect of 100 mg/day was similar to 50 mg/day whereas the efficacy observed with the 10-mg dose was distinctly lower. Serum C-reactive protein and rheumatoid factor levels did not change during or after treatment. In contrast to the trials with the murine CD4 antibody, circulating $CD4^+$ cell numbers, decreasing immediately to an average of 25% of baseline level in all patients, remained abnormally low for several months. CD4 T cells gradually increased but were still at 40% – 60% of baseline levels at 12 months after treatment. The degree of CD4 T cell depression in the individual patient did not correlate with the clinical response. Adverse reactions were mild, usually occuring on the first day of treatment and appeared to be associated with an immediate rise in serum interleukin-6 levels. Besides the mild lymphokine release syndrome the prolonged depression in number of circulating CD4 T cells was the most notable adverse effect in this study. The independent evaluation of clinical responses in the Dutch and German centers gave rather similar results in terms of Ritchie index and number of swollen joints, etc. Most importantly, in neither center a good response was recorded for the group receiving the 10-mg dose of chimeric antibody (van der Lubbe et al. 1992).

Although this notion of a dose-effect relationship was most gratifying, only a placebo-controlled randomized trial performed in a double-blinded fashion can establish clinical efficacy of CD4 antibody in rheumatoid arthritis.

Another phase I trial with incremental doses (10–200 mg) of cM-T412 (Moreland et al. 1992) assessed the efficacy of single and multiple doses of the CD4 antibody in combination with low-dose methotrexate in patients with severe refractory rheumatoid arthritis of at least 6 months' duration. Similar to the results of other multiple-dose trials with cM-T412, levels of circulating $CD4^+$ T cells were decreased in the majority of patients after 6 months of treatment. Although 15 of the 25 patients treated received only a single dose of cM-T412, ranging from 10 to 200 mg intravenously, the authors judged 43% of their patients as showing a significant clinical improvement, defined at least 50% decrease in tender joint counts at 5 weeks compared to baseline. This response appeared to be still present in 33% of the patients 6 months after the antibody infusion. Also in this trial the absence of serious adverse effects was noted for the whole 6-month follow-up period.

In view of these promising results in a notoriously difficult disease such as rheumatoid arthritis a number of different other autoimmune diseases or disorders with an autoimmune background were tackled. It turned out that an autoimmune disease exhibiting a response to cyclosporine A usually also responded to treatment with chimeric CD4 antibody. Table 1 gives an up-date of the indications in which the chimeric CD4 antibody has been used and how the therapeutic effects have been judged. The overall impression gained from clinical experience obtained in the various clinical disorders is that the incidence of intercurrent or opportunistic infections is surprisingly low despite the long-lasting CD4 T cell decrease.

Prompt responses were observed in patients with chronic inflammatory intestinal disease. In patients with Crohn's disease and ulcerative colitis not only acute-phase proteins and other inflammatory laboratory parameters responded to treatment but the prompt clinical and subjective response was

Table 1. Clinical trials in autoimmune disease and preliminary results obtained with chimeric CD4 antibody

Indication	Regimen	*n*	Response
Rheumatoid arthritis	One course of 7 injections, 10–100 mg	32	+
Rheumatoid arthritis	methotrexate weekly + single dose of cM-T412	25	±
Crohn's disease, steroid-dependent patients	Two courses, 20–40 mg/day	13	±
Colitis ulcerosa	Two courses, 20–40 mg/day	4	±
Psoriasis generalisata or severe form	One course, 10–30 mg	3	+
Uveitis posterior	One course	2	±
Myasthenia gravis	One course	1	+
Autoimmune hepatitis	One to three courses, 10–50 mg	14	±

+, Distinct objective response in about 50% of the patients; ±, variable responses.

also supported by objective healing of mucosal defects and granulomas, as demonstrated by endoscopy and histology of biopsies (Mauthe et al. 1992).

In a psoriasis patient presenting with a severe generalized pustular form the CD4 antibody induced a particularly impressive remission (Prinz et al. 1991). Also, in one of the two treated uveitis patients vision improved rapidly, concomitant with ophthalmoscopical signs of improvement (Thurau, personal communication). An objective response was also recorded in a patient with a severe myasthenia gravis in whom a long-lasting electrophysiological improvement as to mean jitter of single fiber EMG and gain in muscle strength was observed after one course of 25 mg cM-T412 daily for 7 days (A. K. Lefvert, personal communication). Other clear positive responses to CD4 treatment have been seen in classical autoimmune hepatitis and a few patients with lupus erythematodes discoides and disseminatus (J. Eisenburg and J. Prinz respectively, personal communication). From the trial at the university of Alabama the impression was gained that a concomitant medication with methotrexate increases the degree and duration of CD4 T cell depletion. Thus it seems advisable to judiciously select the kind and dose of immunosuppressant for a combination regimen (W. Koopman, personal communication).

Another interesting indication for the therapeutic administration of cM-T412 has been reported by Knox et al. (1992) at Stanford. In a phase I trial seven successive patients with mycosis fungoides were treated with doses of 10, 20, 40, and 80 mg cM-T412 twice a week for 3 consecutive weeks.

Although all patients responded to antibody treatment with a reduction in erythema and induration of skin lesions, erythroderma, and/or lymphadenopathy, the responses were rather short-lived, ranging from 9 days to over 12 weeks. The best overall responses occurred in the two patients who received the 80-mg dose, and it was also in these patients that the chimeric antibody was detected in immunostained postinfusion biopsies of characteristic skin lesions. In 11 patients with allogeneic heart transplantion the addition of CD4 antibody to an immunosuppressive combination therapy of prednisone, cyclosporine A, and azathioprine during a 3-week period after transplantation reduced the number of rejection episodes (Meiser et al. 1992).

Toxicity and Adverse Effects

Upon the first infusion of a course of daily doses ranging from 10 to 200 mg cM-T412 a slight and transient fever accompanied by malaise and myalgias was observed in more than half of the patients. In one study (van der Lubbe et al. 1992) the two patients who dropped out of the study because of these immediate adverse effects exhibited a distinct increase in interleukin-6 serum levels. During the subsequent follow-up period of several months to 1 year no major serious adverse effects were noted which could be ascribed to the antibody therapy. Quite notable was the absence of an increase in infectious episodes in CD4 antibody treated patients despite a distinct decrease of circulating CD4 T cells. The marked reduction in circulation $CD4^+$ T cells was the major characteristic finding after chimeric CD4 antibody administration. Delayed-type skin reactions to common bacterial antigens were depressed during the first phase of antibody treatment. When skin tests were performed during a later stage of treatment in patients with Crohn's disease who had received two courses of CD4 antibody therapy, no significant decrease in skin reactivity was detected although circulating CD4 T cells were still depressed at that time.

Mode of Action

While in a few experimental systems univalent CD4 antibodies have appeared to be immunosuppressive, the "blindfolding" hypothesis as explanation for the in vivo reaction mechanism has not found the most ardent supporters. On the other hand, "sterile activation" in the old days of antilymphocytic globulin (ALG), or induction of apoptosis in more recent terms, remains an important mechanism to consider. When the murine M-T412 CD4 antibody was replaced by the chimeric cM-T412, the most striking and consistent finding was the prompt decrease in $CD4^+$ T lymphocytes, lasting in almost all treated patients from several weeks to 1 year. Such a long-lasting decrease in isolated CD4 T cells or all lymphocytes has thus far not been recorded in patients treated with panspecific polyclonal ALG or with monoclonal pan-T-cell antibodies such as anti-CD3 or Campath-I. In the instance of cM-T412, this effect can be clearly related to the constant regions of the human IgG1 molecule since the antigen-binding qualities of the murine and the chimeric antibody have been found to indistinguishable in all tested aspects (Dalesandro et al. 1992; Looney et al. 1992). In functional assays, however, in which Fc receptors of human effector cells were involved the chimeric cM-T412 antibody was by far more efficient than the parental murine antibody.

The question has been raised as to whether the long-lasting depression of circulating $CD4^+$ T cells is the result of an active suppression exerted by a controlling or counterregulatory cell population not affected by the CD4 antibody treatment (Riethmüller et al. 1992). The $CD8^+$ T cell subpopulation increasing slightly after CD4 treatment in absolute size is one candidate for such a counterregulatory subset actively suppressing or retarding maturation of new $CD4^+$ T cells. In vitro experiments have shown that CD8 cells can be readily induced to differentiate into cytotoxic T cells when obtained from patients exhibiting marked CD4 T cell depletion after treatment with CD4 antibodies. Since the long duration of the $CD4^+$ T cell depression clearly outlasts the serum half-life of the adminstered antibodies, either elimination of precursor cells and prolonged maturation of new T cells or an active suppression of CD4 T cell recovery may be considered as possible mechanisms. Thus far remarkably little is known about the homoestatic mechanisms regulating the absolute and relative size of lymphocyte subpopulations. Are there dynamic equilibria operating between the major subpopulations which might control in an interdependent fashion their relative size? It is interesting to note that Pantel et al. (1990) have observed a drastic effect of CD4 antibody treatment on colony-forming hemopoietic stem cells in the spleen of mice recovering from a cytoreductive treatment with cyclophosphamide.

It is evident from the rather limited clinical experience that CD4 antibodies represent an interesting alternative approach to current clinical immunomodulation, but one which requires much more research before it may be considered as an established therapy.

References

Dalesandro M, Pak KY, Tam S, Wilson E, Reiter C, Knight D, Looney J, Ghrayeb J, Rieber EP, Riethmüller G, Daddona P (1991) In vitro efficacy of a mouse/human chimeric CD4 antibody: functional contributions of isotype and Fc. 1991 Keystone Symposia on Molecular and Cellular Biology, March 1991

Dalesandro M, Pak KY, Tam S, Wilson E, Looney DMK, Knight D, Ghrayeb J, Reiter C, Rieber EP, Riethmüller G, Daddona P (1993) Effects of isotype and Fc region on in vitro function of a mouse/human chimeric anti-CD4 antibody. Internat Immunol (in press)

Herzog C, Walker C, Müller W, Rieber P, Reiter C, Riethmüller G, Wassmer P, Stockinger H, Madic O, Pichler WJ (1989) Anti-CD4 antibody treatment of patients with rheumatoid arthritis. I. Effect on clinical course and circulating T cells. J Autoimm 2: 627–642

Horneff G, Burmester G, Emmerich F, Kalden JR (1991) Treatment of rheumatoid arthritis with an anti-CD4 monoclonal antibody. Arthritis Rheum 34: 129–140

Knox SJ, Livy R, Hodgkinson S, Bell R, Brown S, Wood G, Hoppe R, Abel EA, Steinman L, Gaiser C, Young G, Bindl J, Hanham A, Reichert T, Oi V (1992) A clinical trial with chimeric anti-CD4 monoclonal antibody in patients with mycosis fungoides (to be published)

Looney JE, Knight DM, Arevalo-Moore M, Trinh H, Pak KY, Dalesandro MR, Rieber EP, Riethmüller G, Daddona PE, Ghrayeb J (1992) High-level expression and characterization of a mouse/human chimeric CD4 antibody with therapeutical potential. Hum Antibodies Hybridomas (in press)

Meiser B, Reiter C, Ebel M, Überfuhr P, Wenke R, Reichenspurner H, Kreuzer E, Rieber E, Riethmüller G, Reichart B (1992) A new chimeric monoclonal CD4 antibody for prevention of rejection after heart transplantation. Transplant Proc 24 (5): 1734

Mauthe B, Endres N, Reiter C, Riethmüller G, Classen M, Deusch K (1992) Chimeric monoclonal anti-CD4 antibody therapy proves effective for treating inflammatory bowel disease. 8th Frühjahrstagung der Gesellschaft für Immunologie, March 1992

Moreland WW, Bucy RP, Tilden A, Pratt PW, LoBuglio AF, Khazaeli M, Everson M, Daddona P, Ghrayeb J, Kilgarriff C, Sanders ME, Koopman WJ (1992) Use of a chimeric monoclonal anti-CD4 antibody in patients with refractory rheumatoid arthritis (to be published)

Pantel K, Duric Z, Nakeff A (1990) Stem cell recovery from cyclophosphamide-induced myelosuppression requires the presence of $CD4^+$ cells. Br J Haematol 75: 168

Prinz J, Braun-Falco O, Meurer M, Daddona P, Reiter C, Rieber P, Riethmüller G (1991) Chimaeric CD4 monoclonal antibody in treatment of generalised pustular psoriasis. Lancet 338: 320/321

Reiter C, Kakavand B, Rieber EP, Schattenkirchner M, Riethmüller G, Krüger K (1991) Treatment of rheumatoid arthritis with monoclonal CD4 antibody M-T151. Arthritis Rheum 34: 525–536

Riethmüller G, Rieber EP, Kiefersauer S, Prinz J, van der Lubbe P, Meiser B, Breedveld F, Eisenburg J, Krüger K, Deusch K, Sanders M, Reiter C (1992) Immunol Rev 129: 81

van der Lubbe PA, Reiter C, Breedveld FC, Schattenkirchner M, Kakavand B, Sanders ME, Riethmüller G (1993) Chimeric CD4 monoclonal antibody cM-T412 as new therapeutic approach to rheumatoid arthritis. Arthritis Rheum (in press)

van Lambalgen R, Jonker M (1987) Experimental allergic encephalomyelitis in rhesus monkeys. II. Treatment of EAE with anti-T lymphocyte subset monoclonal antibodies. Clin Exp Immunol 67: 305

Waldmann H (1989) Manipulation of T cell responses with monoclonal antibodies. Annu Rev Immunol 7: 407

Walker C, Herzog C, Rieber P, Riethmüller G, Müller W, Pichler WJ (1989) Anti-CD4 antibody treatment of patients with rheumatoid arthritis. II. Effect of in vivo treatment on in vitro proliferative response of CD4 cells. J Autoimmun 2: 643–649

Wofsy D, Seaman WE (1985) Successful treatment of autoimmunity in N2B/N2W F1 mice with monoclonal antibody to L3T4. J Exp Med 161: 387

Molecular Mechanisms of Cyclosporin A

K. Resch and *M. Szamel*

Introduction

Since it was first introduced into clinical medicine in the middle of 1978, the fungal metabolite cyclosporin A has become the standard drug in the management of organ and bone marrow transplantation [1]. In the treatment of various autoimmune diseases the immunosuppressive agent has also proven effective in uveitis and Behçet's disease [2]. Cyclosporin A can cause several side effects, among which nephro- and hepatotoxicity are of most concern. As this toxicity is more pronounced when these organs are already affected by the underlying disease, its use in more generalized autoimmune or chronic inflammatory diseases such as lupus erythematosus or rheumatoid arthritis so far is limited [3]. Finding approaches for minimizing the unwanted side effects while retaining the immunosuppressive potential requires knowledge of the mechanism of action. While the cellular mechanisms have been well established, despite numerous efforts the precise molecular mechanism of immunosuppression by cyclosporin A has not been fully elucidated. Our present knowledge is reviewed here. More recently, two further compounds have been introduced as immunosuppressants, FK 506 and rapamycin, of which FK 506 appears to have the same mechanism of action as cyclosporin A, while that of rapamycin is different [4]. Both are discussed in the context of cyclosporin A.

The Cellular Target of Cyclosporin A

In contrast to cytotoxic drugs such as azathioprine and cyclophosphamide, and antibodies to lymphocytes which decrease the number of circulating lymphocytes, cyclosporin A, FK 506, and rapamycin reversibly prevent their activation without affecting their viability. The activation of both T and B lymphocytes requires the synthesis and action of various cytokines which act as intercellular mediators [5] (Fig. 1). Both cyclosporin A and FK 506

a) act primarily on T lymphocytes,
b) interfere with activation,

c) inhibit the synthesis of several lymphokines at the level of gene transcription [interleukin (IL) 2, 3, 4, 5, and 6, interferon-γ, tumor necrosis factor-α, granulocyte-macrophage colony-stimulating factor], and
d) do not affect the synthesis of tumor necrosis factor-β or the interleukin-2 receptor [6, 7].

Inhibition of the synthesis of these lymphokines secreted by activated T-helper lymphocytes is selective, as the synthesis of other proteins induced in the process of T lymphocyte activation is not inhibited, a notable example being the receptor for interleukin-2 [8]. Rapamycin, on the other hand, interferes with IL-2 receptor dependent events [9].

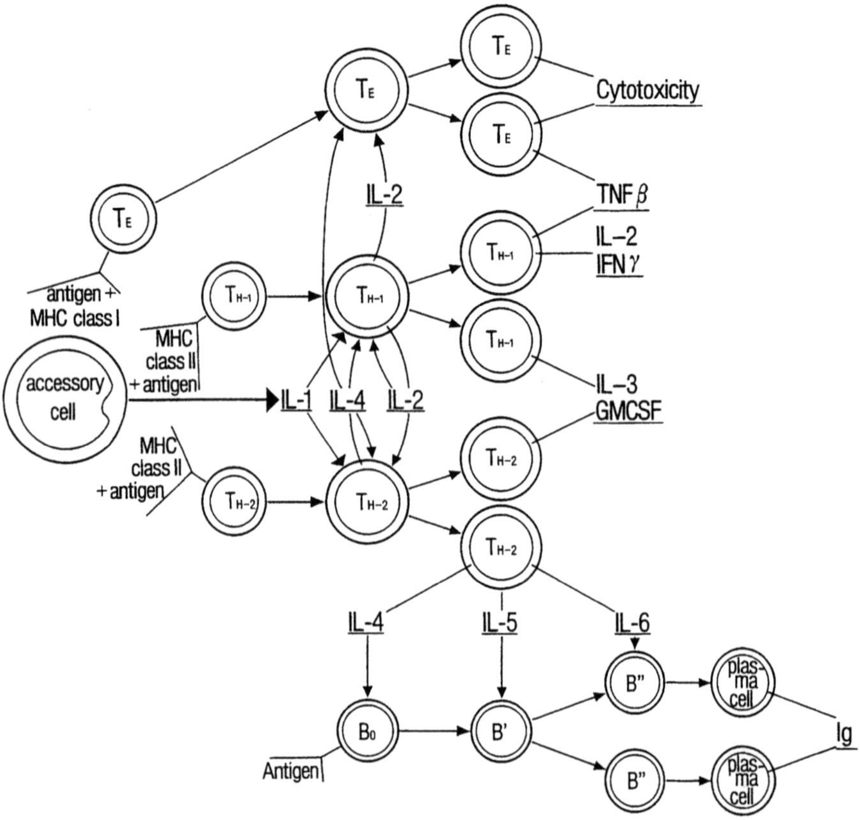

Fig. 1. Activation of T and B lymphocytes. *TNF*, Tumor necrosis fctor; *IL*, interleukin; *IFN*, interferon; *GMCSF*, granulocyte-macrophage colony-stimulating factor

Despite the similarity of their cellular action, cyclosporin A and FK 506 possess completely different structures, cyclosporin A being a cyclic undecapeptide while FK 506 (and rapamycin) belong to the macrolide antibiotics

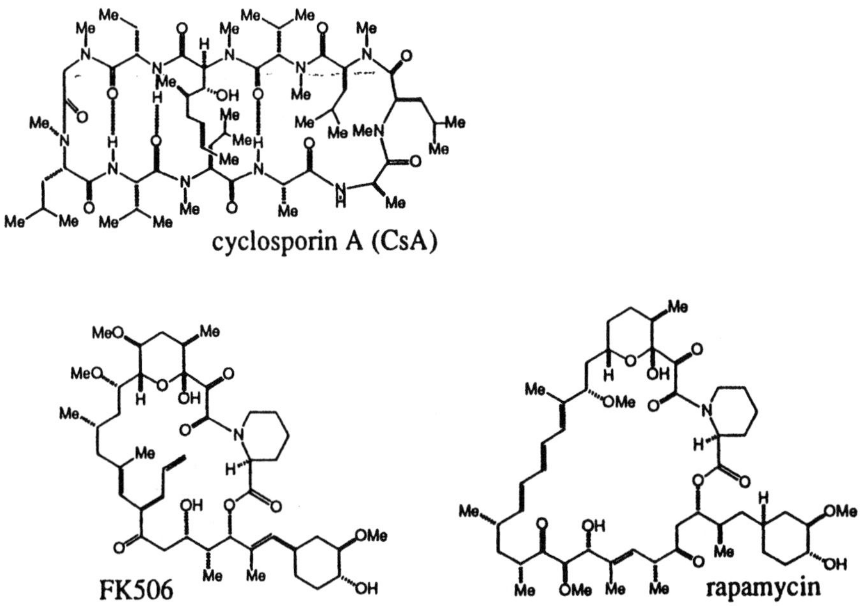

Fig. 2. Structures of cyclosporin A, FK 506, and rapamycin

(Fig. 2). Both, however, bind to cellular cytosolic receptors with similar properties, which have been termed immunophilins, although they are present in eukaryontic cells not belonging to the immune system in similarly high concentrations as in lymphocytes [10]. The immunophilins – including cyclophilin (17 kDA) and FK binding protein (12 kDa) – are peptidyl-prolyl-*cis*-transisomerases (PPIases), enzymes involved in the intracellular processing, especially folding of newly synthesized proteins. As the binding of cyclosporin A or FK 506 inhibits the respective enzyme activity, it has been speculated that this is responsible for the inhibition of activation of T lymphocytes [10]. Mutants of the lower eukaryotes *Neurospora* or *Saccharomyces*, lacking cyclophilin, have proven resistant to the otherwise toxic action of cyclosporin A. These experiments for the first time clearly demonstrated a biological function of the binding of cyclosporin A to cyclophilin [11, 12].

However, although the possibility still exists that PPIase inhibition is relevant for the toxicity of cyclosporin A or FK 506 in clinical situations, a number of experiments suggest a different mechanism underlying their immunosuppressive properties. Thus a number of cyclosporin A or FK 506 analogues which bind to their respective immunophilins and thereby completely abolish PPIase activity have proven ineffective in inhibiting activation or T lymphocytes [13]. Recent experiments with a great number of structural analogues of cyclosporin A have revealed that those domains of the cyclic peptide relevant for immunosuppression are distinct from those interacting with cyclophilin [14]. This suggests a model in which the complex of cyclosporin A with cyclophilin (and similarly of FK 506 with FK binding protein) interacts with a further cellular component and thereby inhibits activation (see Fig. 8).

Molecular Mechanisms Involved in Immunosuppression by Cyclosporin A and FK 506

As outlined above, the cellular mechanism of immunosuppression by cyclosporin A and FK 506 consists in the inhibition of the synthesis of some lymphokines. Of all cytokines so far the regulation of the synthesis of IL-2 has been studied most extensively. The complete gene for IL-2, including the structural and regulatory (enhancer) region have been cloned and sequenced. Experiments in which the regulatory enhancer sequences or parts of it were fused with different reporter genes (such as chloramphenicol acyltransferase) and transfected into T lymphocytes revealed that multiple regulatory elements control the transcription of the IL-2 gene and thus IL-2 synthesis. This includes transcriptional factors active in the regulation of several genes in many cells such as AP-1 and NF-KB and at least one factor which occurs exclusively in T lymphocytes, the nuclear factor of activated T cells (NF-AT; Fig. 3) [15]. Both cyclosporin A and FK 506 inhibited predominantly the activity of NF-AT (Fig. 3), although the activity of other transcription factors has also been shown to be affected by these drugs [16–18].

The obvious possibility that the cyclosporin A–cyclophilin (or FK 506 – FK binding protein) complex binds directly to this nuclear factor and thereby inactivates it, was disproven by several groups [17, 18]. Recent experiments by Crabtree and colleagues suggest that the two immunosuppressive drugs interfere with a modification of NF-AT required for its activation. NF-AT consists of two components, one of which is synthesized during activation but is not affected by cyclosporin A in phorbol myristate acetate ester (PMA) activated cells as used in these experiments. The second is present in an inactive form in the cytosol and is translocated to the nucleus in activated

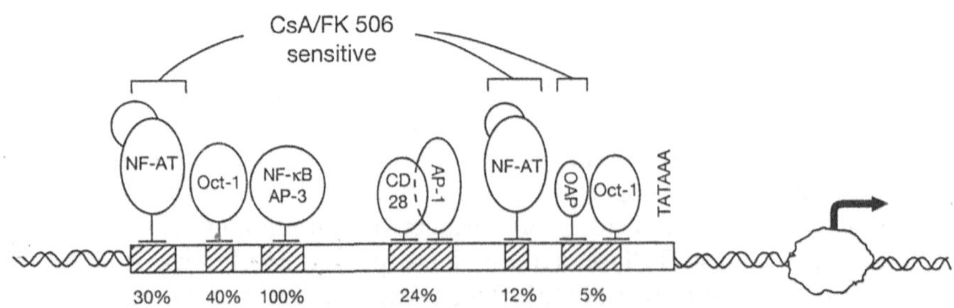

Fig. 3. Transcriptional factors interacting with the interleukin-2 enhancer. *Percentages*, the transcriptional activity after deleting the site. *CsA*, Cyclosporin A. (Modified from [10])

T cells as a consequence of an as yet undefined modification [19] (see Fig. 8). Cyclosporin A (and FK 506) prevent or reverse this modification and thereby block the function of the transcriptionally active NF-AT in the nucleus. Transcriptional factors have been shown to be modified in their activity by phosphorylation or dephosphorylation [20]. The findings by Liu et al. [21] that by affinity chromatography with cyclosporin A–cyclophilin complexes a protein phosphate phosphatase, calcineurin, is purified, thus prompted the idea that this enzyme catalyzes the activating modification of the cytoplasmic NF-AT component, which is blocked by binding of the cyclosporin A–cyclophilin complex (Fig. 8). Very recent experiments with the human T cell line Jurkat in which calcineurin is overexpressed by gene transfer have indeed shown an inverse correlation between calcineurin content and cyclosporin A or FK 506 sensitivity [22, 23].

Cyclosporin A and FK 506 Interfere with Signal Transduction in the Plasma Membrane of T Lymphocytes

Our own results indicate an additional target of the action of cyclosporin A and FK 506, which is more proximal to the induction of cytokine synthesis in activated T lymphocytes, the signal transduction associated with the T lymphocyte receptor. Numerous experiments have well established that the activation of protein kinase C (PKC) activity plays a crucial role in linking the T cell receptor to nuclear events such as the transcription of IL-2 and its high-affinity receptor [24]. One of the key experiments supporting this concept demonstrated a direct activation of PKC by phorbol esters such as PMA together with a rise of cytosolic Ca^{2+} to completely mimic the activation of T lymphocytes in response to activating T cell receptor ligands [24]. Also in our own experiments with human peripheral T lymphocytes, both monoclonal antibodies directed against the T cell receptor/CD3 complex (BMA 030 and BMA 031) and a combination of PMA plus the Ca^{2+} ionophore ionomycin resulted in a similar extent of cell proliferation, as measured by the incorporation of [^{3}H]thymidine into DNA [25, 26] (Fig. 4).

Cyclosporin A, as expected, inhibited the proliferative response in a dose-dependent manner to the stimulating receptor antibody (with an IC_{50} of approximately 10 ng/ml), which was completely reversed when recombinant human IL-2 was supplied exogenously. In contrast, however, the proliferation of T lymphocytes induced by the combination of a high concentration of phorbol ester and the Ca^{2+} ionophore proved completely resistant to inhibition by cyclosporin A [27] (Fig. 5). Together with the finding that cyclosporin A does not interfere directly with the activity of PKC, this suggests that the mechanism by which cyclosporin A interferes with the activation of T lymphocytes must be proximal to the activation of PKC.

In recent years it has become clear that PKC comprises several isoenzymes, of which at least two, PKC-α and PKC-β, are also present in appreciable

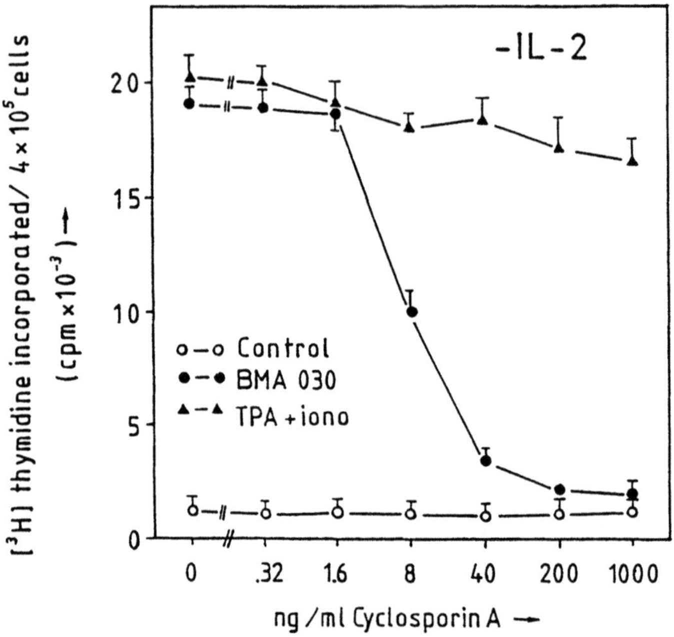

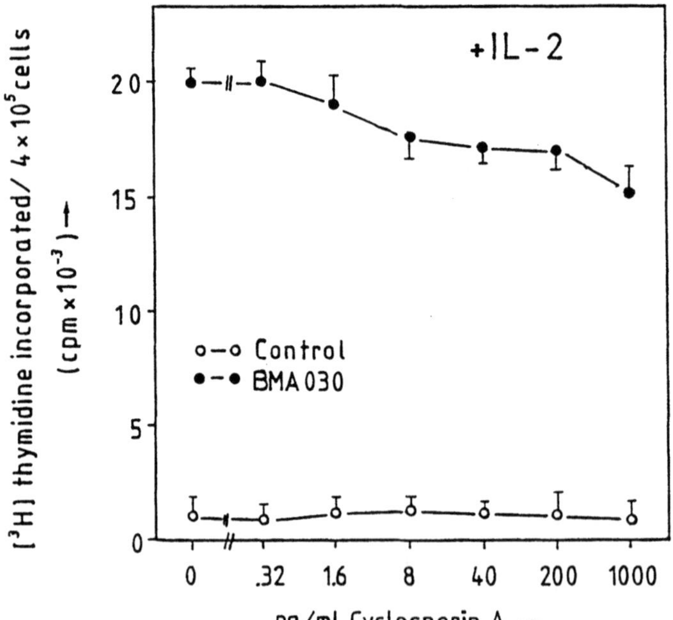

Fig. 4. Inhibition by cyclosporin A of thymidine incorporation in stimulated human lymphocytes. Peripheral blood lymphocytes (4×10^5/0.2 ml) were stimulated for 72 h in microtiter plates with 20 ng/ml BMA 030 (monoclonal antibody against the ε-chain of the T cell receptor/CD3 complex) or 100 ng/ml TPA (= PMA) plus 0.5 μg/ml calcium ionophore ionomycin in the presence or absence of cyclosporin A. When indicated, 20 U/ml human recombinant IL-2 was added. To measure proliferation, for the last 4 h of culture [^{3}H]thymidine was added, and incorporation into DNA was measured [27]

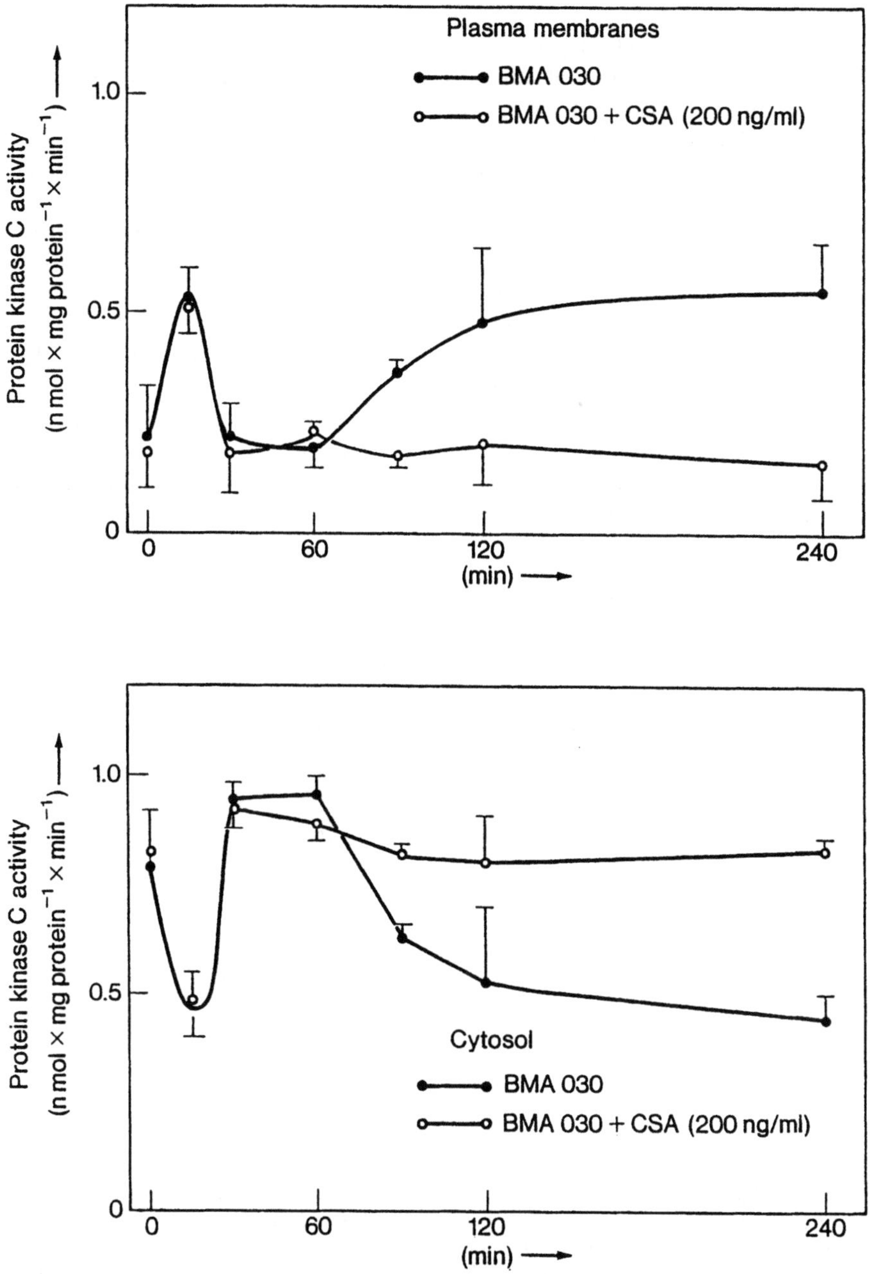

Fig. 5. Inhibition by cyclosporin A of the sustained activation of protein kinase C in stimulated human lymphocytes. Human peripheral blood lymphocytes (2×10^6/ml) were stimulated with 20 ng/ml BMA 030 (see Fig. 4). When indicated, cells were pretreated for 1 h with cyclosporin A. After the times shown the cells were disrupted by nitrogen cavitation, membranes and cytosol separated by ultracentrifugation, and the enzyme activity determined in the individual fractions. Experimental details as in [27]

amounts in T lymphocytes [28, 29]. We have shown previously that activation of human T lymphocytes by some monoclonal antibodies such as BMA 030 or BMA 031 leads to a bimodal activation of PKC activity [25]. In several model experiments, including our own, short-term activation of PKC activity (e.g., by short-lived synthetic diglycerides) leads to the expression of IL-2 receptors; in contrast, a sustained activation proved necessary for the synthesis of the corresponding lymphokine [25, 26].

In unstimulated cells PKC is located in an inactive form in the cytosol. Upon activation it translocates to the plasma membrane. With the availability of monoclonal antibodies to PKC isoenzymes it became clear that the initial transient increase in PKC activity in the plasma membrane is due to the translocation of PKC-α, whereas the long-lasting second wave of PKC activation is due to the translocation of PKC-β to the outer membrane [27] (Fig. 6). Precubation of the T lymphocytes with cyclosporin A does not interfere with the activation and translocation of PKC-α, whereas it completely suppresses the activation and translocation to the plasma membrane of PKC-β [27] (Figs. 5, 6).

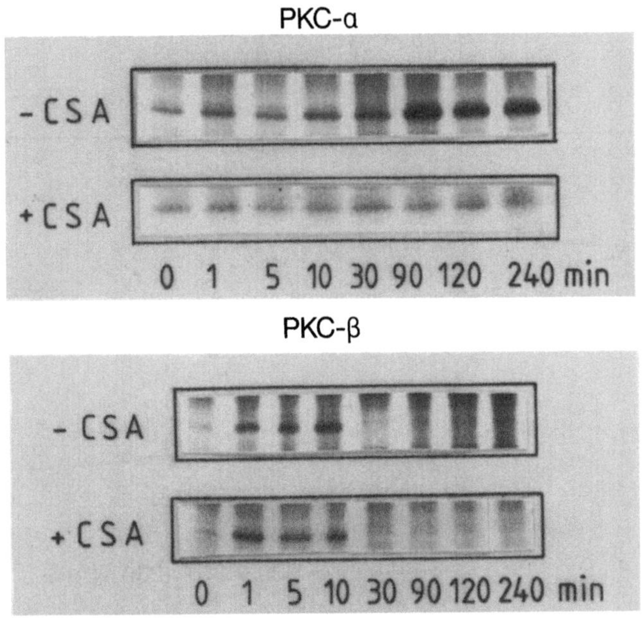

Fig. 6. Inhibition by cyclosporin A of the translocation of protein kinase isoenzymes in stimulated human lymphocytes. Human peripheral blood lymphocytes (2×10^6/ml) were stimulated with 5 μg/ml BMA 031 (monoclonal antibody directed against monomorphic determinants of the T cell receptor). When indicated, the cells were preincubated for 1 h with cyclosporin A (*CsA*). After the times shown the cells were discrupted by nitrogen cavitation and membranes isolated by ultracentrifugation. Membrane proteins were separated by sodium dodecyl sulfate gel electrophoresis and blotted to Immobilon membranes. Areas containing the PKC isoenzymes were developed with monoclonal antibodies to the PKC isoenzymes PKC-α and PKC-β and stained with biotin-streptavidin alkaline, phosphatase-coupled second antibody. Experimental details as in [27]

The result of experiments can well be reconciled with the biological effects of cyclosporin A, i.e., the inhibition of IL-2 synthesis without affecting the expression of its respective receptors in T lymphocytes. For the synthesis and expression of IL-2 receptors a transient activation of PKC-α is sufficient which is resistant to cyclosporin A; transcription of the lymphokine IL-2 requires a long-lasting activation of PKC-β, which is inhibited completely by cyclosporin A. Although the data correlate well, it should be mentioned that the link between the transcriptional control of IL-2, or its receptor, and the PKC isoenzymes has not been formally established.

In physiological receptor-induced cellular responses protein kinase (isoenzymes) is activated by two major known signal transduction pathways, which have in common the generation of diglycerides. Diglycerides formed in the outer membrane by the cleavage of membrane phospholipids translocate, and thereby activate, PKC to the plasma membrane by forming a complex interaction also involving other membrane phospholipids such as phosphatidyl serine and with some PKC isoenzymes Ca^{2+}. Two membrane phospholipids play a predominant role in signal transduction, phosphatidylinositol 1,4-bisphosphate and phosphatidylcholine (Fig. 7). Cleavage of the former, the so-called phosphatidylinositol response, has been established as an initial signal transduction event in T lymphocytes, leading to a transient (within 30 min) generation of inositol 1,4,5-trisphosphate, which raises the levels of cytosolic Ca^{2+} and diglycerides [30]. The mechanism which couples the cleavage enzyme phospholipase Cγ to the T cell receptor was recently

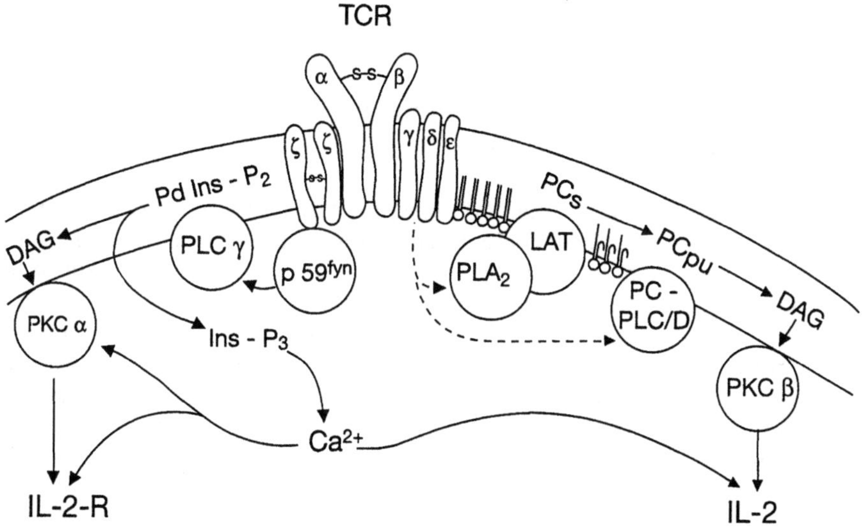

Fig. 7. Signal transduction mechanisms of the T lymphocyte receptor. *LAT*, lysophosphatide acyltransferase; *DAG*, diacylglycerol; *Ins* P_3, inositol 1,4,5 trisposphate; *Pd Ins* P_2, phosphatidylinositol bisphosphate; PLA_2, phospholipase A_2; *PC-PLC/D*, phosphatidyl choline specific phospholipase C/D; PC_s, phosphatidyl choline containing saturated fatty acids; PC_{pu}, phosphatidyl choline containing polyunsaturated fatty acids; $p59^{fyn}$, protein tyrosine kinase encoded by the proto-oncogene fyn; *TCR*, T cell receptor

established as involving phosphorylation by the receptor-associated protein tyrosine kinase $p59^{fyn}$ [31, 32]. Cyclosporin A has been shown not to interfere with this signal transduction pathway in T cell lymphocytes [33]. It was also ineffective in our experiments, as evidenced by an unchanged rise in cytosolic free Ca^{2+} [27].

The signal transduction processes which lead to a sustained activation of PKC-β, and by implication to transcription of the IL-2 gene, are much less understood. Recently, activation of phospholipase C/D, which generates diglycerides from phosphatidylcholine, has been proposed [34]. By this mechanism diglycerides are formed without concomitant rise in Ca^{2+} (as in the case in the phosphatidylinositol response); it is therefore worthwile to reconcile this activation of PKC-β as being less sensitive to Ca^{2+} than PKC-α. Phosphatidylcholine in resting lymphocytes contains predominantly saturated fatty acids [35]; PKC-activating diglycerides, however, must contain polyunsaturated fatty acids [36]. As an early consequence of activation, lymphocytes increase the turnover of the fatty acid moieties of phospholipids, which with time leads to an increase in phospholipid species – predominantly of phosphatidylcholine – with polyunsaturated fatty acids [37].

We have shown that cyclosporin A dose-dependently inhibits the activation of fatty acid turnover, as measured by the incorporation of an exogenously added fatty acid [38]. The drug thus may interfere with the generation of appropriate phosphatidylcholine species from which PKC-activating diglycerides with polyunsatured fatty acids can be formed (see (Fig. 7).

A Model of the Inhibition of Interleukin-2 Gene Expression by Cyclosporin A and FK 506

The interaction of the T lymphocyte receptor with its appropriate antigen – or in model systems with monoclonal antibodies – leads to a chain of events which finally results in the expression of several genes, of which those for cytokines and their receptor play a predominant role in lymphocyte activation (see (Fig. 1). Although some links in the chain between the receptor and gene regulation are still missing for specific cytokines such as IL-2, considerable progress has been made at both ends. Thus it has been well established that a key event in the regulation of the expression of the IL-2 gene consists in a posttranslational modification of a cytosolic component of NF-AT, which then translocates to the nucleus to form the active transcription factor by combining with a second nuclear component, the synthesis of which is induced during activation (Fig. 8). The central event, on the other hand, following receptor occupancy has been established as the activation of protein kinase isoenzymes, of which one, PKC-β, appears to be specifically involved in regulating IL-2 synthesis. The missing link can thus be envisaged as a sequence of phosphorylation/dephosphorylation events. This can lead to

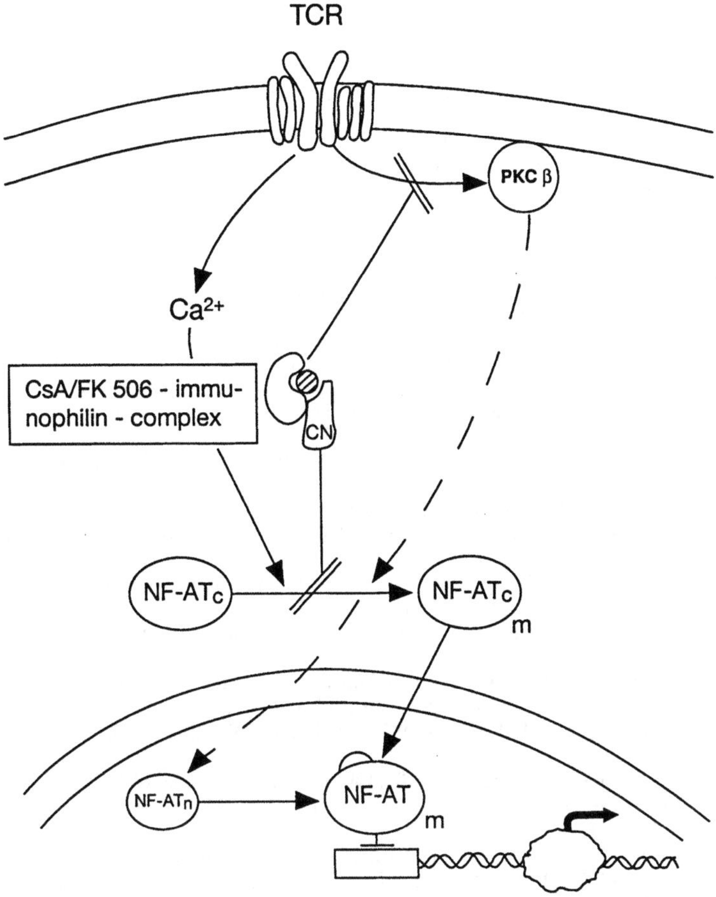

Fig. 8. Model of the inhibition of interleukin-2 gene expression by cyclosporin A (*CsA*) or FK 506. *CN*, calcineurin; *NF-AT$_c$*, cytosolic component of the trancription factor NF-AT; *NF-AT$_n$*, nuclear component of NF-AT; *NF-AT$_m$*, modified NF-AT. (Partly modified from Crabtree [10])

the synthesis of regulatory factors such as the nuclear component of NF-AT; in the case of its preexisting cytosolic component this suggests an alteration in its state of phosphorylation as the activating modification. Cyclosporin A and FK 506 may interfere immediately with the activation of NF-AT by binding and thereby modifying the activity of the Ca^{2+}-dependent protein phosphatase calcineurin.

On the other hand, our own results implicate an (additional) mechanism operating closer to the receptor, the inhibition of the activation of PKC-β, which may also result in an alteration of the phosphorylation of the cytosolic component or, alternatively, prevents the synthesis of the nuclear component of NF-AT.

References

1. Borel JF (1991) Transplant Proc 23: 1867–1874
2. Schindler R (ed) (1985) Ciclosporin in autoimmune diseases. Springer, Berlin Heidelberg New York
3. Kahan D (1989) N Engl J Med 321: 1725–1738
4. Chang JY, Sehgal SN, Bansbach CC (1991) TIPS 12: 218–223
5. Arai K, Lee F, Miyajima A, Shoichiro M, Arai N, Yokota T (1990) Annu. Rev. Biochem. 59: 783–836
6. Sawada S, Suzuki G, Kawase Y, and Takaku F (1987) J Immunol 139: 1797–1803
7. Tocci MJ, Matkovich DA, Collier KA, Kwok P, Dumont F, Lin S, Degudicibus S, Siekierka JJ, Chin J, Hutchinson NI (1989) J Immunol 143: 718–726
8. Ryffel B (1989) Pharmocol Rev 41: 407–422
9. Chang JY (1990) Transplant Immunol Lett 7: 12–15
10. Schreiber SL, Crabtree GR (1992) Immunol Today 13: 136–142
11. Tropschug M, Berthelmess IB, Neupert W (1989) Nature 342: 953–955
12. Heitman J, Movva NR, Hall MN (1991) Science 253: 905–909
13. Schreiber SL (1991) Science 251: 283–287
14. Kallen J, Spitzfaden C, Zurini MG, Wider G, Widmer H, Wuthrich K, Walkinshaw MD (1991) Nature 353: 276–279
15. Crabtree GR (1989) Science 243: 355–361
16. Emmel EA, Verweij CL, Durand DB, Higgins KM, Lazy E, Crabtree GR (1989) Science 246: 1617–1620
17. Mattila PS, Ullman KS, Fiering S, Emmel EA, McCutcheon M, Crabtree GR, Herzenberg LA (1990) EMBO J 9: 4425–4433
18. Randak C, Brabletz T, Hergenröther M, Sobotta I, Serfling E (1990) EMBO J 9: 2529–2536
19. Flanagan WM, Corthesy B, Bram RJ, Crabtree GR (1991) Nature 352: 803–807
20. Karin M (1991) Curr Opin Cell Biol 3: 467–473
21. Liu J, Farmer Jr JD, Lane WS, Friedman J, Weissman I, Schreiber SL (1991) Cell 66: 807–815
22. Clipstone NA, Crabtree GR (1992) Nature 357: 695–697
23. O'Keefe SJ, Tamura J, Kincaid RL, Tocci MJ, O'Neill EA (1992) Nature 357: 692–694
24. Berry N, Nishizuka Y (1990) Eur J Biochem 189: 205–214
25. Szamel M, Rehermann B, Krebs B, Kurrle R, Resch K (1989) J Immunol 143: 2806–2813
26. Szamel M, Kracht M, Krebs B, Hübner U, Resch K (1990) Cell Immunol 126: 117–128
27. Szamel M, Resch K (1992) Eur J Immunol (to be published)
28. Shearman MS, Berry N, Oda T, Ase K, Kikkawa U, Nishizuka Y (1988) FEBS Lett 234: 387–391
29. Lucas S, Marais R, Graves JD, Alexander D, Parker P, Cantrell DA (1990) FEBS Lett 260: 53–56
30. Imboden JB, Stobo JD (1985) J Exp Med 161: 446–456
31. Granja C, Lin LL, Yunis EJ, Relias V, Dasgupta JD (1991) J Biol Chem 266: 16277–16280
32. Samelson LE, Phillips AF, Luong ET, Klausner RD (1990) Proc Natl Acad Sci USA 87: 4358–4362
33. Bijsterbosch MK, Klaus GGB (1985) Immunology 56: 435–440
34. Asaoka Y, Oka M, Yoshida K, Nishizuka Y (1991) Proc Natl Acad Sci USA 88: 8681–8685
35. Goppelt M, Köhler L, Resch K (1985) Biochim Biophys Acta 833: 463–472
36. Sekiguchi K, Tsukuda M, Ase K, Kikkawa U, Nishizuka Y (1988) J Biochem 103: 759–765
37. Resch K, Ferber E (1988) In: Marchalonis JJ (ed) The lymphocyte. Structure and function. Dekker, New York, pp 171–221
38. Szamel M, Berger P, Resch K (1986) J Immunol 136: 264–269

Methotrexate in Rheumatoid Arthritis

M. E. Weinblatt

Studies of Therapeutic Effects

Methotrexate is an established therapy for rheumatoid arthritis. It is also being utilized in a variety of other rheumatological conditions, autoimmune diseases, and inflammatory disorders. Several open studies over the past 20 years have reported efficacy and an acceptable tolerability profile with low-dose methotrexate in rheumatoid arthritis. These open studies report a moderate to marked improvement in selected clinical parameters [1–5]. The results from these uncontrolled trials have generated sufficient interest to initiate randomized placebo-controlled studies. Four randomized placebo controlled trials have been performed (Table 1), and all report efficacy with methotrexate [6–9]. In a 24-week double-blind cross-over study of low-dose weekly methotrexate versus placebo in 35 patients, an improvement in clinical parameters began as early as 3 weeks after initiation of methotrexate [7]. An improvement in the standard rheumatoid arthritis parameters was seen in this study in which the dose of methotrexate ranged from 7.5 to 15.0 mg per week. In this cross-over study an increase in disease activity occurred within 3 weeks after methotrexate discontinuation. A similar clinical response was observed in an 18-week randomized multicenter trial in which 189 patients were randomized to receive oral methotrexate (7.5–15.0

Table 1. Methotrexate: placebo-controlled randomized trials (adapted in part from [100])

	Williams et al. [6]	Weinblatt et al. [7]	Thompson et al. [8]	Andersen et al. [9]
n	189	35	48	15
Design	Parallel	Cross-over	Parallel	Cross-over
Duration (weeks)	18	24	6	26
Methotrexate dose (mg/wk)	7.5–15.0	7.5–15.0	10.0–25.0	5.0–25.0
Administration	Oral	Oral	Intramuscular	Intramuscular
Clinical response	Improvement	Improvement	Improvement	Improvement
Withdrawals due to toxicity	30	1	2	1

mg/week) or placebo [6]. A significant improvement was observed in the methotrexate-treated group in all clinical parameters including the erythrocyte sedimentation rate. A meta-analysis of the four randomized trials confirmed the short-term clinical efficacy of methotrexate in active rheumatoid arthritis [10]. There was a 46% reduction in the duration of morning stiffness, a 27% reduction in the number of painful joints and a 26% reduction in the number of swollen joints achieved in the methotrexate-treated patients. The short-term efficacy of methotrexate was confirmed in these four randomized studies.

The results of several long-term prospective studies have now been published (Table 2). Kremer and Lee reported a long-term open prospective study of rheumatoid patients receiving low-dose weekly methotrexate. In the initial report 27 patients received methotrexate at a maximum dose of 25 mg per week for a mean of 29 months; a significant improvement was observed in the standard clinical parameters [11]. Two patients discontinued therapy due to toxicity, which included one case of pneumonitis and one of gastrointestinal toxicity. Sustained clinical improvement was further reported after 54 months of therapy [12]. An update after 90 months of therapy reported a sustained clinical effect [13]. Similar results have been observed in another long-term prospective study. Twenty-six patients who completed a 24-week cross-over study [7] enrolled in an open long-term prospective study of methotrexate [14]. In this study the maximum dose of oral methotrexate was 15.0 mg per week. In this initial report 16 patients received 36 months of therapy, with a significant improvement observed in all clinical disease parameters. The maximum beneficial effect was achieved by 6 months. A significant reduction in background prednisone dose and a reduction in nonsteroidal anti-inflammatory drug doses was noted. One patient withdrew within the first 36 months of therapy due to a lack of drug efficacy, and there were no withdrawals due to drug toxicity in this time period. After 84 months of treatment 12 patients remained in the study [15]. A significant improvement

Table 2. Methotrexate: long-term studies

	Kremer and Phelps [13]	Weinblatt et al. [15]	Nordstrom et al. [32]	Weinblatt et al. [17]
n	29	26	24	123
Duration (months)	90	84	30	36
Dose (mg/week)	7.5–25.0	2.5–15.0	5.0–30.0	5.0–20.0
Significant improvement	Yes	Yes	Yes	Yes
Steroid reduction	Yes	Yes	No	Yes
Withdrawals:				
Adverse reactions	4	3	2	6
Lack of effect	2	1	3	4
Other	5	10	1	17
Remaining on therapy	18 (62%)	12 (46%)	18 (75%)	96 (78%)

was still observed at 84 months in the number of painful joints, swollen joints, joint pain index, joint swelling index, and physician and patient global assessment; 50% of the patients were able to discontinue prednisone completely. At 84 months, 46% of the patients remained in the study, with 11.5% discontinuing the study due to methotrexate toxicity, which included two cases of pneumonitis. Both of these prospective studies treated patients with methotrexate for over 7 years and reported a sustained clinical improvement and a corticosteroid-sparing effect. Frequent methotrexate dose titrations were required to maintain efficacy and reduce toxicity. Toxicity occurred in these studies, with pneumonitis being the most serious adverse reaction observed.

In another study, 123 patients who successfully completed a 9-month randomized trial comparing auranofin to methotrexate [16] enrolled in a long-term open study of oral methotrexate [17]. The maximum dose of methotrexate in this trial was 20.0 mg per week. Thirty-two patients received at least 36 months of therapy. In this study a significant improvement was observed in all standard parameters of rheumatoid arthritis activity. In addition, a significant reduction in prednisone dose was achieved. Of the 27 patients who withdrew during the study, 4 (3%) withdrew due to a lack of efficacy, and 6 (5%) did so due to clinical or laboratory adverse experiences. It was projected that 72% of the patients would remain on methotrexate therapy for 48 months. Several retrospective studies reported a similar percentage of patients being maintained on chronic methotrexate therapy. Of 124 patients treated at one institution with methotrexate, 60 patients (48%) at 2 years continued to receive methotrexate with a sustained clinical benefit [18]. Of 152 rheumatoid patients treated with methotrexate at another academic institution, the probability of remaining on methotrexate at 1 year was 71%, and at 6 years it was projected at 49% [19]. In this study the major reason for withdrawal was drug toxicity. These projections are similar to those observed in the study by Kremer and Phelps [13], in which after a mean of 90 months of treatment 66% of patients remained on therapy, and the study by Weinblatt et al. [15], in which at 84 months 46% of patients remained on treatment.

There have been several studies comparing methotrexate to other approved second-line therapies. Methotrexate was superior to auranofin in efficacy and tolerability in a 9-months, multicenter trial involving 282 patients [16]. Three smaller studies comparing methotrexate to intramuscular gold reported similar improvements in disease activity, with both drugs achieving a clinical effect [20–22]. There was, however, a trend toward greater toxicity in the gold-treated population.

Several studies have compared methotrexate to azathioprine. In two small studies comparing methotrexate to azathioprine no difference was observed in clinical response between the two drugs [23, 24]. In a 48-week multicenter trial of 64 patients methotrexate was found to be superior to azathioprine in improving disease activity [25]. There were also fewer withdrawals due to toxicity in the methotrexate group compared to the azathioprine group.

Methotrexate has been used in combination with several second-line therapies. In a randomized trial of methotrexate used in combination with auranofin no difference was observed in either efficacy or toxicity with the combination treatment compared to either therapy alone [26]. It should be noted that the maximum dose of methotrexate in this study for the combination group and the monotherapy group was only 7.5 mg per week. This dose of methotrexate is lower than that usually used to treat rheumatoid arthritis. In a combination study of intramuscular gold and methotrexate no greater efficacy was achieved than with methotrexate alone [27]. An open study of methotrexate and sulfasalazine reported a beneficial effect with this combination [28]. The combination of methotrexate and azathioprine did not yield greater efficacy than methotrexate alone in a randomized multicenter double-blind trial [29]. The drop-out rate due to side effects was greater in the azathioprine group than in the methotrexate group or in the group receiving the combination therapy.

It has been well established that methotrexate must be continued for clinical response to be maintained. Two short-term cross-over studies [7, 9] reported an abrupt flare-up of disease activity with methotrexate discontinuation. Two longer term studies [30, 31] confirmed this flare-up of arthritis activity following methotrexate discontinuation. This flare-up generally occurs after methotrexate has been discontinued for at least 3 weeks.

The effects of methotrexate on radiographic progression are variable. After 29 months of therapy one study [11] reported a healing of erosions in several of the patients. The follow-up report of these patients after a mean of 54 months of therapy, however, observed new erosion formation [12]. In another prospective study, after 28 months of therapy a worsening of the radiographs was observed in 6 of 14 patients, whereas an improvement in the number and size of erosions was seen in 5 of the 14 patients [14]. This improvement in erosions was associated with a marked narrowing of the joint space. After 81 months of therapy it is of interest that 3 of these patients showed no further radiographic progression with no new erosions [15]. One patient continued to demonstrate erosion healing with associated joint space narrowing. In a study comparing the rate of radiographic progression in 18 patients who received radiographs prior to receiving methotrexate and while on methotrexate, a progression was observed despite 30 months of methotrexate treatment [32]. In the two patients who achieved a clinical remission on methotrexate there was no radiographic progression. Several other studies suggested a slowing of radiographic progression in a subset of patients receiving methotrexate [33–35]. In the study comparing methotrexate to azathioprine a difference was observed in the rate of progression between the methotrexate group and the azathioprine group, with less progression observed with methotrexate therapy [36].

Methotrexate has also been utilized in a variety of other rheumatological illnesses, including Reiter's syndrome [37], Felty's syndrome [38], corticosteroid-resistant polymyalgia rheumatica and giant cell arteritis [39], systemic lupus erythematosus [40], scleroderma [41, 42], and juvenile rheumatoid arthritis [43, 44]. A preliminary report of the United States – Russian Cooperative Study of methotrexate in juvenile rheumatoid arthritis reported that methotrexate at a dose of 10 mg per m^2 per week was more effective than placebo [45].

Methotrexate is also being used and studied in a number of other inflammatory illnesses, including sarcoidosis [46], primary biliary cirrhosis [47], inflammatory bowel disease [48], asthma [49–51], and sclerosing cholangitis [52].

Biochemistry/Pharmacology

Methotrexate is a structural analog of folic acid and is classified as an antimetabolite. It is a potent inhibitor of the enzyme dihydrofolate reductase, which is a critical enzyme in the reduction of folic acid to metabolically active reduced folates. Reduced folates are important in the synthesis of purines, in the biosynthesis of thymidylate which is required for DNA synthesis, and in protein biosynthesis.

The mechanisms of action of methotrexate in rheumatoid arthritis remain unknown. Methotrexate has been demonstrated in vitro and in vivo to have multiple effects on a variety of systems. Neither a global suppression of T cell function nor global changes in T cell subsets have been reported with methotrexate in rheumatoid arthritis [7, 9, 14]. In vitro rheumatoid factor production was attenuated with methotrexate administration [53]. In vivo suppression of IgM and IgA rheumatoid factor as measured by an enzyme-linked immunosorbent assay has been noted after methotrexate therapy [54]. Inhibition by methotrexate of selected interleukin-1 activities has been reported in vitro, but the results of in vivo studies are inconclusive [55]. An antiproliferative effect on peripheral blood mononuclear cells in vitro [56] and an inhibition of in vitro vascular epithelial cell proliferation [57] have also been observed with methotrexate. Methotrexate also increases adenosine release in vitro [58]. Adenosine is a potent inhibitor of stimulated neutrophil function. A suppression of leukotriene B_4 generation ex vivo has been observed in patients receiving chronic methotrexate [59]. This effect has also been observed after the first dose of methotrexate [60]. Methotrexate does not affect, however, cyclo-oxygenase function or activity [61]. Research is undergoing to determine more precise sites of activity of methotrexate in rheumatoid arthritis.

Pharmacokinetics

Methotrexate is administered *weekly* either orally or by parenteral injection. The bioavailability with low doses is reasonably good, with a mean reported bioavailability of 0.67 [62]. Patients not responding to oral methotrexate should be given a trial of parenteral methotrexate to ensure complete bioavailability. Both intramuscular and subcutaneous methotrexate are rapidly absorbed with a similar pharmacokinetic profile [63]. Oral doses of greater than 20 mg per week may be associated with decreased absorption; parenteral therapy is recommended for doses in excess of 20 mg per week. Methotrexate is 50% – 60% bound to plasma protein. It undergoes a limited metabolism to the 7-hydroxymethotrexate metabolite. Methotrexate and its metabolites are excreted by the kidney both by glomerular filtration and proximal tubular secretion. The plasma half-life of methotrexate is less than 10 hours but increases in the presence of renal insufficiency.

Drugs that are highly protein bound, such as aspirin, nonsteroidal anti-inflammatory drugs and sulfonamides, may displace methotrexate from the binding protein. Several kinetic studies have failed to note a significant interaction between low-dose methotrexate and a variety of nonsteroidal anti-inflammatory drugs [64, 65]. One kinetic study reported an interaction between aspirin and methotrexate, with higher concentrations of methotrexate occurring with aspirin therapy [66]. With high-dose methotrexate, as used in cancer chemotherapy, coadministration of nonsteroidal anti-inflammatory drugs or aspirin may be toxic and should be avoided. Drugs with antifolate activity such as trimethoprim/sulfamethoxyzole and drugs which affect tubular function such as probenecid should be used with great caution due to an increased risk of toxicity.

Dose and Drug Administration

Methotrexate must only be given on a *weekly* basis. More frequent administration of methotrexate has been associated with a greater incidence of acute and chronic toxicity. Oral methotrexate can be taken as one dose, or it can be cycled over a 24-hour period once a week. Parenteral methotrexate at low doses can be administered by subcutaneous or intramuscular injection. The initial dose of methotrexate in rheumatoid arthritis is generally 7.5 mg per week, but occasionally lower doses may be used. If a positive response has not been observed in 4–8 weeks, and there has been no toxicity, the dose may be increased. Although an optimal dose is unknown, most studies have utilized doses of 7.5–20.0 mg per week. One dose response study suggested a greater clinical response at 10.0 mg/m^2 than at 5 mg/m^2 [67]. Doses above 20.0 mg per week should be administered parenterally due to decreased oral bioavailability at these higher doses. The maximum dose to be used in rheumatoid arthritis is unknown, but one study reported efficacy and tolerability at a dose of 40 mg/m^2 [68] whereas another study reported increased toxicity at doses of 50 mg/week [5]. Once a clinical response has been observed, the dose of methotrexate may be slowly reduced. Some patients, however, may require dose escalations over time to maintain a positive clinical response.

Toxicity

Adverse experiences with low-dose methotrexate have been reported frequently in clinical trials. Despite the high frequency of reported adverse experiences, serious toxicity has fortunately been rare. The most common toxicity associated with methotrexate is gastrointestinal intolerance, including nausea, anorexia, vomiting, diarrhea, and weight loss [69]. This toxicity may improve with dose reduction or change in method of administration and may diminish with chronic therapy. Stomatitis may also occur and varies in severity. Folic acid [70] and folinic acid (leucovorin) [71, 72] may improve the nausea and stomatitis associated with methotrexate.

Hematologic toxicity including leukopenia, thrombocytopenia, megaloblastic anemia, and pancytopenia is unusual with low-dose methotrexate, occurring in fewer than 5% of patients [69]. There are definite risk factors for hematologic toxicity, which include renal insufficiency, folic acid deficiency, concomitant use of selected drugs including probenecid and trimethoprim/sulfamethoxyzole, dosing errors, and the use of the drug during a superimposed infection [73, 74]. An elevation in mean corpuscular volume might be a predictor of impending hematologic toxicity [75]. Folinic acid (leucovorin) should be administered immediately in cases of suspected methotrexate overdose or hematologic toxicity.

Renal toxicity with low-dose methotrexate has not generally been reported. Higher doses of methotrexate can be associated with renal toxicity due to crystalization of the drug in the renal tubules. Due to the excretion of methotrexate, however, renal insufficiency from any cause can lead to sustained and toxic levels of methotrexate. Regular monitoring of renal function is required with methotrexate use.

Skin rashes including urticaria, cutaneous vasculitis, and reactivation of ultraviolet light induced erythema and alopecia may occur with low-dose methotrexate [69, 76]. An increase in the number and the size of rheumatoid nodules has occasionally been observed in rheumatoid patients receiving methotrexate despite an improvement in the articular disease [14, 77].

Ovarian dysfunction has not been reported with methotrexate [78]; however, the drug is a definite teratogenic agent. Methotrexate should not be administered to women of childbearing potential without the use of adequate birth control measurcs. Women should discontinue use of methotrexate at least one ovulatory cycle before attempting conception. Transient but reversible decreases in the sperm count have been reported with high-dose methotrexate in cancer chemotherapy [78] and low-dose therapy in psoriasis [79]. There have been no reports of males who received methotrexate and subsequently conceived abnormal children. It is recommended that males, however, discontinue methotrexate at least 90 days before attempting conception.

There are no published trials which demonstrate that methotrexate is a carcinogenic agent. In several animal species treated with methotrexate a carcinogenic effect was not observed [80]. In patients receiving high-dose methotrexate for choriocarcinoma an increased risk for a second malignancy was not noted [81]. A carcinogenic effect has also not been reported in studies of psoriasis patients receiving low-dose methotrexate [82, 83].

Acute and chronic pulmonary toxicity has been observed with low-dose weekly methotrexate. The clinical presentation includes nonproductive cough, fever, and progressive dyspnea. Several studies reported a 3% – 5% incidence of rheumatoids developing a pulmonary reaction while on methotrexate [84, 85]. Definite risk factors for this toxicity have not been confirmed, but underlying pulmonary disease including interstitial fibrosis has been suggested as a risk factor [86]. Chest radiographs may initially be normal but generally progress to interstitial and occasionally aveolar infiltrates. The lung pathology is consistent with a hypersensitivity reaction with inflammatory infiltrates primarily of mononuclear cells, giant cells, granuloma formation, and varying degrees of bronchiolitis and fibrosis. This pathology may be indistinguishable from that of rheumatoid lung disease. Occasionally the fibrosis may progress and lead to chronic interstitial lung disease [87]. Treatment has included discontinuation of methotrexate, respiratory support, and administration of systemic corticosteroids. Opportunistic organisms must be excluded; there are reports of *Pneumocystis carini* infection and fungal infections occurring in rheumatoids receiving methotrexate [88, 89]. The outcome of methotrexate-associated lung disease is variable, but most patients have recovered.

Liver toxicity in rheumatoid arthritis patients receiving methotrexate has been to date uncommon. In a review of 714 patients who underwent liver biopsy after approximately 1.5-g therapy mild fibrosis was noted in 8% [90]. In many of these patients fibrosis was seen only with a more sensitive trichrome stain. Moderate fibrosis was observed in only four (0.5%) of the patients. In a prospective liver biopsy study of 27 patients mild fibrosis was noted in 52% of patients after a mean of 52 months of therapy [91]. In a study of 23 rheumatoid patients who had received methotrexate for over 10 years there were no cases of cirrhosis [92]. There are, however, isolated reports of cirrhosis [93, 94] and acute decompensated liver disease [95, 96] in rheumatoid patients receiving methotrexate. A recent study which included a survey of members of the American College of Rheumatology identified and confirmed 24 cases of serious liver disease occurring in rheumatoid patients receiving methotrexate [97]. A case-control study identified two independent risk factors for toxicity; age and duration of therapy. The estimated risk of developing serious liver disease after 5 years of therapy was projected at 1 in 1000. In this study isolated elevations in serum transaminases and a decrease in serum albumin occurred more frequently within the year prior to the acute event in the patients who developed liver disease compared to the control population. Recommendations regarding surveillance liver biopsies have still not been developed. Based on the available data some rheumatologists recommend liver biopsy after approximately 3–5 years of therapy unless the patient is in a higher risk group, which could include insulin-dependent diabetes. Earlier biopsies might be recommended in patients who develop serial elevations in serum transaminases or a decreasing serum albumin. The drug should not be administered to patients with a history of significant alcohol ingestion or in patients with underlying liver disease. A baseline liver biopsy is not indicated unless there is a history of alcoholism, underlying liver disease, positive hepatitis B serology, or extreme morbid obesity. The risk of the liver biopsy must be considered and discussed with the patient.

Other side effects that have been associated with low-dose weekly methotrexate include headache, weight loss, fatigue, mood alterations, depression, dizziness, fever, polyarthralgias, and rarely opportunistic infections [88, 89, 98].

Methotrexate is currently being used in patients with active rheumatoid arthritis who do not respond to anti-inflammatory medicine and generally a trial of at least one second-line therapy. However, there is increasing use of methotrexate as the first of the second-line treatments due to its rapid onset of action. Patients with renal insufficiency, women of childbearing potential, untreated folate deficiency, active liver disease, excessive alcohol consumption, noncompliance, or serious medical illness should be excluded from receiving therapy. Baseline laboratory parameters should generally include a complete blood count, serum creatinine, liver blood tests, and a chest radiograph. After initiation of therapy a complete blood count should be monitored monthly, and there should be regular monitoring of renal function and liver blood tests. Decisions about the need for liver biopsy should be discussed between the rheumatologist and the patient. Methotrexate should be temporarily discontinued during acute infections and for major surgical procedures. Appropriate patient selection, patient education, and rigorous monitoring are required with methotrexate to reduce the potential for adverse reactions.

Methotrexate has become a major therapy in the treatment of rheumatoid arthritis. It is considered one of the significant advances over the past decade in the treatment of rheumatoid arthritis [99].

References

1. Hoffmeister RT (1972) Methotrexate in rheumatoid arthritis. Arthritis Rheum 15: 114 (abstract)
2. Willkens RF, Watson MA (1982) Methotrexate: a perspective of its use in the treatment of rheumatic diseases. J Lab Clin Med 100: 314–321
3. Steinsson K, Weinstein A, Korn J, Abeles M (1982) Low dose methotrexate in rheumatoid arthritis. J Rheumatol 9: 860–866
4. Weinstein A, Marlowe S, Korn J, Farouhar F (1985) Low-dose methotrexate treatment of rheumatoid arthritis. Long-term observations. Am J Med 79: 331–337
5. Michaels RM, Nashel DJ, Leonard A, Sliwinski AJ, Derbes SJ (1982) Weekly intravenous methotrexate in the treatment of rheumatoid arthritis. Arthritis Rheum 25: 339–341
6. Williams HJ, Willkens RF, Samuelson CO Jr, Alarcon GS, Guttadauria M, Yarboro C, Polisson RP, Weiner SR, Luggen ME, Billingsley LM et al. (1985) Comparison of

low-dose oral pulse methotrexate and placebo in the treatment of rheumatoid arthritis. A controlled clinical trial. Arthritis Rheum 28: 721–730

7. Weinblatt ME, Coblyn JS, Fox DA, Fraser PA, Holdsworth DE, Glass DN, Trentham DE (1985) Efficacy of low-dose methotrexate in rheumatoid arthritis. N Engl J Med 312: 818–822
8. Thompson RN, Watts C, Edelman J, Esdaile J, Russell AS (1984) A controlled two-centre trial of parenteral methotrexate therapy for refractory rheumatoid arthritis. J Rheumatol 11: 760–763
9. Andersen PA, West SG, O'Dell JR, Via CS, Claypool RG, Kotzin BL (1985) Weekly pulse methotrexate in rheumatoid arthritis. Clinical and immunologic effects in a randomized, double-blind study. Ann Intern Med 103: 489–496
10. Tugwell P, Bennett K, Gent M (1987) Methotrexate in rheumatoid arthritis. Indications, contraindications, efficacy, and safety. Ann Intern Med 107: 358–366
11. Kremer JM, Lee JK (1986) The safety and efficacy of the use of methotrexate in long-term therapy for rheumatoid arthritis. Arthritis Rheum 29: 822–831
12. Kremer JM, Lee JK (1988) A long-term prospective study of the use of methotrexate in rheumatoid arthritis. Update after a mean of fifty-three months. Arthritis Rheum 31: 577–584
13. Kremer JM, Phelps CT (1992) Long-term prospective study of the use of methotrexate in rheumatoid arthritis: update after a mean of 90 months. Arthritis Rheum 35: 138–145
14. Weinblatt ME, Trentham DE, Fraser PA, Holdsworth DE, Falchuk KR, Weissman BN, Coblyn JS (1988) Long-term prospective trial of low-dose methotrexate in rheumatoid arthritis. Arthritis Rheum 31: 167–175
15. Weinblatt ME, Weissman BN, Holdsworth DE, Fraser PA, Maier AL, Falchuk KR, Coblyn JS (1992) Long-term prospective study of methotrexate in the treatment of rheumatoid arthritis eighty-four-month update. Arthritis Rheum 35: 129–137
16. Weinblatt ME, Kaplan H, Germain BF, Merriman RC, Solomon SD, Wall B, Anderson L, Block S, Irby R, Wolfe F et al. (1990) Low-dose methotrexate compared with auranofin in adult rheumatoid arthritis. A thirty-six-week, double-blind trial. Arthritis Rheum 33: 330–338
17. Weinblatt ME, Kaplan H, Germain BF, Merriman RC, Solomon SD, Wall B, Anderson L, Block S, Small R, Wolfe F, Gall E, Torretti D, Polisson R (1991) Methotrexate in rheumatoid arthritis: Effects on disease activity in a multicenter prospective study. J Rheumatol 18: 334–338
18. Fehlauer CS, Carson CW, Cannon GW, Ward JR, Samuelson CO, Williams HJ, Clegg DO (1989) Methotrexate therapy in rheumatoid arthritis: 2-year retrospective followup study. J Rheumatol 16: 307–312
19. Alarcon GS, Tracy IC, Blackburn WD Jr. (1989) Methotrexate in rheumatoid arthritis. Toxic effects as the major factor in limiting long-term treatment. Arthritis Rheum 32: 671–676
20. Morassut P, Goldstein R, Cyr M, Karsh J, McKendry RJ (1989) Gold sodium thiomalate compared to low dose methotrexate in the treatment of rheumatoid arthritis – a randomized, double blind 26-week trial. J Rheumatol 16: 302–306
21. Suarez-Almazor ME, Fitzgerald A, Grace M, Russell AS (1988) A randomized controlled trial of parenteral methotrexate compared with sodium aurothiomalate (Myochrysine) in the treatment of rheumatoid arthritis. J Rheumatol 15: 753–756
22. Rau R, Herborn G, Karger T, Menninger H, Elhardt D, Schmitt J (1991) A double blind randomized parallel trial of intramuscular methotrexate and gold sodium thiomalate in early erosive rheumatoid arthritis. J Rheumatol 18: 328–333
23. Hamdy H, McKendry RJ, Mierins E, Liver JA (1987) Low-dose methotrexate compared with azathioprine in the treatment of rheumatoid arthritis. A twenty-four-week controlled clinical trial. Arthritis Rheum 30: 361–368
24. Arnold MH, O'Callaghan J, McCredie M, Beller EM, Kelly DE, Brooks PM (1990) Comparative controlled trial of low-dose weekly methotrexate versus azathioprine in rheumatoid arthritis: 3-year prospective study. Br J Rheumatol 29: 120–125

25. Jeurissen MEC, Boerbooms AMT, van de Putte LBA, Doesburg WH, Mulder J, Rasker JJ, Kruijsen MWM, Haverman JF, van Beusekom HJ, Muller WH, Franssen MJAM, De Rooy D-JRAM (1991) Methotrexate versus azathioprine in the treatment of rheumatoid arthritis: A forty-eight-week randomized, double-blind trial. Arthritis Rheum 34: 961–972
26. Williams HJ, Ward JR, Reading JC (1990) Comparison of auranofin, methotrexate, and the combination of both in the treatment of rheumatoid arthritis. Arthritis Rheum 33: S10 (abstract)
27. Rau R, Herborn G, Scleusser B, Elhard D (1991) Prospective open longterm observation of RA-patients treated with methotrexate or MTX + gold. Arthritis Rheum 34: S92 (abstract)
28. Shiroky JB, Watts CS, Neville C (1989) Combination methotrexate and sulfasalazine in the management of rheumatoid arthritis: case observations. Arthritis Rheum 32: 1160–1164
29. Willkens RF, Urowitz MB, Stablein DM (1991)A randomized multicenter controlled trial comparing a combination of methotrexate (MTX) and azathioprine (AZA) to MTX plus placebo and AZA plus placebo. Arthritis Rheum 34: S53 (abstract)
30. Kremer JM, Rynes RI, Bartholomew LE (1987) Severe flare of rheumatoid arthritis after discontinuation of long-term methotrexate therapy. Double-blind study. Am J Med 82: 781–786
31. Szanto E (1986) Low-dose methotrexate in rheumatoid arthritis: effect and tolerance. An open trial and a double-blind randomized study. Scand J Rheumatol 15: 97–102
32. Nordstrom DM, West SG, Andersen PA, Sharp JT (1987) Pulse methotrexate therapy in rheumatoid arthritis. A controlled prospective roentgenographic study. Ann Intern Med 107: 797–801
33. Hanrahan PS, Scrivens GA, Russell AS (1989) Prospective long term follow-up of methotrexate therapy in rheumatoid arthritis: toxicity, efficacy and radiological progression. Br J Rheumatol 28: 147–153
34. Reykdal S, Steinsson K, Sigurjonsson K, Brekkan A (1989) Methotrexate treatment of rheumatoid arthritis: effects on radiological progression. Scand J Rheumatol 18: 221–226
35. Rau R, Herborn G, Karger T, Werdier D (1991) Retardation of radiologic progression in rheumatoid arthritis with methotrexate therapy: A controlled study. Arthritis Rheum 34: 1236–1244
36. Jeurissen MEC, Boerbooms AMT, van de Putte LBA, Doesburg WH, Lemmens AM (1991)Influence of methotrexate and azathioprine on radiologic progression in rheumatoid arthritis. A randomized, double-blind study. Ann Intern Med 114: 999–1004
37. Lally EV, Ho G Jr (1985) A review of methotrexate therapy in Reiter syndrome. Semin Arthritis Rheum 15: 139–145
38. Fiechtner JJ, Miller DR, Starkebaum G (1989) Reversal of neutropenia with methotrexate treatment in patients with Felty's syndrome. Correlation of response with neutrophil-reactive IgG. Arthritis Rheum 32: 194–201
39. Krall PL, Mazanec DJ, Wilke WS (1989) Methotrexate for corticosteroid-resistant polymyalgia rheumatica and giant cell arteritis. Cleve Clin J Med 56: 253–257
40. Rothenberg RJ, Graziano FM, Grandone JT, Goldberg JW, Bjarnason DF, Finesilver AG (1988) The use of methotrexate in steroid-resistant systemic lupus erythematosus. Arthritis Rheum 31: 612–615
41. Bode BY, Yocum DE, Gall EP, Yee D, Mann CC, Ko M, Boyer J, Maricic M (1990) Methotrexate (MTX) in scleroderma: Experience in ten patients. Arthritis Rheum 33: S66 (abstract)
42. van den Hoogen F, Boerbooms A, Rasker J, van Venrooij W, van de Putte L (1990) Treatment of systemic sclerosis with methotrexate: results of a one-year open study. Arthritis Rheum 33: S66 (abstract)

43. Truckenbrodt H, Hafner R (1986) Methotrexate therapy in juvenile rheumatoid arthritis: a retrospective study. Arthritis Rheum 29: 801–807
44. Wallace CA, Bleyer WA, Sherry DD, Salmonson KL, Wedgwood RJ (1989) Toxicity and serum levels of methotrexate in children with juvenile rheumatoid arthritis. Arthritis Rheum 32: 677-681
45. Giannini EH, Brewer EJ, Shaikov A, Kuzmina N, Maximov A (1991) Low dose methotrexate in recalcitrant JRA – results of the USA-USSR randomized controlled trial. Arthritis Rheum 34: S53 (abstract)
46. Toews GB, Lynch JP III (1990) Methotrexate in sarcoidosis. Am J Med Sci 300: 33–36
47. Kaplan MM, Knox TA, Arora SA (1988) Primary biliary cirrhosis treated with low-dose oral pulse methotrexate. Ann Intern Med 109: 429–431
48. Kozarek RA, Patterson DJ, Gelfand MD, Botoman VA, Ball TJ, Wilske KR (1989) Methotrexate induces clinical and histologic remission in patients with refractory inflammatory bowel disease. Ann Intern Med 110: 353–356
49. Mullarkey MF, Blumenstein BA, Andrade WP, Bailey GA, Olason I, Wetzel CE (1988) Methotrexate in the treatment of corticosteroid-dependent asthma. A double-blind crossover study. N Engl J Med 318: 603–607
50. Shiner RJ, Nunn AJ, Chung KF, Geddes DM (1990) Randomised, double-blind, placebo-controlled trial of methotrexate in steroid-dependent asthma. Lancet 336: 137–140
51. Mullarkey MF, Lammert JK, Blumenstein BA (1990) Long-term methotrexate treatment in corticosteroid-dependent asthma. Ann Intern Med 112: 577–581
52. Kaplan MM, Arora S, Pincus SH (1987) Primary sclerosing cholangitis and low-dose oral pulse methotrexate therapy. Clinical and histologic response. Ann Intern Med 106: 231–235
53. Olsen NJ, Callahan LF, Pincus T (1987) Immunologic studies of rheumatoid arthritis patients treated with methotrexate. Arthritis Rheum 30: 481–488
54. Alarcón GS, Schrohenloher RE, Bartolucci AA, Ward JR, Williams HJ, Koopman WJ (1990) Suppression of rheumatoid factor production by methotrexate in patients with rheumatoid arthritis: Evidence for differential influences of therapy and clinical status on IgM and IgA rheumatoid factor expression. Arthritis Rheum 33: 1156–1161
55. Segal R, Mozes E, Yaron M, Tartakovsky B (1989) The effects of methotrexate on the production and activity of interleukin-1. Arthritis Rheum 32: 370–377
56. Olsen NJ, Murray LM (1989) Antiproliferative effects of methotrexate on peripheral blood mononuclear cells. Arthritis Rheum 32: 378–385
57. Hirata S, Matsubara T, Saura R, Tateishi H, Hirohata K (1989) Inhibition of in vitro vascular endothelial cell proliferation and in vivo neovascularization by low-dose methotrexate. Arthritis Rheum 32: 1065–1073
58. Cronstein BN, Eberle MA, Gruber HE, Levin RI (1991) Methotrexate inhibits neutrophil function by stimulating adenosine release from connective tissue cells. Proc Natl Acad Sci USA 88: 2441–2445
59. Sperling RI, Coblyn JS, Larkin JK, Benincaso AI, Austen KF, Weinblatt ME (1990) Inhibition of leukotriene B_4 synthesis in neutrophils from patients with rheumatoid arthritis by a single oral dose of methotrexate. Arthritis Rheum 33: 1149–1155
60. Sperling RI, Benincaso AI, Anderson RJ, Coblyn JS, Austen KF, Weinblatt ME (1992) Acute and chronic suppression of leukotriene B_4 synthesis ex vivo in neutrophils from patients with rheumatoid arthritis beginning treatment with methotrexate. Arthritis Rheum (in press)
61. Welles WL, Silkworth J, Oronsky AL, Kerwar SS, Galivan J (1985) Studies on the effect of low dose methotrexate on rat adjuvant arthritis. J Rheumatol 12: 904–906
62. Herman RA, Veng-Pedersen P, Hoffman J, Koehnke R, Furst DE (1989) Pharmacokinetics of low-dose methotrexate in rheumatoid arthritis patients. J Pharm Sci 78: 165–171

63. Brooks PJ, Spruill WJ, Parish RC, Birchmore DA (1990) Pharmacokinetics of methotrexate administered by intramuscular and subcutaneous injections in patients with rheumatoid arthritis. Arthritis Rheum 33: 91–94
64. Stewart CF, Fleming RA, Arkin CR, Evans WE (1990) Coadministration of naproxen and low-dose methotrexate in patients with rheumatoid arthritis. Clin Pharmacol Ther 47: 540–546
65. Ahern M, Booth J, Loxton A, McCarthy P, Meffin P, Kevat S (1988) Methotrexate kinetics in rheumatoid arthritis: is there an interaction with nonsteroidal antiinflammatory drugs? J Rheumatol 15: 1356–1360
66. Stewart CF, Fleming RA, Germain BF, Seleznick MJ, Evans WE (1991) Aspirin alters methotrexate disposition in rheumatoid arthritis patients. Arthritis Rheum 34: 1514–1520
67. Furst DE, Koehnke R, Burmeister LF, Kohler J, Cargill I (1989) Increasing methotrexate effect with increasing dose in the treatment of resistant rheumatoid arthritis. J Rheumatol 16: 313–320
68. Gabriel S, Creagan E, O'Fallon WM, Jaquith J, Bunch T (1990) Treatment of rheumatoid arthritis with higher dose intravenous methotrexate. J Rheumatol 17: 460–465
69. Weinblatt ME (1985) Toxicity of low dose methotrexate in rheumatoid arthritis. J Rheumatol 12 [Suppl 12]: 35–39
70. Morgan SL, Baggott JE, Vaughn WH, Young PK, Austin JV, Krumdieck CL, Alarcon GS (1990) The effect of folic acid supplementation on the toxicity of low-dose methotrexate in patients with rheumatoid arthritis. Arthritis Rheum 33: 9–18
71. Tishler M, Caspi D, Fishel B, Yaron M (1988) The effects of leucovorin (folinic acid) on methotrexate therapy in rheumatoid arthritis patients. Arthritis Rheum 31: 906–908
72. Buckley LM, Vacek PM, Cooper SM (1990) Administration of folinic acid after low dose methotrexate in patients with rheumatoid arthritis. J Rheumatol 17: 1158–1161
73. Kerwar SS, Oronsky AL (1989) Methotrexate in rheumatoid arthritis: studies with animal models. Adv Enzyme Regul 29: 247–265
74. Maricic M, Davis M, Gall EP (1986) Megaloblastic pancytopenia in a patient receiving concurrent methotrexate and trimethoprim-sulfamethoxazole treatment. Arthritis Rheum 29: 133–135
75. Weinblatt ME, Fraser P (1989) Elevated mean corpuscular volume as a predictor of hematologic toxicity due to methotrexate therapy. Arthritis Rheum 32: 1592–1596
76. Marks CR, Willkens RF, Wilske KR, Brown PB (1984) Small-vessel vasculitis and methotrexate (letter). Ann Intern Med 100: 916
77. Segal R, Caspi D, Tishler M, Fishel B, Yaron M (1988) Accelerated nodulosis and vasculitis during methotrexate therapy for rheumatoid arthritis. Arthritis Rheum 31: 1182–1185
78. Shamberger RC, Rosenberg SA, Seipp CA, Sherins RJ (1981) Effects of high-dose methotrexate and vincristine on ovarian and testicular functions in patients undergoing postoperative adjuvant treatment of osteosarcoma. Cancer Treat Rep 65: 739–746
79. Sussman A, Leonard JM (1980) Psoriasis, methotrexate, and oligospermia. Arch Dermatol 116: 215–217
80. Rustia M, Shubik P (1973) Life-span carcinogenicity tests with 4-amino-N10-methylpteroylglutamic acid (methotrexate) in Swiss mice and Syrian golden hamsters. Toxicol Appl Pharmacol 26: 329–338
81. Rustin GJ, Rustin F, Dent J, Booth M, Salt S, Bagshawe KD (1983) No increase in second tumors after cytotoxic chemotherapy for gestational trophoblastic tumors. N Engl J Med 308: 473–476
82. Bailin PL, Tindall JP, Roenigk HH Jr, Hogan MD (1975)Is methotrexate therapy for psoriasis carcinogenic? A modified retrospective-prospective analysis. JAMA 232: 359–362

83. Stern RS, Zierler S, Parrish JA (1982) Methotrexate used for psoriasis and the risk of noncutaneous or cutaneous malignancy. Cancer 50: 869–872
84. St Clair EW, Rice JR, Snyderman R (1985) Pneumonitis complicating low-dose methotrexate therapy in rheumatoid arthritis. Arch Intern Med 145: 2035–2038
85. Carson CW, Cannon GW, Egger MJ, Ward JR, Clegg DO (1987) Pulmonary disease during the treatment of rheumatoid arthritis with low dose pulse methotrexate. Semin Arthritis Rheum 16: 186–195
86. Searles G, McKendry RJ (1987) Methotrexate pneumonitis in rheumatoid arthritis: potential risk factors. Four case reports and a review of the literature. J Rheumatol 14: 1164–1171
87. Kaplan RL, Waite DH (1978) Progressive interstitial lung disease from prolonged methotrexate therapy. Arch Dermatol 114: 1800–1802
88. Perruquet JL, Harrington TM, Davis DE (1983) Pneumocystis carinii pneumonia following methotrexate therapy for rheumatoid arthritis (letter) Arthritis Rheum 26: 1291–1292
89. Altz-Smith M, Kendall LG Jr, Stamm AM (1987) Cryptococcosis associated with low-dose methotrexate for arthritis. Am J Med 83: 179-181
90. Weinblatt ME, Kremer JM (1988) Methotrexate in rheumatoid arthritis. J Am Acad Dermatol 19: 126–128
91. Kremer JM, Lee RG, Tolman KG (1989) Liver histology in rheumatoid arthritis patients receiving long-term methotrexate therapy. A prospective study with baseline and sequential biopsy samples. Arthritis Rheum 32: 121–127
92. Aponte J, Petrelli M (1988) Histopathologic findings in the liver of rheumatoid arthritis patients treated with long-term bolus methotrexate. Arthritis Rheum 31: 1457-1464
93. Phillips C, Cera P, Mangan T, Newman E (1990) Liver disease in rheumatoid arthritis (RA) patients on methotrexate (MTX). Arthritis Rheum 33: S60 (abstract)
94. Augur NA, Anderson LC, Cogen L, Miller M, Morton GL (1990) Prospective study of hepatotoxicity in patients receiving methotrexate for rheumatoid arthritis. Arthritis Rheum 33: S60 (abstract)
95. Clegg DO, Furst DE, Tolman KG, Pogue R (1989) Acute, reversible hepatic failure associated with methotrexate treatment of rheumatoid arthritis. J Rheumatol 16: 1123–1126
96. Kujala GA, Shamma'a JM, Chang WL, Brick JE (1990) Hepatitis with bridging fibrosis and reversible hepatic insufficiency in a woman with rheumatoid arthritis taking methotrexate. Arthritis Rheum 33: 1037–1041
97. Weinblatt M, Walker AM, Funch D, Dreyer NA, Alarcón G, Klippel J, Kremer J, Lee R, Tolman K (1991) Serious liver disease in methotrexate-treated rheumatoid arthritis patients. Arthritis Rheum 34: S49 (abstract)
98. Wernick R, Smith DL (1989) Central nervous system toxicity associated with weekly low-dose methotrexate treatment. Arthritis Rheum 32: 770–775
99. Fries JF (1989) Advances in management of rheumatic disease 1965 to 1985. Arch Intern Med 149: 1002–1011
100. Weinblatt ME (1988) Aggressive therapy of rheumatoid arthritis. Postgraduate advances in rheumatology. Forum Medicum

Intravenous Immunoglobulins in the Treatment of Autoimmune Diseases

V. Hurez and *M. D. Kazatchkine*

Intravenous immunoglobulins (IVIg) have been used increasingly over the past 10 years in the treatment of a large number of autoimmune and systemic inflammatory diseases [1]. A recent consensus conference conducted by the National Institute of Health [2] has emphasized the need for a better understanding of the mechanisms by which IVIg modulate autoimmune responses. As discussed in this review, the immunomodulatory effects of IVIg may depend on interactions between the Fc portion of infused IgG with Fc receptors on inflammatory cells and lymphocytes and/or on the modulation of the expressed antibody repertoire through the interaction of variable regions of IVIg with circulating immunoglobulins and antigen receptors on immunocompetent cells.

Intravenous Immunoglobulins

IVIg are prepared from large pools of plasma of more than 15 000 healthy blood donors. Most preparations that are currently available contain almost exclusively intact IgG. The subclass distribution is that of normal serum, and the half-life of infused immunoglobulins is 3 weeks. The most commonly used preparations of IVIg contain less than 5% of Fc-dependent IgG aggregates, 0% – 7% of $F(ab')_2$ fragments, and traces of IgA and IgM.

Therapeutic Effect of IVIg in Autoimmune and Systemic Inflammatory Diseases

A beneficial role of IVIg has been discribed in several autoimmune and systemic inflammatory diseases [1, 3]. Those in which a clinical improvement and/or decrease in autoantibody titer has been established in clinical trials or suggested by open trials or preliminary reports include the following:

Idiopathic thrombocytopenic purpura
Autoimmune hemolytic anemias
Autoimmune neutropenia

Anti-factor VIII autoimmune disease
Autoimmune erythroblastopenia

Myasthenia gravis
Guillain-Barré syndrome
Chronic inflammatory demyelinating polyneuropathy
Antineutrophil cytoplasmic autoantibody positive systemic vasculitis
Systemic lupus erythematosus
Rheumatoid arthritis

Birdshot retinopathy
Juvenile diabetes
Multiple sclerosis

Kawasaki's disease
Refractory polymyositis

Graft-versus-host disease

The diseases are tentatively classified into autoantibody-mediated peripheral autoimmune cytopenias, autoimmune diseases in which there is evidence for a pathogenic role of autoantibodies, autoimmune diseases in which there is evidence for a pathogenic role of autoreactive T cells, and inflammatory diseases for which there is little or no evidence for an autoimmune origin. Some of these diseases are clearly of autoimmune origin, mediated by autoantibodies or autoreactive T cells; for other diseases, the autoimmune origin is only presumptive.

The first report of a beneficial effect of IVIg in autoimmune disease was in patients with ITP, a bleeding disorder characterized by an accelerated splenic removal of platelets opsonized with autoantibodies. In the acute form of ITP, IVIg therapy has a short-lived beneficial effect in the majority of patients [4, 5]. Administration of IVIg (0.4 g/kg body weight for 5 days) is followed by an increase in platelet counts occuring within 24–76 h and often lasting for 15–25 days. In the chronic forms of ITP, a long-term improvement is achieved in more than 60% of patients if the treatment is started within 6 months from the onset of the disease [4]. As in the case of other peripheral autoimmune cytopenias, the short-term effect of IVIg in acute ITP has been attributed to a transient blockade of Fc receptor function of splenic macrophages and to the subsequent decrease in the splenic clearance of antibody-coated platelets [5]. Mechanisms of action of IVIg other than Fc receptor blockade such as anti-idiotype mediated inhibition of antiplatelet antibodies [6] may also contribute to the beneficial effect of IVIg treatment.

Severe bleeding complications are often associated with the occurence of anti-factor VIII autoantibodies. Several reports have demonstrated that the administration of IVIg may suppress anti-factor VIII autoantibody activity within the first 2 days of treatment [7]. In a few patients the suppressive effect of IVIg has lasted for several years. In vitro studies have demonstrated that IVIg and $F(ab')_2$ from IVIg inhibit anti-factor VIII autoantibody activity in patients' serum, IgG, and $F(ab')_2$ fragments of IgG. The ability of IVIg to neutralize anti-factor VIII autoantibodies in vitro has correlated with the therapeutic effect in vivo in several patients [8].

Idiopathic systemic vasculitides are frequently associated with ANCA. Preliminary studies performed on patients who did not respond to conventional immunosuppressive therapy have indicated that IVIg may be effective in ANCA-positive vasculitides, and that the clinical therapeutic effect is associated with a decrease in ANCA activity in serum [9]. IVIg and $F(ab')_2$ from IVIg have been shown to inhibit the binding of ANCA to the autoantigens [10].

The therapeutic effect of IVIg in human autoimmune diseases has been reviewed in detail in the recent article by Dwyer [3].

Mechanisms of Action of IVIg in Autoimmune and Systemic Inflammatory Diseases

IVIg may be effective in autoimmune diseases by mechanisms involving the Fc portion of IgG and/or variable regions of infused antibodies.

Fc-Dependent Mechanism of Action of IVIg

The blockade of Fc receptor on splenic macrophages probably plays a critical role in the short-term beneficial effect of IVIg therapy in peripheral autoimmune cytopenias. Administration of IVIg is followed by a decrease in the clearance of autologous erythrocytes coated with anti-D antibodies in vivo [5]; peripheral blood monocytes from IVIg-treated patients with ITP exhibit a decreased ability to form rosettes with IgG-coated erythrocytes in vitro [11]; a similar effect to that of IVIg on platelet counts may be achieved in ITP patients by blocking Fc receptors with anti-D antibodies [12] or with monoclonal antibodies directed against FcγRIII [13].

Some of the immunomodulatory effects of IVIg may be mediated by the binding of IVIg to Fcγ receptors of B and/or T cells. Aggregated or complexed IgG has been shown to inhibit antibody synthesis by B cells; in addition, the suppressive effect of anti-idiotypic antibodies on B cells has been shown to require binding of the antibody to the target cell via both the antibody combining site and the Fc portion [14].

The anti-inflammatory effect of IVIg may depend on the ability of IVIg to down-regulate the synthesis and/or release of proinflammatory mediators and cytokines by monocyte and macrophages. IVIg was shown to inhibit the release of interleukin (IL) 1, tumor necrosis factor-α, and IL-6 from lipopolysaccharide-stimulated cultures of human monocytes [15]. The binding of IVIg to Fc receptors on monocytes also induces the synthesis and release of an antagonist molecule of IL-1 (IL-1 Ra). These effects explain the antipyretic activity of IVIg in patients with systemic inflammatory diseases (e.g., Kawasaki's disease) and in experimental animals [16].

Another postulated Fc-dependent mechanism of action of IVIg is the interaction of the Fc with complement components in the fluid phase and/or on the targets of complement activation. IVIg was shown to protect guinea pigs from shock induced by lethal doses of anti-Forssman antibodies [17]. The effect of IVIg was mediated by covalent binding of C3b and C4b to the infused IgG, preventing the activated components from binding to antibody-coated endothelial cells.

V Region Dependent Mechanisms of Action of IVIg

Infusion of IVIg results in changes in the expressed antibody repertoire. These may depend on interactions between variable regions of infused IgG and antibodies and/or antigen receptors on lymphocytes and in subsequent alterations in the regulatory function of immune networks. Immunomodulatory effect of IVIg may also depend on the presence of natural antibodies to functional surface molecules of B and T lymphocytes other than surface immunoglobulin or T cell receptor.

The presence in IVIg of an anti-idiotypic activity directed against pathological autoantibodies was first demonstrated in patients with autoantibodies to factor VIII in whom infusion of IVIg had resulted in decreased autoantibody titers [7]. Incubation of $F(ab')_2$ fragments of the patients' IgG with $F(ab')_2$ fragments of IVIg resulted in a dose-dependent neutralization of autoantibody activity in vitro. In further studies IVIg were shown to interact with the combining site of a variety of other autoantibodies [6, 10, 18–22]. Three additional lines of evidence contribute to demonstrate that IVIg interact with autoantibodies through idiotypic interactions: (a) Autoantibody activity in $F(ab')_2$ fragments of patients' IgG is specifically retained on affinity columns of Sepharose-bound $F(ab')_2$ of IVIg. (b) IVIg do not contain antibodies against allotypes in the $F(ab')_2$ region of human IgG [20]. (c) IVIg recognize idiotypes on autoantibodies that are defined targets for heterologous anti-idiotypic antibodies. One such idiotype was shown to be an alpha, immunodominant cross-reactive idiotype expressed by anti-thyroglobulin antibodies from patients with autoimmune thyroiditis, but not by natural anti-thyroglobulin antibodies from healthy individuals [22]. Anti-idiotypic activity of IVIg against cross-reactive idiotypes on disease-specific autoantibodies may be relevant for the suppressive effect of IVIg on autoantibodies from some but not all patients with a given autoimmune disease; this suggests that normal human IgG contains regulatory anti-idiotypes which prevent expansion of pathogenic autoantibody clones under physiological conditions.

The presence in IVIg of antibodies interacting idiotypically with disease-associated antibodies is related to the large number of donors contributing to the pool. Increasing the number of donors increases the probability that "privileged" donors with high titer of anti-idiotypes against autoantibodies contribute to the pool; such donors could be, for example, individuals who have recovered from autoimmune diseases through autologous idiotypic suppression of autoantibodies [8, 22]. Pools of IVIg may also be enriched in

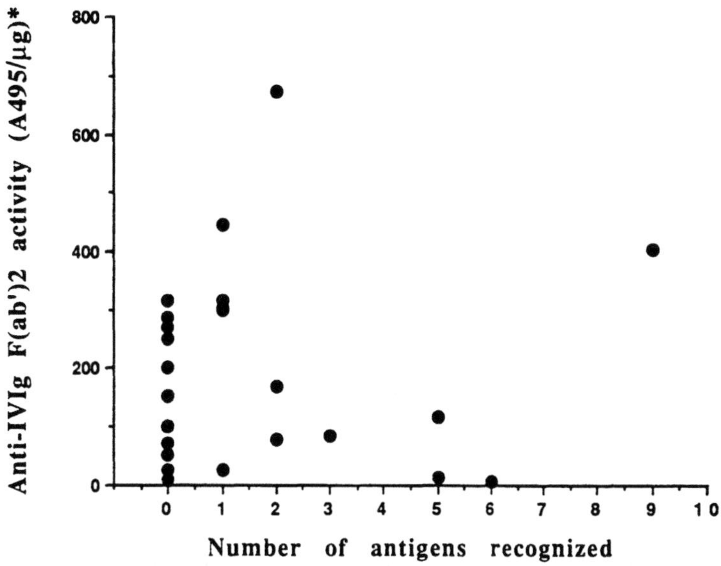

Fig. 1. Binding of IgM antibodies from Epstein-Barr virus (EBV) transformed human B cells to $F(ab')_2$ fragments from IVIg. The figure shows the lack of correlation between the binding activity of natural IgM antibodies to $F(ab')_2$ from IVIg and the relative degree of polyreactivity of the IgM. *Abcissa*, the number of antigens recognized by IgM antibodies. The specific anti-IVIg $F(ab')_2$ activity (A495/µg) was measured by enzyme-linked immunosorbent assay on microtiter plates coated with $F(ab')_2$ from IVIg using a 1:5 dilution of EBV-transformed cell culture supernatants

anti-idiotypic activity against autoantibodies because of a synergistic effect resulting from mixing antibodies together so that a pool of IVIg may express anti-idiotypic activity that is not detectable in the IgG of individual donors contributing to the pool [23]. Thus the content of an IgG pool in complementary pairs of antibodies increases with the number of donors in the pool. This is consistent with the observations by Roux and Tankersley of $F(ab')_2$ – $F(ab')_2$ dimers in large pools of IgG [24].

We have shown that, in addition to idiotypes on pathogenic autoantibodies, IVIg recognize idiotypic determinants on natural autoantibodies from healthy individuals. Thus, IVIg interacts idiotypically with IgM autoantibodies secreted by EBV-transformed normal peripheral blood B cells (Fig. 1) [25] and natural IgG antibodies such as those present within the IVIg preparation itself (Fig. 2). The presence in IVIg of natural IgG autoantibodies and complementary IgG molecules indicates that normal human serum IgG contains an autoreactive idiotypically connected subfraction [26]. Our current working hypothesis is that autoimmune disease is associated with a primary or acquired defect in regulatory antibody networks, and that infusion of IVIg suppress autoimmune responses by restoring a physiological control of autoreactivity by bringing to the patient normal elements of the network in which he is deficient. Direct evidence for this hypothesis comes from the

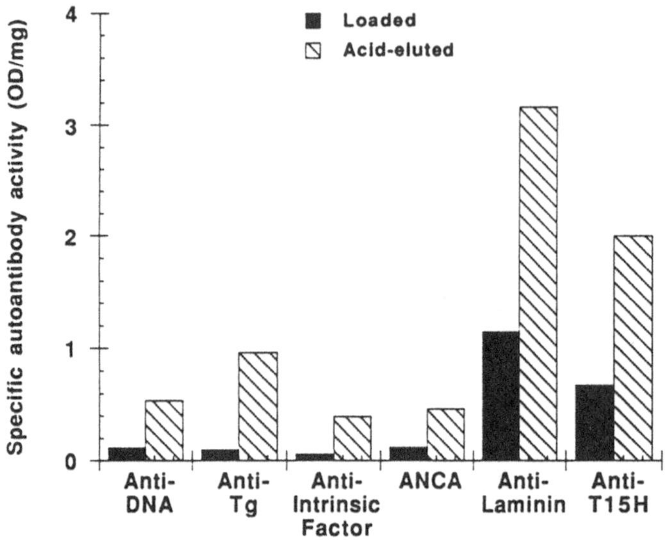

Fig. 2. Affinity chromatography of $F(ab')_2$ fragments from IVIg on Separose-bound $F(ab')_2$ fragments from IVIg. The figure depicts the specific autoantibody activity (OD/mg) of IVIg (loaded, *black bars*) and of IgG capable of binding to $F(ab')_2$ fragments of IVIg (acid-eluted, *hatched bars*). The autoantibody activity was assessed by enzyme-linked immunosorbent assay on microtiter plates coated with DNA, thyroglobulin (*Tg*), intrinsic factor, neutrophil cytoplasmic antigens (*ANCA*), laminin, and the T15H(50-73) self-binding peptide [29]

analysis of spontaneous changes in the expression of the autoreactive repertoire in healthy individuals and patients with autoimmune diseases treated with IVIg. In healthy individuals, autoantibody activity fluctuates with a well-defined periodicity, indicating that expression of the autoreactive repertoire is under the constraint of a functional regulatory network. The kinetics of spontaneous fluctuations of autoantibodies is perturbed in patients with autoimmune diseases and in autoimmune animals [27]. Preliminary results from our laboratory indicate that infusion of IVIg restores a normal kinetic pattern of expression of autoantibodies in serum of patients with autoimmune diseases. In addition, IVIg has been shown to modify the VH family gene usage in animal models, indicating that circulating immunoglobulins contribute to select the expressed preimmune repertoire [28].

Infusion of high amounts of normal IgG results in modulation of cellular functions of immunocompetent cells and alterations in the expressed immune repertoire. IVIg may thus provide a substitutive therapy for the quantitative and/or qualitative defect in network regulation that are associated with autoimmune diseases [29].

Acknowledgements. This work was supported by Institut National de la Santé et de la Recherche Médicale (INSERM), France, and the Central Laboratory of the Swiss Red Cross Blood Transfusion Service, Bern, Switzerland.

References

1. Kaveri SV, Dietrich G, Hurez V, Kazatchkine MD (1991) Intravenous immunoglobulins (IVIg) in the treatment of autoimmune diseases. Clin Exp Immunol 86: 192–198
2. Department of Health and Human Services (1990) Intravenous immune globulin: consensus statement. NIH Consensus Developement Conference May 1990, vol 8 (5). Department of Health and Human Services, Bethesda, pp 21–23
3. Dwyer MD (1992) Manipulating the immune system with immune globulin. N Engl J Med 326: 107–116
4. Imbach P, Muller B, Imholz B et al. (1986) Intravenous immunoglobulin therapy in immune thrombocytopenic purpura (ITP) and other immune related haemorrhagic disorders in childhood. In: Morell A, Nydegger UE (eds) Clinical use of intravenous immunoglobulins. Academic, London, pp 177–186
5. Fehr J, Hofmann V, Kappeler U (1982) Transient reversal of thrombocytopenia in idiopathic thrombocytopenic purpura by high dose intravenous gammaglobulin. N Engl J Med 306: 1254–1258
6. Berchtold P, Dale GL, Tani P et al. (1989) Inhibition of autoantibody binding to platelet glycoprotein IIb/IIa by anti-idiotypic antibodies in intravenous immunoglobulins. Blood 74: 2414–2417
7. Sultan Y, Kazatchkine MD, Maisonneuve P et al. (1984) Anti-idiotypic suppression of autoantibodies to factor VIII (anti-haemophilic factor) by high-dose intravenous immunoglobulin. Lancet ii: 765–768
8. Sultan Y, Rossi F, Kazatchkine MD (1987) Recovery from anti-VIIIc (anti-hemophilic factor) autoimmune disease is dependent on generation of anti-idiotypes against anti-VIIIc autoantibodies. Proc Natl Acad Sci USA 84: 828–831
9. Jayne DRW, Davies MJ, Fox CJV et al. (1991) Treatment of systemic vasculitis with pooled intravenous immunoglobulin. Lancet 337: 1137–1139
10. Rossi F, Jayne DRW, Lockwood CM et al. (1991) Anti-idiotypes against anti-neutrophil cytoplasm antigen autoantibodies in normal human polyspecific IgG for therapeutic use and in the remission sera of patients with systemic vasculitis. Clin Exp Immunol 83: 1–6
11. Kimberly RP, Salmon JE, Bussel JB et al. (1984) Modulation of mononuclear phagocyte function by intravenous gammaglobulin. J Immunol 132: 745–750
12. Salama A, Mueller-Eckhart C, Kiefel V (1983) Effect of intravenous immunoglobulin in immune thrombocytopenia. Competitive inhibition of the reticuloendothelial system function by sequestration by autologous red blood cells. Lancet ii: 193–195
13. Clarkson SB, Bussel JB, Kimberly RP et al. (1986) Treatment of refractory immune thrombocytopenic purpura with an anti Fc gamma receptor antibody. N Engl J Med 314: 1236–1239
14. Uher F, Dickler HB (1986) Cooperativity between B lymphocyte membrane molecules: independent ligand occupancy and cross-linking of antigen receptors and Fcγ receptors down regulates B lymphocyte function. J Immunol 137: 3124–3129
15. Shimozato T, Iwata M, Kawada H et al. (1991) Human immunoglobulin preparation for intravenous use induces elevation of cellular cyclic adenosine 3':5'-monophosphate levels, resulting in suppression of tumor necrosis factor alpha and interleukin-1 production. Immunology 72: 497–501
16. Iwata M, Shimozato T, Tokiwa H, Tsubura E (1987) Antipyretic activity of a human immunoglobulin preparation for intravenous use in an experimental model of fever in rabbits. Infect Immun 55: 547–552
17. Basta M, Langlois PF, Marques M et al. (1989) High-dose intravenous immunoglobulin modifies complement-mediated in vivo clearance. Blood 74: 326–333
18. Van Doorn PA, Rossi F, Brand A et al. (1990) On the mechanism of high dose intravenous immunoglobulin treatment of patients with chronic inflammatory demyelinating polyneuropathy. J Neuroimmunology 29: 57–64

19. McGuire WA, Yang HH, Bruno E et al. (1987) Treatment of antibody-mediated pure red-cell aplasia with high-dose intravenous gammaglobulin. N Engl J Med 317: 1004–1008
20. Rossi F, Sultan Y, Kazatchkine MD (1988) Anti-idiotypes against autoantibodies and alloantibodies to factor VIIIc (anti-hemophilic factor) are present in therapeutic polyspecific normal immunoglobulins. Clin Exp Immunol 74: 311–316
21. Rossi F, Kazatchkine MD (1989) Antiidiotypes against autoantibodies in pooled normal human polyspecific Ig. J Immunol 143: 4104–4109
22. Dietrich G, Kazatchkine MD (1990) Normal immunoglobulin G (IgG) for therapeutic use (intravenous Ig) contain antiidiotypic specifities against an immunodominant, disease-associated, cross-reactive idiotype of human anti-thyroglobulin autoantibodies. J Clin Invest 85: 620–625
23. Dietrich G, Algiman M, Sultan Y et al. (1992) Origin of anti-idiotypic activity against autoantibody in pools of normal human immunoglobulin G (IVIg). Blood 79: 1–5
24. Roux KH, Tankersley DL (1990) A view of the human idiotypic repertoire: electron microscopic and immunologic analysis of spontaneous idiotype – anti-idiotype dimers in pooled human IgG. J Immunol 144: 1387–1395
25. Rossi F, Guilbert B, Tonnelle C et al. (1990) Idiotypic interactions between normal human polyspecific IgG and natural IgM antibodies. Eur J Immunol 20: 2089–2094
26. Dietrich G, Kaveri SV, Kazatchkine MD (1992) A V region-connected subfraction of normal human serum immunoglobulin G. Eur J Immunol 22: 1701–1706
27. Varela F, Anderson A, Dietrich G et al. (1991) The population dynamics of antibodies in normal and autoimmune individuals. Proc Natl Acad Sci USA 88: 5917–5921
28. Freitas AA, Viale AC, Sundblad A et al. (1991) Normal serum immunoglobulins participate in the selection of peripheral B-cell repertoires. Proc Natl Acad Sci USA 88: 5640–5644
29. Dietrich G, Kaveri SV, Kazatchkine MD (1992) Modulation of autoimmunity by intravenous immunoglobulins (IVIg) through interactions with the function of the immune/idiotypic network. Clin Immunol Immunopathol 62: S73–S81

Plasmapheresis and Subsequent Pulse Cyclophosphamide in Systemic Lupus Erythematosus

H.H. Euler

Cyclophosphamide in SLE

Cyclophosphamide (Ctx) is activated in the liver. It alkylates DNA during the cell cycle G_2 phase and inhibits mitotic activity. Its major side effects are amenorrhea, alopecia, infections during leukocytopenia, hemorrhagic cystitis, lung fibrosis [35], and secondary malignancies [2, 3, 26, 45, 68]. Ctx was introduced for treating systemic lupus erythematosus (SLE) in 1964 [56]. Early controlled trials in lupus nephrotic syndrome revealed a significant reduction in relapse frequence [7]. Double-blind trials showed a tendency toward improved kidney function during Ctx therapy [105]. A meta-analysis [44] indicated that oral Ctx or azathioprine led to reduced mortality and reduced incidence of kidney failure as compared with prednisone (Prd) alone. Since then, several reports have described Ctx as effective for most SLE manifestations [44, 89]. Ctx is usually given orally, either in a constant dosage (e.g., 100–150 mg/day) or adjusted to reduce the white blood cell (WBC) count to approximately 2.0 to 4.0/nl.

Intravenous pulse Ctx (0.5–1 g/m^2 every 3–12 weeks) was introduced in SLE in 1982 [34], and in some centers it is increasingly replacing oral Ctx [2, 45, 87]. In a controlled long-term study (lasting up to 13 years) on 107 patients with lupus nephritis [2] (update: [106]) pulse Ctx tended to induce better long-term results and fewer side effects (neoplasia and infection). The latter may have been due to the lower cumulative Ctx dose [3]. The survival rate was not higher in patients treated with pulse Ctx; however, fatal courses were observed in 23/107 patients [87, 106]. Serious side effects have been reported following pulse Ctx [48, 66]. Uncontrolled studies in which pulse Ctx was administered have led to positive results in CNS lupus [45, 72], SLE-associated thrombocytopenia [10], aplastic anemia [37], and lupus transverse myelitis [5] but not in lupus myositis [9]. When cytotoxic drugs have been administered previously, bone marrow recovery before pulse Ctx is mandatory [66]. An advantage of pulse Ctx is its more rapid initial effect. A problem might be the intervals between pulses. During these intervals not only the bone marrow but also disease activity may recover. Possibly, the most intensive initial effect should be achieved with a maximum pulse prior to oral maintenance treatment [26, 100].

Whether and how the administration of supplementary drugs might influence the efficacy of pulse Ctx has not yet been evaluated. Since it is

M. M. Eibl, C. Huber, H. H. Decker, U. Wahn (Eds.)
Symposium in Immunology I
Symposium in Immunology II

thought that Ctx has its predominant effect on proliferating lymphocytes, especially T-helper lympocytes [29], and since experimentally the presence of Prd retards this proliferation [25, 31, 36, 83, 97, 102], the efficacy of Ctx might be increased by avoiding Prd prior to, during, and immediately after pulse Ctx.

Plasmapheresis in SLE

The basic concept of plasmapheresis was first described in 1902 [53]. In 1974–1975 the procedure was applied by Jones et al. in SLE [62] and by Lockwood et al. in Goodpasture's syndrome [77]. This was followed by a large number of case reports and small patients series. The prevailing result was that the effect was beneficial in the short term, but that without accompanying immunosuppression relapses occurred soon [60, 61, 63, 65, 73, 98]. Again, treatment-free long-term remissions were not achieved.

A controlled double-blind study [121] revealed no difference between plasmapheresis and sham plasmapheresis with continued immunosuppression in 20 cases of mild lupus. The French Cooperative Study Group [8, 46] compared steroids plus plasmapheresis versus steroids alone in 39 patients over a period of 29 months and did not detect a significant difference. The Dutch Cooperative Study Group published similar results: 20 patients were treated eiher with Prd and plasmapheresis or with Prd and cytotoxic drugs. Neither protocol was superior [32]. A further randomized study of 86 patients with lupus nephritis was performed in 1981–1986 and was published recently [74]. No significant difference was found between Ctx and Prd plus plasmapheresis versus Ctx and Prd alone. In a randomized trial [22] better results tended to be achieved in 39 patients with lupus nephritis by combining Prd and cytotoxic drugs with plasmapheresis and by substitution with human albumin. Wallace et al. [120] analyzed a number of variables in 27 patients with severe lupus nephritis. Compared with treatments that did not involve plasmapheresis, plasmapheresis was associated with a more rapid improvement of laboratory parameters, and all 7 patients who had the best response (resolution of nephrotic syndrome and normalization of creatinine) had been subjected to plasmapheresis. Thus, the currently generally accepted view tends to skip plasmapheresis procedures from treatment protocols of SLE [16] despite the fact that most case reports describe rapid improvement in life-threatening situations (which are hardly investigable by controlled trials) and the fact that all previous trials have combined plasmapheresis with preexisting and continued immunosuppressive treatment, which might be the wrong approach for dealing with the basic immunologic mechanisms induced by antibody depletion.

Antibody Kinetics Following Antibody Depletion

In these previous investigations a long-term reduction of autoantibody levels generally was not possible [13], although each exchange of one plasma volume eliminates approximately 50% of circulating IgG. When no long-term depletion is achieved, despite multiple repetitions and parallel immunosuppression, it must be assumed that there is a feedback cycle that counterbalances the losses. Within this feedback cycle between antibodies and their resynthesis, the term "antibody rebound" is used to describe enhanced antibody synthesis (or excretion) following antibody depletion [13–15, 116]. This mechanism might have played a crucial role in the previous negative results with therapeutic plasmapheresis. On the other hand, it may be possible to use it to increase clonal deletion if pulse cytotoxic drugs are administered during the period of increased lymphocyte activity and vulnerability. Evidence of the existence of this feedback cycle is discussed below.

Antibody Rebound: Theoretical Considerations

In closed biological systems a feedback between a product and the producing cell is the rule. The opposite – a productive mechanism that is not influenced by its product – has rarely been demonstrated in nonneoplastic diseases. It can be assumed that antibody production is subject to a regulatory mechanism since it does not end abruptly with the disappearance of the corresponding antigenic stimulus. Another argument favoring the existence of a regulatory mechanism is the observation that initial titers are reached again within a reasonable period of time. This becomes even more evident when we consider the individual components of antibody resynthesis following antibody elimination.

One component is redistribution from the extravascular space. Approximately 50% of IgG is distributed in the extravascular space [70]. Redistribution is largely completed within 24 h [21]. Thus, following exchange of one plasma volume eliminating 50% of intravascular IgG [67], a rapid reincrease to 75% of the initial titer can be expected. The second component is the basic synthesis rate, which must initially be assumed to be constant. Assuming steady-state conditions and a 50% turnover rate for human IgG of 20 (18–23) days [70], 2.5% is resynthesized within 24 h. The third component is decreasing catabolism. Normally, resynthesis is balanced by the respective catabolism rate. Catabolism diminishes to compensate for protein depletion [21, 70]. Assuming catabolism were to halt completely, decreased catabolism might induce a daily IgG increase of up to 2.5%. Enhanced clearance of the reticuloendothelial system following plasmapheresis [78] represents a fourth component. In contrast to the mechanisms described above, this aspect tends to retard reincreasing antibody titers, but it is difficult to quantify. Any further increase indicates enhanced neosynthesis or enhanced excretion

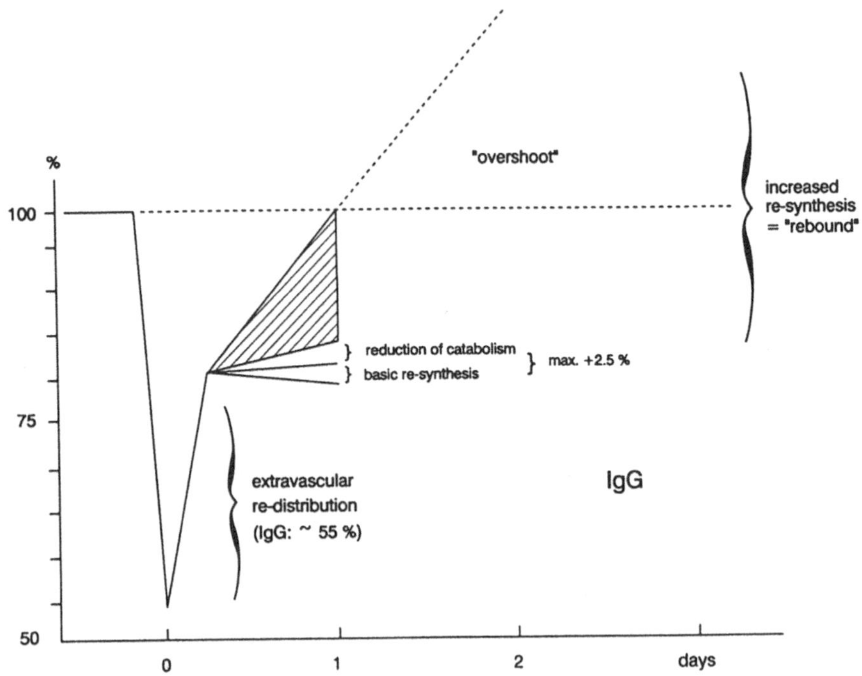

Fig. 1. Components of reincreasing antibody titers following plasmapheresis (one plasma volume)

(Fig. 1). It is important to note that there is still a considerable difference between the renewed increase due to redistribution, basic resynthesis, and altered catabolism, on the one hand, and the initial titer, on the other. This difference represents the "scope" in which enhanced compensatory synthesis, i.e., the "rebound," can take place. Although rebound kinetics overshooting the baseline have been described [14, 33, 111], rebound without overshoot should be more frequent. Possibly, the discussion of the existence of rebound kinetics has not come to final conclusions because of early experimental data [14, 15, 40, 111] that were partially modified later [42], and that did not take these more detailed calculations into account, leading to expect drastic overshoot kinetics following antibody depletion.

Another important aspect might be the following calculation: the basic synthesis rate of an IgG antibody is approximately 2.5% of the amount of this antibody in circulation. A 100% increase in the synthesis rate represents a scarcely measurable 2.5% increase in the antibody titer. Despite this small absolute difference, however, this 100% increase should correspond to a 100% increase in lymphocyte proliferation and thus a 100% increase in vulnerability.

Antibody Rebound: Experimental Evidence

Experimental evidence suggesting that circulating antibodies are a component of a feedback mechanism regulating antibody synthesis has long been available [14, 15, 50, 111, 115]. Uhr and Baumann [115] and others [12, 18, 19, 90, 116, 122] have shown in animal models that antibody synthesis can be specifically suppressed by passive administration of complete antibodies as well as of Fab' of F(ab')$_2$ fragments of the same specificity before or during immunization with various antigens. The expected reverse effect, i.e., stimulation of resynthesis following antibody depletion, was demonstrated by Graf and Uhr [50] in 1969 by means of immunoadsorption in the rabbit. This was later confirmed to be clonally specific by exchange transfusion with reduction of specific antibodies [15]. In recent studies as well, antibodies in the rat could not be decreased to below 50% of the values of untreated controls despite elimination of several plasma volumes [119]. Furthermore, levels rose to the values of untreated controls within 7 days despite repeated plasmaphereses that lowered antibody levels by 75% – 87.5% [92]. In addition, an overshooting rebound of naturally occurring xenoantibodies was observed beginning on day +2 and reaching a 16-fold increase 3 days after plasma removal [91]. By contrast, however, another immunization schedule using bovine insulin did not result in an IgG rebound following 4 weeks of plasmapheresis in rabbits [20]. Activation by antibody depletion at the cellular level has been reported only once [109]. The observation of more pronounced activation after an initial immunization than after a second immunization [11] remains unconfirmed.

Despite this ostensibly clear picture some critical remarks are necessary. Measured against the clinical significance of this issue, it has been dealt with by very few groups. Sham controls to dinstinguish between nonspecific polyclonal effects and specific clonal effects have seldom been performed. Factors influencing lymphocyte kinetics by substitution media have not been investigated, although in vitro proof exists of B cell stimulation in rats, for example, by dextran sulfate [84]. Whether the antibody kinetics following depletion are dependent of the antigen [86], and – of special importance – whether resting and active clones are subject to the same compensatory mechanism, are aspects that have scarcely been examined.

The molecular mechanism controlling lymphocyte activation following antibody depletion is only partially known. It may include clonal stimulation through antigen liberation [112, 116], shifting antigen/antibody ratios within circulating immune complexes toward antigen-rich, B cell stimulating complexes [17, 108] and/or coelimination of suppressive anti-idiotypes [23, 94].

Antibody Rebound: Clinical Evidence

As early as 1957 it was noticed that in immunized plasma donors specific antibody levels remained more clearly elevated than in controls without plasma donation [103]. This is in accordance with routine laboratory knowledge that high antibody titers are best obtained by starting bloodletting shortly after immunization.

In SLE, evidence of increased production of immune complexes and autoantibodies following depletion has been reported [60, 63, 65, 71, 98]. This led to a warning against plasmapheresis without accompanying immunosuppression [63, 98]. Similar evidence also exists for rhesus incompatibility and morbus hemolyticus neonatorum [4, 59], diabetes mellitus [81], rheumatoid arthritis [118], and pemphigus vulgaris [95].

On the whole, however, clinical examples of rebound effects are few. There may be several reasons for this. Principally, simultaneous immunosuppression [24, 101] exerts a mitigating effect on these kinetics. Furthermore, the lack of extreme overshoot kinetics may have been interpreted as an absence of rebound. In addition, inferences drawn from observations in healthy controls may have led to false conclusions; in the former circulating immunoglobulins should originate from resting clones, which are only slightly subject to rebound kinetics [33], whereas pathogenic clones should exhibit a higher degree of activity and be easier to stimulate. Finally, Nasca et al. [86] found evidence that different clones react differently to depletion, depending on the antigen. This could explain the differences in kinetics between various autoimmune diseases.

The Synchronization Concept

If depletion induces a compensatory increase in antibody synthesis, the resulting enhanced vulnerability of the activated lymphocytes could be utilized to increase their deletion by large doses of Ctx. The efficacy of cytotoxic agents rests on the basic principle that slowly proliferating cells are not injured as much as rapidly proliferating cells [64, 76, 113]. Inducing maximum proliferation of pathogenic clones improves the chances that they will be eliminated semiselectively by high-dose Ctx [30]. Experimental data show that Ctx clearly has an inhibitory influence on B cells if it is applied early following stimulation and at high doses [1, 47, 107]. This sequence has been well documented in studies inducing proliferation by readministration of antigen and subsequently administering Ctx [1, 55]. Optimization of the time sequence makes the experimental induction of immunologic tolerance feasible [82]. The critical factors in Ctx-induced tolerance to sheep red blood cells have been very precisely determined experimentally [1]. Crucial for the induction of tolerance was (a) an exact schedule, calling for administration of Ctx in the brief "window" a few days before or after clonal stimulation [1], (b) a high Ctx dosage [1], (c) maximum clonal stimulation through high doses of antigen [1], and (d) the absence of steroids [36].

Clinically, this principle has seldom been applicable. Pathogenic antigens are seldom known, and their readministration would pose major ethical problems. One exception is the successful combination of reimmunization with factor VIII and subsequent Ctx in factor VIII antibody hemophilia [88]. Similar approaches have attempted to improve transplant tolerance in allogeneic transplantation by clonal stimulation with donor antigens prior to immunosuppression [38, 43, 51]. The principles involved in timing antigenic stimulation and drug administration were recently summarized from the perspective of transplantation medicine in an excellent review [82].

Applied to stimulation by means of antibody depletion, this concept was termed "stimulation/deletion" [60] or "synchronization" [41, 100]. It has been tested experimentally [15, 111] and repeatedly discussed as an improved therapeutic option [30, 42, 60, 95]. In the first case report in myasthenia gravis [27] plasmapheresis with subsequent pulse Ctx (up to 0.7 g) led to clinical remission under Prd for 10 weeks. In SLE [63] plasmapheresis and subsequent pulse Ctx (1 g) induced a symptom-free remission under Prd and azathioprine for 2 years. Pulse Ctx (1.8 g) following plasmapheresis induced a complete remission in Goodpasture's syndrome [39] without maintenance treatment, which has now lasted for more than 10 years. In pemphigus vulgaris [96] plasmapheresis with subsequent Ctx (0.3 g) led to clinical remission under Prd. In 26 cases of refractory SLE, Barr et al. [6] applied plasmapheresis and subsequent pulse Ctx (up to 1 g/m^2). The course was lethal in three patients while stable remissions occurred in 58%. In three patients antinuclear antibodies could no longer be demonstrated. In some cases treatment-free remissions were observed. Zielinski et al. [123] compared three treatment options in ten SLE patients: up to eight plasmaphereses in 3 weeks versus one plasmapheresis per week combined with Prd and oral Ctx for several months versus one or two plasmaphereses with subsequent pulse Ctx (up to 1 g). In six cases that did not respond to either of the first two approaches symptoms, hematologic parameters and organ function improved following treatment with the third option. Finally, pulse Ctx (0.75 g/m^2) alone was compared with plasmapheresis and subsequent pulse Ctx in 20 patients. At 3-month follow-up, decreasing serum creatinine levels (+50% versus –48%) were observed only in the latter group [58].

In these reports, the details of the protocols vary considerably. In our view, and based on available experimental evidence, a treatment protocol that aims at optimum utilization of the antibody rebound mechanism should include the following principles (Fig. 2).

a) The basic rationale combines antibody depletion with subsequent pulse alkylating agents.
b) Repeated initial large volume plasmaphereses at short intervals achieve extensive elimination of intravascular and extravascular antibodies [70].
c) Any influence that might be capable of retarding lymphocyte proliferation should be avoided. Thus, Prd [25, 31, 36, 83, 97, 102] and other substances that might retard lymphocyte proliferation (e.g., morphins [54]) should be withdrawn during the period of plasmapheresis and pulse Ctx. Nevertheless Prd withdrawal is often neglected, mainly because dangerous disease

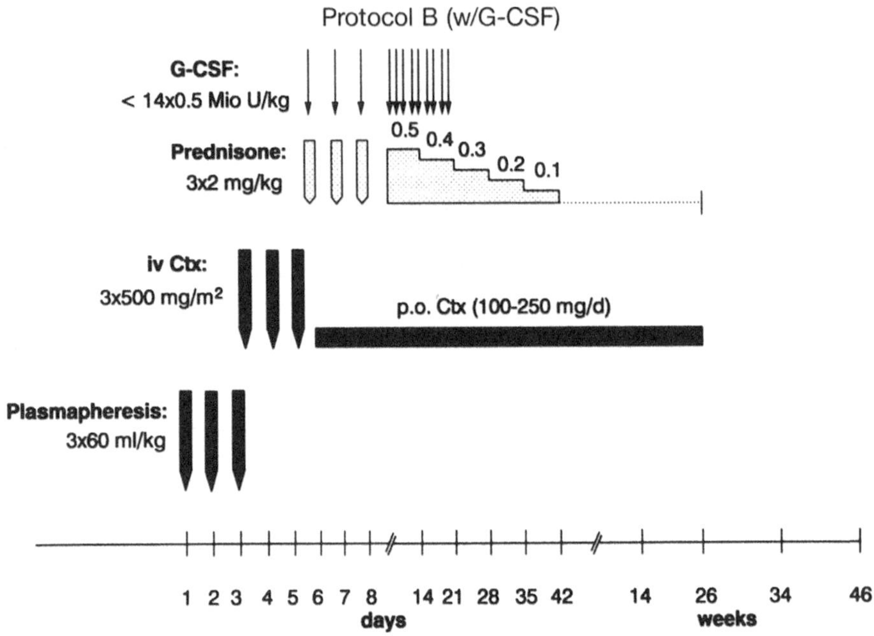

Fig. 2. Protocol combining plasmapheresis with subsequent pulse Ctx

exacerbation is feared. According to our experience, the immediate relief induced by plasmapheresis outweighs possible exacerbations. Another argument against Prd withdrawal is the short turnover time of Prd that is thought to enable renewed lymphocyte stimulation during the next plasmapheresis. A major rationale for repeated plasmaphereses in short intervals is, however, to achieve maximum lymphocyte activation step by step, and any interruption of this activation by administering Prd might obstruct this goal.

d) Again, to accomplish maximum lymphocyte proliferation, substitution fluids containing immunoglobulin should be avoided [80, 94].

A proposal for the comprehensive utilization of these principles is the following protocol. It has been applied in patients with SLE [99, 100] and other autoimmune diseases [41, 42]. Some aspects of this protocol (Prd and repeated cycles of pulse Ctx alone versus Prd and repeated cycles of plasmapheresis and subsequent pulse Ctx) are currently being investigated in a randomized trial by the Lupus Plasmapheresis Study Group [79].

Initially, the protocol starts with a wash-out period during which immunosuppressive drugs are discontinued: cytotoxic agents 3 weeks prior to the first plasmapheresis and Prd 2 days before. This wash-out period is followed by three large-volume (60 ml/kg) plasmaphereses with 4% human albumin substitution on subsequent days. Pulse Ctx (3 days, 12 mg/kg each day; total dose, 36 mg/kg) is started 6 h after the third plasmapheresis begins. Prd is readministered 6 h after the third part of the Ctx pulse. Granulocyte colony-stimulating factor may be administered additionally, starting on day +4 and being continued until recovery from the lower WBC nadir (approximately day +14) [104]. During the next 6 months Ctx and Prd are given orally. In accordance with the results of weekly WBC counts, the Ctx dosage is closely modified, the strict aim being an uninterrupted immunosuppressive effect by maintaining WBC counts between 2.0 and 4.0/nl.

Results

To date, 14 patients with severe and refractory SLE have been treated according to this synchronization protocol in the framework of an uncontrolled pilot study within the recruitment period from February 1986 to January 1990 [99, 100] (Fig. 3). All 14 patients (women; mean age 28, range 18–56 years) had severe SLE, fulfilling a mean of seven (5–8) American Rheumatism Association criteria [110]. Disease activity, as measured by the systemic lupus activity measure (SLAM) [75] was 28.4 (13–37) points. The minimum lupus activity criteria count (LACC) [117] was 5 points, and the

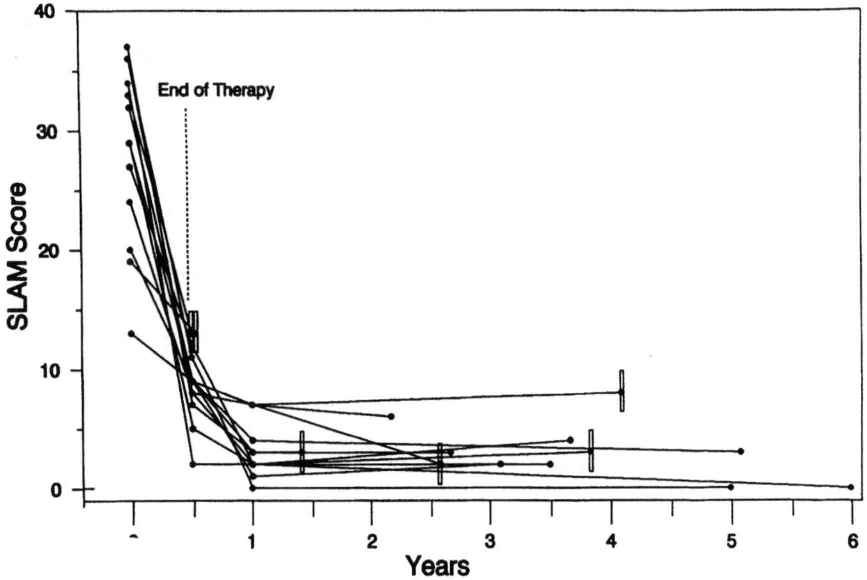

Fig. 3. Reduction of the systemic lupus activity measure (*SLAM*) in 14 patients with severe SLE following "synchronized" treatment with plasmapheresis and subsequent pulse CTX. *End of treatment*, withdrawal of all immunosuppressive drugs, including corticosteroids (12/14 patients); *vertical bars*, reinstitution of immunosuppressive treatment (4/12 patients). Eight of 14 patients remain currently under treatment-free follow-up

mean pretreatment disease duration was 48 (4–138) months. All patients had positive tests for antinuclear antibodies and for anti-double stranded DNA antibodies, and all have had insufficient attempts at controlling disease activity with at least two immunosuppressive drugs: long-term oral Prd over 0.5 mg/kg per day, pulse methylprednisolone, hydroxychloroquine, azathioprine, Ctx, and/or cyclosporin A without achieving remission. The presence of a florid infection (including pneumonia, septicemia, mycosis, infectious hepatitis, toxoplasmosis, borreliosis, cytomegalovirus, Epstein-Barr virus, human immunodeficiency virus, and herpes zoster) either had to be ruled out, or the infection had to have been successfully treated. Since all patients presented with cytopenia (thrombocytopenia, anemia, and/or leukocytopenia), a bone marrow biopsy was performed in each case to exclude bone marrow hypoplasia. A hyperregenerative or normal bone marrow was found in all patients. Patients at risk were advised to use adequate nonhormonal contraception. Six patients underwent renal biopsy, revealing lupus nephritis of World Health Organization grade III or IV with an activity index higher than 4 and a chronicity index below 7 [52]. Informed consent to all aspects of the protocol, which has been approved by the Ethics Committee of Christian Albrecht University in Kiel, was obtained in writing in the presence of a witness.

All patients clearly improved within 8 weeks. The distinctly elevated pretreatment SLAM of 28.4 (13–37) decreased to 14.7 (5–19) 4 weeks after treatment. One patient with severe lupus pneumonitis initially requiring assisted ventilation could be extubated after 5 days [100]. On day 16 after the start of treatment her chest radiograph was nearly normal. In another case of CNS involvement with coma, hemiparesis, and seizures consciousness was regained at day 4, and a normal neurological status was noted at week 3. Anemia (< 100 g/l) was initially present in eight patients, with a mean hemoglobin level of 97 g/l (69–144; all patients). At month 6, hemoglobin had increased to 114 g/l (92–140). Five patients had thrombocytopenia with more than 100 000 cells/μl, with a mean platelet count (all patients) of 154 000 cells/μl (37 000–306 000). The limit of 100 000 cell/μl was passed in all cases by day 30, with a mean platelet count at month 6 of 240 000 cells/μl (100 000–435 000). Arthralgia, reported by 12 patients, improved during the initial plasmaphereses in the majority of cases. Signs of renal involvement were present in all patients, with increased creatinine in nine patients. The mean creatinine level in these patients was 176.8 μmol/l (132.6–256.4) and normalized (< 133 μmol/l) after 4 weeks in all cases. Proteinura was found in 13 patients, with a mean of 5.8 g/day (1.0–22.7). At month 6, 11 patients still were proteinuric, with a decline to 2.7 g/day (0.6–7.0).

After 6 months the median SLAM had decreased to 8.9 (2–13) points. Low-dose Prd was continued in two patients because of persistent arthralgia or incompletely healed ulcers of the fingers. In 12 patients clinical remission was so extensive that immunosuppression (including Prd) could be stopped completely.

At the time of this assessment (August 1991), eight patients had neither relapsed nor were they under treatment with immunosuppressive drugs. They remained in clinical remission after a follow-up of 35 months (14–60) after initiation of the protocol. Their mean SLAM was 2.9 (0–7) points (Fig. 2). The patient with the longest remission (residual SLAM: 1) is now stable for 54 months without treatment [99, 100]. This patient initially had a high pretreatment SLAM of 34. Residual SLE manifestations resulting in the accumulation of SLAM points were predominantly laboratory parameters, such as slight proteinuria of at least 0.1 g/day (5/8), elevated erythrocyte sedimentation rate of at least 25 mm (2/8), elevated diastolic blood pressure at least 90 mmHg (3/8), or lymphopenia of less than 1.5/nl (2/8).

Three relapses occurred following treatment-free intervals of 12, 25, and 39 months, and identical retreatment was initiated. Another patient died at month 49 of a preexisting liver cirrhosis of unclear (SLE-related?) origin without evidence of SLE activity. An oropharyngeal squamous cell carcinoma was diagnosed in one patient at month 17. It cannot be excluded that this was induced by the treatment, although in view of the brief latency period this seems unlikely. The cumulative Ctx dosage of the protocol is approximately 25 g Ctx, well below the 80 g considered to be potentially carcinogenic [3].

Shaking chills occurred in five patients during the plasmapheresis. A segmental herpes zoster was observed in five patients and was treated with intravenous acyclovir. The WBC nadir following pulse Ctx occurred on the 12th day. Six patients had WBC counts under the limit of 2.0 WBC/nl for a mean of 9 days. Patients with fever were treated early with antibiotics [57].

Comparison of IgG-isotype antinuclear antibodies with total serum IgG during treatment showed a rapid drop in both parameters during plasmapheresis followed by a subsequent rise to near pretreatment levels. Three to five months later the two curves separated; whereas total serum IgG remained nearly normal, the antinuclear antibody IgG titers decreased. The synchronization concept may have to be extended by the assumption that active or disease-associated clones are more clearly subject to stimulation/deletion kinetics than resting clones, which comprise the larger portion of the total IgG pool. This semiselective principle may explain why the treatment does not induce severe humoral immunodeficiency. An additional explanation may be provided by observations of increasing numbers of lymphocytes with suppressor activity following treatment [28, 29].

Basically, the fact that disease-associated lymphocyte clones in SLE react highly to stimulation [49, 114] might make this disease especially suitable for the synchronized approach.

In summary, these results demonstrate that in SLE the optimized combination of plasmapheresis with subsequent pulse Ctx consistently led to rapid relief, and that for the first time long-term treatment-free remissions can be achieved at least in some patients.

Conclusion and Prospects

The synchronization concept applies plasmapheresis both to eliminate pathogenic antibodies and to enhance lymphocyte proliferation. The latter should likewise by achievable by the administration of cytokines [49], and future protocols for patients with moderate disease activity might substitute the administration of interferon or interleukins for plasmapheresis prior to pulse Ctx. For patients with severe disease activity, however, future protocols might consist in a sequence of plasmapheresis, then interleukins, and finally pulse Ctx.

Possibly, other alkylating agents are more effective then Ctx. Thus, ifosfamide has been described as being superior to Ctx in terms of inducing immunologic tolerance [85]. Additionally, colony-stimulating factors should provide leeway for either reduced granulocytopenia or improved therapeutic effects through the administration of higher doses of Ctx [104].

An extended synchronization concept for severe SLE might encompass the sequence: more selective immunoadsorption, cytokines, pulse alkylating agents, and granulocyte colony-stimulating factor. Intensive experimental and clinical investigations are, however, necesary to evaluate the individual steps, dose, and time schedule.

Thus, the established treatment of severe SLE consists of Prd and Ctx. According to controlled trials, the additional application of plasmapheresis in the usual combination with long-term immunosuppression is no longer justified. New perspectives may be opened up by exploiting the antibody rebound mechanism, if pulse immunosuppression is applied shortly after plasmapheresis. Whether or not this concept leads to improved therapeutic results must be confirmed in randomized trials. Initial uncontrolled results are encouraging. First reports of treatment-free, long-term remissions in severe SLE may offer new hope, and it would be worthwile to investigate carefully their extent.

References

1. Aisenberg AC (1967) Studies on cyclophosphamide-induced tolerance to sheep erythrocytes. J Exp Med 125: 833–845
2. Austin HA, Klippel JH, Balow JE, LeRiche NGH, Steinberg AD, Plotz PH, Decker JL (1986) Therapy of lupus nephritis. Controlled trial of prednisone and cytotoxic drugs. N Engl J Med 314: 614–619
3. Baker GL, Kahl LE, Zee BC, Stolzer BL, Agarwal AK, Medsger TA Jr (1987) Malignancy following treatment of rheumatoid arthritis with cyclophosphamide. A long-term case-control follow-up study. Am J Med 83: 1–9
4. Barclay GR, Greiss AM, Urbaniak SJ (1980) Adverse effects of plasma exchange on anti-D production in rhesus immunisation owing to removal of inhibitory factors. Br Med J 280: 1569–1571
5. Barile L, Lavalle C (1992) Transverse myelitis in systemic lupus erythematosus – the effect of iv pulse methylprednisolone and cyclophosphamide. J Rheumatol 19: 370–372

6. Barr WG, Hubbell EA, Robinson JA (1987) Persistently active lupus erythematosus treated with intermittent plasmapheresis and bolus cyclophosphamide. In: Oda T, Shiokawa Y, Inoue N (eds) Proceedings of 1st international congress of the World Apheresis Association: therapeutic plasmapheresis IV. ISAO, Cleveland, pp 79–94
7. Barrat TM, Soothill JF (1970) Controlled trial of cyclophosphamide in steroid-sensitive relapsing nephrotic syndrome of childhood. Lancet 2: 479–482
8. Belghiti-Deprez D, Sobel P (1988) A controlled trial of plasma exchange in severe acute systemic lupus erythematosus. In: Immunointervention in autoimmune diseases. Abstracts. Maison de la Chimie, Paris
9. Boulware DW, Makkena R (1991) Monthly cyclophosphamide in lupus pneumonitis and myositis (letter). J Rheumatol 18: 153
10. Boumpas DT, Barez S, Klippel JH, Balow JE (1990) Intermittent cyclophosphamide for the treatment of autoimmune thrombocytopenia in systemic lupus erythematosus. Ann Intern Med 112: 674–677
11. Branda RF, Moldow CF, McCullough JJ, Jacob HS (1975) Plasma exchange in the treatment of immune disease. Transfusion 15: 570–576
12. Brody NJ, Walker GJ, Siskind GW (1967) Studies on the control of antibody synthesis. Interaction of antigen competition and suppression of antibody formation by passive antibody on the immune response. J Exp Med 126: 81–90
13. Bystryn JC (1988) Plasma exchange in pemphigus. Arch Dermatol 124: 1702–1704
14. Bystryn JC, Graf MW, Uhr JW (1970) Regulation of antibody formation by serum antibody. II. Removal of specific antibody by means of exchange transfusion. J Exp Med 132: 1279–1287
15. Bystryn JC, Schenkein I, Uhr JW (1971) A model for regulation of antibody synthesis by serum antibody. In: Amos B (ed) Progress in immunology. Academic, New York, pp 627–636
16. Campion EW (1992) Desperate diseases and plasmapheresis. N Engl J Med 326: 1425–1427
17. Caulfield MJ, Shaffer D (1987) Immunoregulation by antigen/antibody complexes. I. Specific immunosuppression induced in vivo with immune complexes formed in antibody excess. J Immunol 138: 3680–3683
18. Cerottini JC (1969) The immunosuppressive effect of passively administered antibody Ig-fragments. J Immunol 102: 1008–1011
19. Chang H, Schneck S, Brody NI, Deutsch A, Siskind GW (1969) Studies on the mechanism of the suppression of active antibody synthesis by passively administered antibody. J Immunol 102: 37–41
20. Charlton B, Antony G, Cooper SG, Schindhelm K (1988) A comparison of the effects of plasma exchange and immunoadsorption on anti-insulin antibodies in rabbits. Clin Exp Immunol 72: 326–329
21. Charlton B, Schindhelm K, Smeby LC, Farrel PC (1985) Analysis of immunoglobulin G kinetic in the non-steady-state. J Lab Clin Med 105: 312–320
22. Clark WF, Lindsay RM, Ulan RA, Cordy PE, Linton AL (1981) Chronic plasma exchange therapy in SLE nephritis. Clin Nephrol 16: 20–23
23. Corvetta A, Della Bitta R, Gabrielli A, Spaeth PJ, Danieli G (1989) Use of high-dose intravenous immunoglobulin in systemic lupus erythematosus: report of three cases. Clin Exp Rheumatol 7: 295–299
24. Council on Scientific Affairs (1985) Current status of plasmapheresis and related techniques. J Am Med Assoc 253: 819–825
25. Cupps TR, Edgar LC, Thomas CA, Fauci AS (1984) Multiple mechanisms of B cell immunoregulation in man after administration of in vivo corticosteroids. J Immunol 132: 170–175
26. Cupps TR (1990) Cyclophosphamide: to pulse or not to pulse. Am J Med 89: 399–402
27. Dau PC (1980) Plasmapheresis therapy in myasthenia gravis. Muscle Nerve 3: 468–482

28. Dau PC (1990) Increased proliferation of blood mononuclear cells after plasmapheresis treatment of patients with demyelinating disease. J Neuroimmunol 30: 15–21
29. Dau PC, Callahan J, Parker R, Golbus J (1991) Immunologic effects of plasmapheresis synchronized with pulse cyclophosphamide in systemic lupus erythematosus. J Rheumatol 18: 270–276
30. Dau PC, Lindstrom JM, Cassel CK, Denys EH, Shev EE, Spitler L (1977) Plasmapheresis and immunosuppressive drug therapy in myasthenia gravis. N Engl J Med 297: 1134–1140
31. Dennis GJ, Mond JJ (1986) Corticosteroid-induced suppression of murine B cell immune response antigens. J Immunol 136: 1600–1604
32. Derksen RH, Hene RJ, Kallenberg CG, Valentijn RM, Kater L (1988) Prospective multicentre trial on the short-term effects of plasma exchange versus cytotoxic drugs in steroid-resistant lupus nephritis. Neth J Med 33: 168–177
33. Derksen RHWM, Schuurman HJ, Meyling GFHJ, Struyvenberg A, Kater L (1984) Rebound and overshoot after plasma exchange in humans. J Lab Clin Med 104: 35–43
34. Dinant HJ, Decker JL, Klippel JH, Balow JE, Plotz PH, Steinberg AD (1982) Alternative modes of cyclophosphamide and azathioprine therapy in lupus nephritis. Ann Intern Med 96: 728–736
35. Díaz-González F, Castaneda-Sanz S, López-Robledillo JC, García-Vicuna R (1992) Lung fibrosis in a patient with polyarteritis nodosa receiving cyclophosphamide therapy. J Rheumatol 19: 325–327
36. Dukor P, Dietrich FM (1970) Prevention of cyclophosphamide-induced tolerance to erythrocytes by pretreatment with cortisone. Proc Soc Exp Biol Med 133: 280–285
37. ElMouzan MI, Ahmad MAM, Saleh MAF, Sohaibani MOA, Gindan YMA (1988) Myelofibrosis and pancytopenia in systemic lupus erythematosus. Acta Haematol 80: 219–221
38. Eto M, Mayumi H, Tomita Y, Yoshika Y, Nishimura Y, Maeda T, Ando T, Nomoto K (1991) Specific destruction of host-reactive mature T cells of donor origin prevents graft-versus-host disease in cyclophosphamide-induced tolerant mice. J Immunol 146: 1402–1409
39. Euler HH, Kleine L, Gutschmidt HJ, Herrlinger JD (1982) Effect of early plasmapheresis and high-dose cyclophosphamide therapy in Goodpasture's syndrome. In: Beyer JH, Borberg H, Fuchs C, Nagel GA (eds) Plasmapheresis in immunology and oncology. Karger, Basel, pp 238–246
40. Euler HH, Krey U, Schroeder JO, Löffler H (1985) Membrane plasmapheresis technique in rats. Confirmation of antibody rebound. J Immunol Methods 84: 313–319
41. Euler HH, Löffler H, Christophers E (1987) Synchronization of plasmapheresis and pulse cyclophosphamide in pemphigus vulgaris. Arch Dermatol 123: 1205–1210
42. Euler HH, Schroeder JO, Löffler H (1987) The antibody rebound as a rationale for synchronizing plasmapheresis with pulse cytotoxic drugs. In: Oda T, Shiokawa Y, Inoue N (eds) Proceedings of the 1s international congress of the World Apheresis Association; therapeutic plasmapheresis VI. ISAO, Cleveland, pp 200–207
43. Fauchald P, Leivestad T, Bratlie A, Jakobsen A, Flatmark A (1987) Plasma exchange and immunosuppressive therapy before renal transplantation. Transplant Proc 19: 727–728
44. Felson DT, Anderson J (1984) Evidence for the superiority of immunosuppressive drugs and prednisone over prednisone alone in lupus nephritis: results of a pooled analysis. N Engl J Med 311: 1528–1533
45. Fox DA, McCune WJ (1989) Immunologic and clinical effects of cytotoxic drugs used in the treatment of rheumatoid arthritis and systemic lupus erythematosus. In: Cruse IM, Lewis RE (eds) Therapy of autoimmune diseases. Karger, Basel, pp 20–78
46. French Cooperative Study Group (1985) A randomised trial of plasma exchange in severe acute systemic lupus erythematosus. Plasma Ther Transfus Tech 6: 535–539

47. Gagnon RF, Maclennan ICM (1981) The effect of chronic daily cyclophosphamide administration on established antibody responses. Clin Exp Immunol 46: 178–184
48. Gibbons RB, Westermann E (1988) Acute nonlymphocytic leukemia following short-term, intermittent, intravenous cyclophosphamide in the treatment of lupus nephritis. Arthritis Rheum 31: 1552–1554
49. Golbus J, Salata M, Greenwood J, Hudson J, Richardson BC (1988) Increased immunoglobulin response to gamma-interferon by cultured lymphocytes from subjects with systemic lupus erythematosus. Clin Immunol Immunopathol 46: 129–140
50. Graf MW, Uhr JW (1969) Regulation of antibody formation by serum antibody. I. Removal of specific antibody by means of immunoadsorption. J Exp Med 130: 1175–1186
51. Grailer AP, Sollinger HW, Kawamura T, Burlingham WJ (1991) Donor-specific cytotoxicT lymphocyte hyporesponsiveness following renal transplantation in patients pretreated with donor-specific transfusions. Transplantation 51: 320–324
52. Hayslett JP, Kashgarian M (1988) Nephropathy of systemic lupus erythematosus. In: Schrier RW, Gottschalk CW (eds) Diseases of the kidney. Little Brown, Boston, pp 2253–2271
53. Hedon E (1902) Sur l'hemolyse par les glycosides, globulicides et les conditions de milieu qui la favorisent ou l'empechent. Arch Internist Pharmacol Gand Paris 7: 381–385
54. Heijnen CJ, Bevers C, Kavelaars A, Ballieux RE (1986) Effect of alpha-endorphin on the antigen-induced primary antibody response of human blood B cells in vitro. J Immunol 136: 213–216
55. Herrlinger JD, Müller-Ruchholtz W (1978) Different suppressive effects of combined cyclophosphamide-antigen treatment compared with exclusive cyclophosphamide treatment of primary and secondary humoral immune reactivity. Int Arch Allergy Appl Immunol 57: 82–89
56. Hill RD, Scott GW (1964) Cytotoxic drugs for systemic lupus (letter). Br Med J 1: 370
57. Hughes WT, Amstrong D, Bodey G, Feld R, Mandell GL, Meyers JD, Pizzo PA, Schimpf SC, Shenep JL, Wade J, Young LS, Yow MD (1990) Guidelines for the use of antimicrobial agents in neutropenic patients with unexplained fever. J Infect Dis 161: 381–396
58. Huston DP, Bressler RB, Suki WN, Huston MM, Andrew SL, Kavanaugh AF (1988) A controlled trial of pulse cyclophosphamide and plasmapheresis therapy of lupus nephritis. Arthritis Rheum 31 [Suppl]: s55, no A106 (abstract)
59. Isbister JP, Ting A, Seeto KM (1977) Development of Rh-specific maternal autoantibodies following intensive plasmapheresis for Rh immunisation during pregnancy. Vox Sang 33: 353–358
60. Jones JV (1982) Plasmapheresis in SLE. Clin Rheum Dis 8: 243–260
61. Jones JV, Cumming RH, Bacon PA, Evers J, Fraser ID, Bothamley J, Tribe CR, Davis P, Hughes GR (1979) Evidence for a therapeutic effect of plasmapheresis in patients with systemic lupus erythematosus. Q J Med 48: 555–576
62. Jones JV, Cumming RH, Bucknall RC, Asplin CM, Fraser ID, Bothamley J, Davis P, Hamblin TJ (1976) Plasmapheresis in the management of acute systemic lupus erythematosus. Lancet I: 709–710
63. Jones JV, Robinson MF, Parciany RK, Layfer LF, McLeod B (1981) Therapeutic plasmapheresis in systemic lupus erythematosus. Effect on immune complexes and antibodies to DNA. Arthritis Rheum 24: 1113–1120
64. Kakiuchi T, Watanabe M, Hozumi N, Nariuchi H (1990) Differential sensitivity of specific and nonspecific antigen-presentation by B cells to a protein synthesis inhibitor. J Immunol 145: 1653–1658
65. Kater L, Derksen RH, Houwert FA, Hene RJ, Struyvenberg A, Gmeling Meyling FHJ, Verroust P (1981) Effect of plasmapheresis in active systemic lupus erythematosus. Neth J Med 24: 209–216

66. Kattwinkel N, Cook L, Agnello V (1991) Overwhelming fatal infection in a young woman after intravenous cyclophosphamide therapy for lupus nephritis. J Rheumatol 18: 79–81
67. Kellogg RM, Hester JP (1988) Kinetics modelling of plasma exchange. J Clin Apheresis 4: 183–187
68. Klippel JH (1990) Systemic lupus erythematosus. Treatment-related complications superimposed on chronic disease. J Am Med Assoc 263: 1812–1815
69. Klippel JH (1990) Survival in SLE. In: Hai CT (ed) Proceedings of the 2nd international conference on systemic lupus erythematosus. Professional Postgraduate Services, Singapore, pp 187–189
70. Kramer GC, Harms BI, Demling RH, Renkin EM (1982) Mechanisms for redistribution of plasma-proteins following acute protein depletion. Am J Physiol 243: 803–809
71. Krapf F, Manger B, Koch B, Krauledat P, Kalden JR (1985) The estimation of circulating immune complexes, C3d, and anti-ds-DNA-antibody serum levels in the monitoring of therapeutic plasmapheresis in a patient with systemic lupus erythematosus. A case report. Clin Exp Rheumatol 3: 159–162
72. LaRochelle G, Lacks S, Borenstein D (1985) Iv cyclophosphamide therapy of steroid resistant neuropsychiatric SLE. Clin Exp Rheumatol 3: 159–162
73. Leaker BR, Becker GJ, Dowling JP, Kincaid-Smith PS (1986) Rapid improvement in severe lupus glomerular lesions following intensive plasma exchange associated with immunosuppression. Clin Nephrol 25: 236–244
74. Levey AS, Lan SP, Corwin HL, Kasinath BS, Lachin JL, Neilson EG, Hunsicker LG, Lewis ES, LNCS Group (1990) Progression and remission in the Lupus Nephritis Collaborative Study (LNCS). J Am Soc Nephrol 1: 310 (abstract)
75. Liang MH, Socher SA, Larson MG, Schur PH (1989) Reliability and validity of six systems for the clinical assessment of disease activity in systemic lupus erythematosus. Arthritis Rheum 32: 1107–1118
76. Lin H (1973) Differential lethal effect of cytotoxic agents on proliferating and nonproliferating lymphoid cells. Cancer Res 33: 1716
77. Lockwood CM, Boulton-Jones JM, Lowenthal RM, Simpson IJ, Peters DK, Wilson CB (1975) Recovery from Goodpasture's syndrome after immunosuppressive treatment and plasmapheresis. Br Med J 2: 252–254
78. Lockwood CM, Worlledge S, Nicholas A, Cotton C, Peters DK (1979) Reversal of impaired splenic function in patients with nephritis or vasculitis (or both) by plasma exchange. N Engl J Med 300: 524–530
79. Lupus Plasmapheresis Study Group, Clark WF, Dau PC, Euler HH, Guillevin L, Hasford J, Heer AH, Jones JV, Kashgarian M, Knatterud G, Lockwood CM, Pusey CD, Rifle G, Robinson JA, Schroeder JO, Tan EM, Wallace DJ, Weiner SR (1991) Plasmapheresis and subsequent pulse cyclophosphamide versus pulse cyclophosphamide alone in severe lupus: Design of the LPSG trial. J Clin Apheresis 6: 40–47
80. Macey MG, Newland AC (1990) CD4 and CD8 subpopulation changes during high dose intravenous immunoglobulin treatment. Br J Haematol 76: 513–520
81. Marner B, Lernmark A, Ludvigsson J, MacKay P, Matsuba I, Nerup J, Rabinovitch A (1985) Islet cell antibodies in insulin-dependent (type 1) diabetic children treated with plasmapheresis. Diabetes Res 2: 231–236
82. Mayumi H, Tokunaga K (1990) Cyclophosphamide-induced chimera-type tolerance to allografts: an overview of drug-induced immunological tolerance. Fukuoka Acta Med 81: 20–40
83. McMillan R, Longmire R, Yelenosky R (1976) The effect of corticosteroids on human IgG synthesis. J Immunol 116: 1592–1595
84. Minchin SA, Leitenberg D, Stunz LL, Feldbush TL (1990) Polyclonal activation of rat B cells. II. Dextran sulfate as a cofactor in mitogen-induced and antigen-induced differentiation of rat B lymphocytes. J Immunol 145: 2427–2433

85. Müller-Ruchholtz W (1974) The influence of cyclophosphamide and other homologue oxazaphosphorine-2-oxides on transplantation-immunologic reactions. Drug Res 24: 1160–1167
86. Nasca TJ, Muder RR, Thomas DB, Schrecker JC, Ruben FL (1990) Antibody response to pneumococcal polysaccharide vaccine in myasthenia gravis: effect of therapeutic plasmapheresis. J Clin Apheresis 5: 133–139
87. NIH Conference, Balow JE, Austin HA, Tsokos GC, Antonovych TT, Steinberg AD, Klippel JH (1987) Lupus nephritis. Ann Intern Med 106: 79–94
88. Nilsson IM, Berntorp E, Zettervall O (1988) Induction of immune tolerance in patients with hemophilia and antibodies to factor VIII by combined treatment with intravenous IgG, cyclophosphamide, and factor VIII. N Engl J Med 318: 947–950
89. Perez MC, Wilson WA, Scopelitis E (1989) Cyclophosphamide use in a young woman with antiphospholipid antibodies and recurrent cerebrovascular accident. South Med J 82: 1421–1424
90. Pierce CW (1969) Immune responses in vitro. II. Suppression of the immune response in vitro by specific antibody. J Exp Med 130: 365–379
91. Reding R, White DJG, Davies HS, Calne RY (1987) Successful removal of immune and preformed xeno-antibodies by plasma exchange in rats. Eur Surg Res 19: 74–75
92. Reding R, White DJG, Davies HS, Calne RY (1988) Plasma exchange technique in the unheparinized, unanaesthetized rat. Lab Anim 22: 293–296
93. Reveille JD, Barolucci A, Alarcón-Segovia G (1990) Prognosis in systemic lupus erythematosus. Negative impact of increasing age at onset, black race, and thrombocytopenia, as well as causes of death. Arthritis Rheum 33: 37–48
94. Rossi F, Kazatchkine MD (1989) Antiidiotypes against autoantibodies in pooled normal polyspecific IgG. J Immunol 143: 4104–4109
95. Roujeau JC, Andre C, Revuz J, Touraine R (1983) Effects of various immunosuppressive regimens on the "rebound phenomenon" induced by plasma exchange in pemphigus. In: Nosé Y, Malchesky PS, Smith JW, Krakauer RS (eds) Plasmapheresis. Therapeutic applications and new techniques. Raven, New York, pp 285–292
96. Ruocco V, Astarita C, Pisani M (1984) Plasmapheresis as an alternative or adjunctive therapy in problem cases of pemphigus. Dermatologica 168: 219–223
97. Saxon A, Stevens RH, Ramer SJ, Clements PJ, Yu DTY (1977) Glucocorticosteroids in vivo inhibit human suppressor cell function and diminish B lymphocyte responsiveness in in-vitro immunoglobulin synthesis. J Clin Invest 61: 922–925
98. Schlansky R, de Horatius RJ, Pincus T, Tung KS (1981) Plasmapheresis in systemic lupus erythematosus. A cautionary note. Arthritis Rheum 24: 49–53
99. Schroeder JO, Euler HH (1989) Treatment combining plasmapheresis and pulse cyclophosphamide in severe systemic lupus erythematosus. In: Hörl WH, Schollmeyer PJ (eds) New perspectives in hemodialysis, peritoneal dialysis, arteriovenous hemofiltration, and plasmapheresis. Plenum, New York, pp 203–213
100. Schroeder JO, Euler HH, Löffler H (1987) Synchronization of plasmapheresis and pulse cyclophosphamide in severe systemic lupus erythematosus. Ann Intern Med 107: 344–346
101. Shumak KH, Rock GA (1984) Therapeutic plasma exchange. N Engl J Med 310: 762–771
102. Smith KA, Crabtree GR, Kennedy SJ, Munck AV (1977) Glucocorticoid receptors and glucocorticoid sensitivity of mitogen stimulated and unstimulated human lymphocytes. Nature 267: 523–526
103. Smolens J, Stokes J, Vogt AB (1957) Human plasmapheresis and its effect on antibodies. J Immunol 79: 434–439
104. Stein RS (1992) G-CSF for fever and neutropenia induced by chemotherapy. N Engl J Med 326: 269
105. Steinberg AD, Kaltreider HB, Staples PJ, Goetzl EJ, Talal N, Decker JL (1971) Cyclophosphamide in lupus nephritis: a controlled trial. Ann Intern Med 75: 165–171

106. Steinberg AD, Steinberg SC (1991) Long-term preservation of renal function in patients with lupus nephritis receiving treatment that includes cyclophosphamide versus those treated with prednisone only. Arthritis Rheum 34: 945–950
107. Stevenson HC, Fauci AS (1979) Activation of human B lymphocytes. XII. Differential effects of in vitro cyclophosphamide on human lymphocyte subpopulations involved in B cell activation. Immunology 39: 391–397
108. Stockinger B, Lemmel EM (1978) Fc receptor dependency of antibody mediated feedback regulation: on the mechanism of inhibition. Cell Immunol 40: 395–403
109. Sturgill BC, Worzniak MJ (1970) Stimulation of proliferation of 19S antibody forming cells in the spleens of immunized guinea-pigs after exchange transfusion. Nature 228: 1304–1305
110. Tan EM, Cohen AS, Fries JF, Masi AT, McShane DJ, Rothfield NF, Schaller JG, Talal N, Winchester RJ (1982) The 1982 revised criteria for the classification of systemic lupus erythematosus. Arthritis Rheum 25: 1271–1277
111. Terman DS, Garcia-Rinaldi R, Dannemann B, Moore D, Crumb C, Tavel A, Poser R (1978) Specific suppression of antibody rebound after extracorporal immunoadsorption. I. Comparison of single versus combination chemotherapeutic agents. Clin Exp Immunol 34: 32–41
112. Tew JG, Phipps RP, Mandel TE (1980) The maintenance and regulation of the humoral immune response: persisting antigen and the role of follicular antigen-binding dendritic cells as accessory cells. Immunol Rev 53: 175–201
113. Turk JC, Poulter CW (1972) Selective depletion of lympoid tissue by cyclophosphamide. Clin Exp Immunol 10: 285–296
114. Ueda Y, Sakane T, Tsunematsu T (1989) Hyperreactivity of activated B cells to B cell growth factor in patients with systemic lupus erythematosus. J Immunol 143: 3988–3993
115. Uhr JW, Baumann JB (1961) Antibody formation: the suppression of antibody formation by passively administered antibodies. J Exp Med 113: 935–957
116. Uhr JW, Moeller G (1968) Regulatory effect of antibody on the immune response. Adv Immunol 8: 81–127
117. Urowitz MB, Gladman DD, Tozman ECS, Goldsmith CH (1984) The lupus activity criteria count. J Rheumatol 11: 783–787
118. Van Wanghe P, Dequeker J (1982) Effect of intravenous cyclophosphamide as an adjuvant to therapeutic plasma exchange in rheumatoid arthritis. Plasma Ther Transf Technol 3: 171–176
119. Vendeville B, Baran D, Imbert F, Kuhn J, Vial MC, Hibbard J, Paris M, Mahieu P, Druet P (1988) Plasma exchange in a rat model of autoimmune glomerulonephritis. Nephrol Dial Transplant 3: 405–411
120. Wallace DJ, Goldfinger D, Savage G, Nichols S, Goodman D, Fichman M, Stewart M, Klinenberg JR (1987) Controlled study of the use of plasmapheresis in steroid/immunosuppressive resistant systemic lupus erythematosus with nephrotic syndrome. In: Oda T, Shiokawa Y, Inoue N (eds) Proceedings of the 1st international congress of the World Apheresis Association: therapeutic plasmapheresis (IV). ISAO, Cleveland, pp 91–102
121. Wei N, Klippel JH, Huston DP, Hall RP, Lawley TJ, Balow JE, Steinberg AD, Decker JL (1983) Randomised trial of plasma exchange in mild systemic lupus erythematosus. Lancet I: 17–22
122. Wigzell H (1966) Antibody synthesis at the cellular level: antibody induced suppression of 7s-antibody synthesis. J Exp Med 124: 953–975
123. Zielinski C, Mueller C, Smolen J (1988) Plasmapheresis in the treatment of systemic lupus erythematosus: a controlled study. Acta Med Austriaca 15: 155–158

The CD2 Molecular Complex: An Accessory Receptor Mediating Secondary Signals for Human T Cell Activation

S. C. Meuer, Y. Samstag, and *B. Schraven*

Two Kinds of Lymphocyte Receptors Mediate T Cell Activation

A large number of surface structures on cells of the human immune system have been identified in the past decade. Mainly due to the availability of monoclonal antibodies it has been possible to define their molecular characteristics. Based on genetic and structural relationships many of these molecules that are expressed by immunocompetent cells form superfamilies such as the immunoglobulin superfamily, the integrins, and the selectins (for review see Springer 1990; Hemler 1990; Meuer 1992). Functional investigations have suggested that most if not all cell surface molecules function as receptors capable of transmitting signals from the extracellular environment into the inner cell compartments and thereby influencing the functional cell behavior. Among approximately 100 different receptors identified in the surface of human T lymphocytes so far only one receptor type possesses variable regions. Expression of this clonally restricted T cell antigen receptor – a member of the immunoglobulin superfamily – provides the molecular basis of antigen-specific lymphocyte activation by clonal selection (Meuer et al. 1984 a, b). No additional cell surface receptors express variable regions, and they are therefore structurally identical among all circulating T lymphocytes. They are termed accessory receptors in the present report.

Given the exquisitely fine specificity of immunological reactions in vivo, a number of predictions could be made:

a) under physiologic conditions, accessory receptors do not function independent of the T cell receptor;
b) the T cell receptor must therefore be capable of exerting control over accessory receptors; and
c) intracellular signals produced by the T cell antigen receptor should differ, at least in part, from those induced via accessory receptors.

Antibodies that Exert Ligandlike Functional Effects

The molecular mechanisms underlying these considerations can now be experimentally addressed. The most convenient and decisive tools for this purpose are monoclonal antibodies which react with individual receptor structures and exert ligandlike agonistic functional effects (Reinherz et al.

1982; Meuer et al. 1983, 1984 b; Meuer and Meyer zum Büschenfelde 1986). Thus, it is now possible to examine highly purified cellular systems and, with the use of monoclonal antibodies, each receptor selectively.

Monoclonal antibodies directed at variable or constant subunits of the T cell antigen receptor have been shown to produce antigenlike functional effects in vitro (Meuer et al.1983). Fortuitously, particular monoclonal antibodies directed at an additional receptor of the Ig superfamily, namely CD2, exist which when combined can induce the expression of the functional T cell repertoire in vitro as well (Meuer et al. 1984c). Besides activation through the T cell antigen receptor the CD2 complex provides the only alternative triggering mechanism for inducing T cell activation in vitro. Thus, one can regard CD2 as a representative accessory receptor and compare its structural and functional characteristics as a signaling molecule vis-à-vis the antigen receptor/CD3 complex (TCR/CD3).

Besides representing an excellent model system for experimental in vitro analysis, it is now clear that the interaction between CD2 and its natural ligand, CD58, is involved in many important functional processes in vivo, including thymic selection, T cell activation in the peripheral compartment, effector functions of cytotoxic T lymphocytes, and interactions between T lymphocytes and endothelial cells (Bierer and Burakoff 1988; Hughes et al. 1990; Moingeon et al. 1989; Albert-Wolf et al. 1991).

T Cell Receptor Triggering Alone Does Not Lead to Clonal T Cell Expansion

A number of earlier experiments in which monoclonal antibodies were employed as single ligands for the T cell receptor clearly demonstrated that engagement of the antigen receptor complex in the absence of additional (secondary) signals mediated by accessory molecules was not sufficient to induce clonal T cell expansion and lymphocyte activation (Reinherz et al. 1982; Meuer et al. 1983, 1984 c; Mueller et al. 1989; Schwartz 1990; Jenkins 1992). However, such treatment produced profound functional changes. Thus, T cell receptor triggering by a single ligand resulted in acquisition of a state of unresponsiveness/anergy/tolerance in which T lymphocytes no longer responded to mitogenic signals mediated by CD2 (Meuer et al. 1984 c). This finding was the first evidence to suggest that the T cell receptor can exert functional control over accessory receptors, although the molecular basis of this phenomenon remained elusive.

Nevertheless, these experiments demonstrated an important principle underlying immunological reactions, namely, that they require more than one signal to be complete. Thus, T cell receptor engagement provides a primary signal for lymphocyte activation, which determines the specificity of an immune response whereas secondary signals transmitted by accessory receptors are responsible for the functional outcome or the "kind" of an immune response (reviewed by Schwartz 1990; Jenkins 1992). Depending on the kinetics and the types of accessory receptors that are engaged following antigen receptor triggering immune reactions can range from clonal expansion and expression of the full immune repertoire to total unresponsiveness and/or specific clonal deletion. The former reactions occur when T cell receptor and accessory receptor(s) are concomitantly engaged within a certain time frame while the latter response results when primary signals are delivered and secondary signals prohibited (Fig. 1).

These basic rules also seem to apply to situations in vivo (Waldmann 1989; Gückel et al. 1991) and can be employed to establish novel strategies for

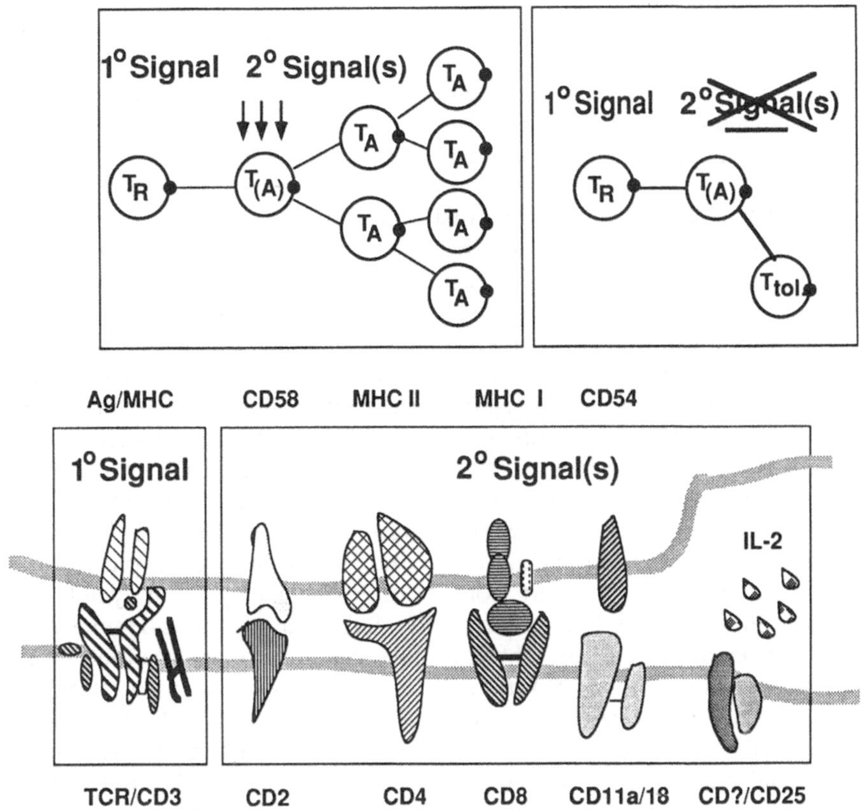

Fig. 1. The two signal hypothesis of T cell activation. *Upper panel,* T cell receptor dependent (primary) signals determine the specificity of an immune response whereas secondary signals dictate the "kind" of an immune reaction. Importantly, while the simultaneous delivery of primary and secondary signls induces clonal T cell expansion and lymphocyte activation, situations in which the primary signal is received yet secondary signals are not provided or prohibited lead to clonal anergy and unresponsiveness. *Lower panel,* besides the TCR/CD3 complex, which is uniquely responsible for delivering the primary signal in T cell activation, some central secondary signal receptors and their respective ligands have recently been identified. Given the multitude of accessory receptors by which secondary signals can be transmitted for T cell activation, it seems likely to expect a considerable degree of redundancy at this level (see text)

clinical immune modulation, for example, with the goal of specific tolerance induction.

The Signaling Machinery Associated with CD2

Incubation of human T lymphocytes with monoclonal antibodies directed at the TCR/CD3 complex induces transient modulation and loss of TCR/CD3 from the cell surface in the absence of proliferation (Reinherz et al. 1982; Meuer et al. 1984 a, b). Importantly, while untreated T cells grow and differentiate in vitro following incubation with monoclonal CD2 antibodies, following TCR/CD3 modulation they do not respond with proliferation and cytokine production when triggered by CD2 (Meuer et al. 1984 c). Since CD2 does not comodulate with the T cell receptor and remains surface expressed even at higher density, this unresponsiveness must be attributed to changes in the intracellular signal transducing mechanisms that are linked to activation via CD2.

To address this question, it was first necessary to define potential signaling molecules that are linked to CD2 in human T cells. That such molecules must exist can be concluded from the fact that CD2 itself (e.g., when transfected into nonlymphoid cells) cannot serve as a signaling molecule (Moingeon 1991). Moreover, when mutant CD2 molecules which were truncated in the intracellular domain were transfected into murine T cell hybridomas, it became clear that particular regions of the intracellular CD2 sequence are relevant for signal transduction (Bierer and Burakoff 1988; Moingeon et al. 1989). The conclusion from these two findings was that CD2 must interact with other signaling components through its intracellular portion.

The first clues on CD2-related signaling molecules resulted from functional studies in which monoclonal antibodies directed at the tyrosine phosphatase CD45 were shown to exert potent comitogenic effects on lymphocyte activation via CD2 (Schraven et al. 1989). Subsequently it was demonstrated that CD45 and CD2 are physically associated with each other in the lymphocyte membrane (Schraven et al. 1990). Such an association was reported to exist in mouse T cells as well (Altevogt et al. 1990) and even in murine T lymphocytes expressing a human CD2 transgene (there, human CD2 and murine CD45 associate physically and functionally; unpublished results). Thus, under cross-linking conditions the CD45 molecules coprecipitate with CD2 and vice versa. Moreover, tyrosine phosphatase activity was demonstrated in CD2 immunoprecipitates. Recently, a molecular phosphoprotein complex (pp29-32) was discovered which is linked to CD45 and CD2 in human T lymphocytes (Schraven et al. 1991). Since the pp29-32 molecules are also present in immunoprecipitates employing antisera against the lymphocyte-specific tyrosine kinase $p56^{lck}$ (Telfer and Rudd 1991), it was suggested that pp29-32 might form a functional complex with CD45 and $p56^{lck}$ and perhaps even represent their natural substrate, which is probably influenced in a reciprocal fashion by these two antogonistic enzymes. In fact,

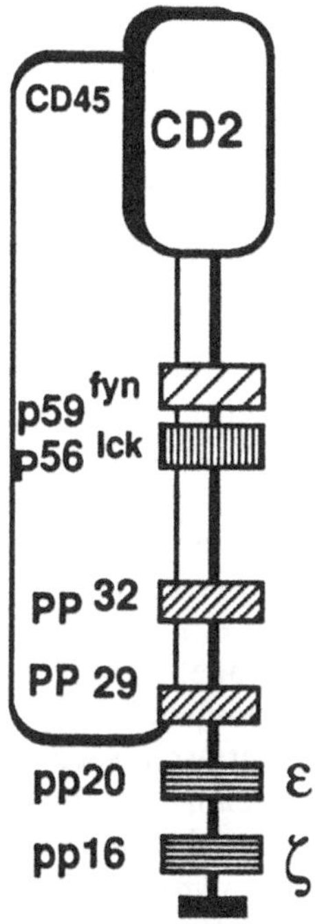

Fig. 2. The CD2 molecular complex. A number of potential signaling molecules have been identified which are linked with CD2 in untransformed resting human T lymphocytes. Since accessory receptors – under physiologic conditions – should not function independently, the mere presence of these molecules cannot constitute a functional signaling receptor

following lymphocyte activation the CD45-associated pp29-32 molecules rapidly change their molecular features, suggesting that they may play an important role in lymphocyte activation (Schraven et al. 1992 a). Findings suggesting that the pp29-32 molecules react with anti-G protein sera (Telfer and Rudd 1991; Schraven et al. 1992 a), and that under certain circumstances in vitro these molecules can hydrolize GTP provide the first hints as to their functional nature.

Besides $p56^{lck}$, a second tyrosine kinase of the src family, namely $p59^{fyn}$, can be detected in CD2 immunoprecipitates. It is not known at present which of a number of molecules that are phosphorylated on tyrosine following T cell triggering represent substrates for $p56^{lck}$ versus $p59^{fyn}$ (Fig. 2).

Most importantly, a physical relationship between the TCR/CD3 complex and CD2 was recently substantiated (Brown et al. 1989) by detecting the ζ and ε chains of the T cell antigen receptor in CD2 immunoprecipitates (Beyers 1992; Schraven et al. 1992 b).

Induction of T cell Unresponsiveness Is Accompanied by Uncoupling of the ζ and ε Chains from the CD2 Molecular Complex

In a next series of experiments it was investigated whether engagement of the TCR/CD3 complex and subsequent modulation from the T cell surface (and the associated T cell unresponsiveness) correlates with alterations in the composition of CD2-associated signaling proteins. To this end, freshly prepared untransformed human T lymphocytes were exposed to a CD3 monoclonal antibody known to efficiently induce TCR/CD3 modulation. As shown in Fig. 3, following incubation overnight the antigen receptor complex is completely removed from the T cell surface, as determined by means of indirect immunofluorescence employing monoclonal antibodies directed at CD3-ε or, alternatively, the α/β heterodimer. Cell surface expression of CD2 is not affected by this treatment (if anything, the surface density of CD2 is slightly enhanced). Subsequently, T cells were lysed in the nonionic detergent BRIJ58 and CD2 immunoprecipitates obtained. These immunoprecipitates were then subjected to in vitro phosphorylation and loaded onto sodium dodecyl sulfate gels, and following electrophoresis dried gels were exposed to autoradiography. Functional T cell responses with regard to DNA synthesis (determined by means of $[^3H]$thymidine incorporation) were analyzed in parallel. As shown in Fig. 3, CD2 immunoprecipitates from TCR/CD3 modulated T lymphocytes were completely depleted of the ζ and ε chains. In contrast, associations between CD2 and the tyrosine kinases $p56^{lck}$ and $p59^{fyn}$ remained unaffected. This finding provides strong support for the notion that not only ζ and ε chains are associated with CD2 in physiologic T cells, but that the *same* ζ and ε chains which are believed to represent an integral part of a functional T cell receptor complex are also linked with CD2.

A number of early signaling events have been identified and found to be common for T cell activation by both TCR/CD3 and CD2. These include phosphorylation of a number of intracellular proteins on tyrosine residues, the activation of phospholipase C, generation of diacylglycerol and IP3, mobilization of intracellular calcium, and activation of protein kinase C (Altmann et al. 1990). Interestingly, as described in a number of previous reports, these molecular changes can no longer be induced in TCR/CD3 modulated cells. Similarly, characteristic molecular weight changes of $p56^{lck}$ and pp29-32 which represent common events following activation by either TCR/CD3 or CD2 do not occur in TCR/CD3 modulated cells where ζ and ε are no longer linked to the CD2 molecular complex (Schraven et al. 1993). Thus, one might conclude that common signaling events which result from either TCR/CD3 or CD2 activation of T cells are linked to the coupling of these cell surface receptors with the ζ and ε chains, although this must be substantiated further.

T Cell Receptor Independent Signaling Events Inducible by CD2

The fact that incubation of T lymphocytes with CD3 monoclonal antibodies leads to complete uncoupling of the CD3/TCR complex from the CD2 molecular complex now allows investigation of whether triggering by the CD2 molecule can produce its own characteristic intracellular signaling events toward the nucleus. Despite the fact that T cell proliferation and

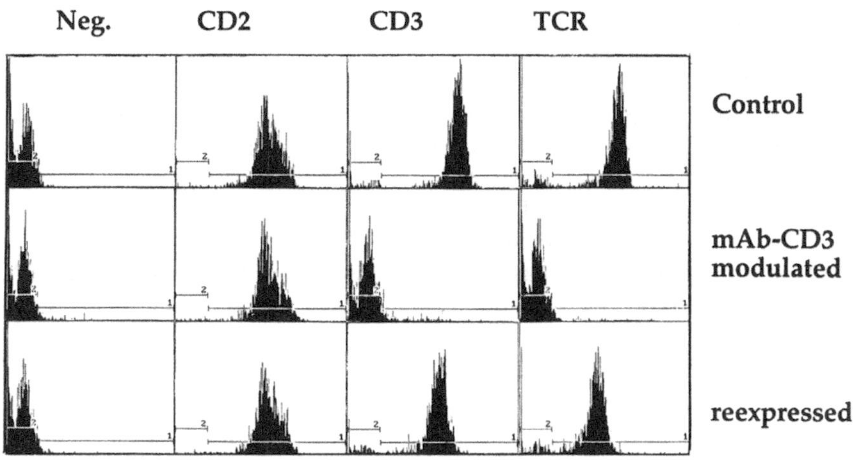

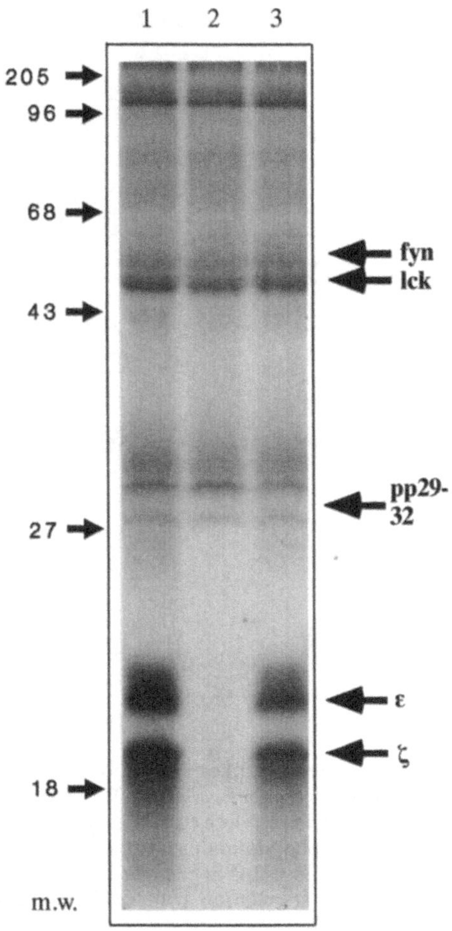

Fig. 3 a, b. TCR modulation leads to uncoupling of the ζ and ε chains from the CD2 molecular complex. **a** Incubation of T cells with monoclonal CD3 monoclonal antibodies leads to transient modulation and loss of the TCR/CD3 complex from the cell surface. In this state T cells can no longer proliferate to CD2 dependent stimuli. **b** CD2 immunoprecipitates in TCR modulated versus unmodulated T cells. Immunoprecipitates were obtained under mild detergent conditions, subjected to in vitro phosphorylation and run on sodium dodecyl sulfate polyacrylamide gel electrophoresis under reducing conditions. The identity of the various CD2-associated proteins (compare Fig. 2) was confirmed by reprecipitation analysis employing specific antisera (not shown)

interleukin-2 production are no longer inducible in the TCR/CD3 modulated state, other functional responses which are independent of T cell growth might still be detectable. Such a view is supported by results from two further experiments. Comparison of tyrosine phosporylated proteins in untreated versus TCR/CD3 modulated cells clearly demonstrates that some proteins become no longer phosporylated whereas others are clearly phosphorylated similarly as in the untreated state (Fig. 4).

Perhaps even more characteristic, a 19-kDa serine phosphorylated cytosolic protein (pp19) which has been identified recently (Samstag et al. 1991) and shown to be become dephosphorylated by a serine phosphatase

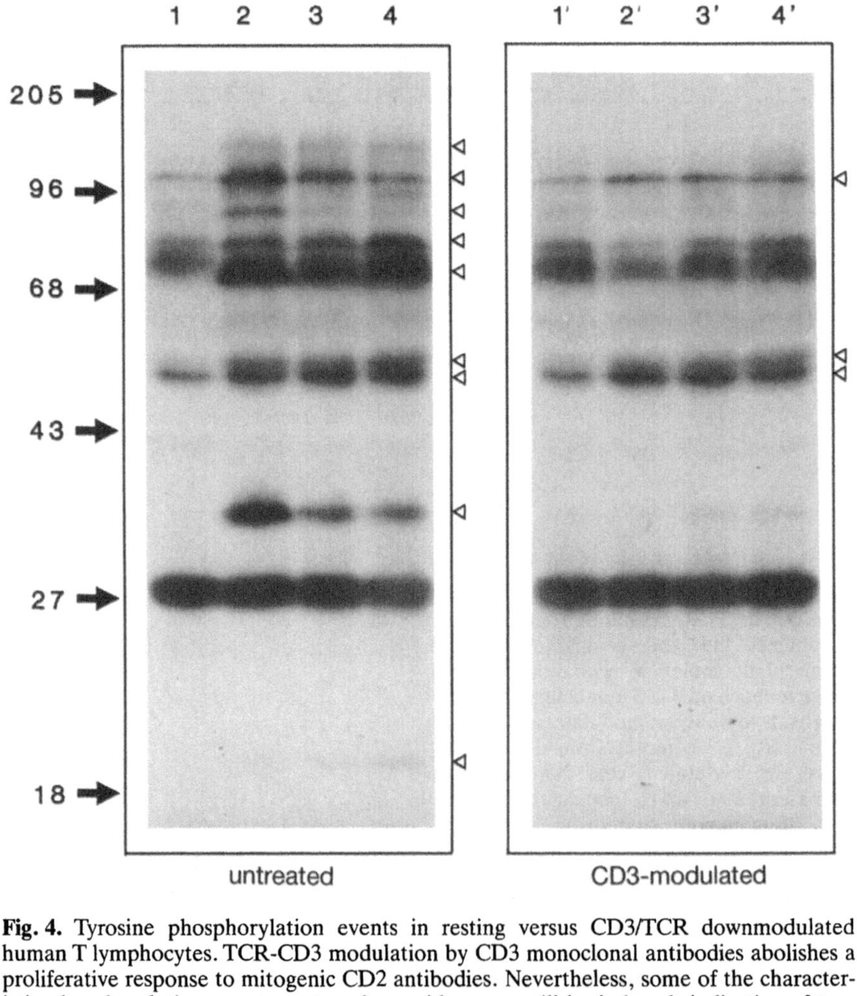

Fig. 4. Tyrosine phosphorylation events in resting versus CD3/TCR downmodulated human T lymphocytes. TCR-CD3 modulation by CD3 monoclonal antibodies abolishes a proliferative response to mitogenic CD2 antibodies. Nevertheless, some of the characteristic phosphorylation events on tyrosine residues can still be induced, indicative of true accessory receptor dependent (secondary) signals (*open arrows*). *Numbers,* time points following stimulation with CD2 monoclonal antibodies: (*1*,0 min; *2*, 2 min; *3*, 4 min; *4*, 15 min)

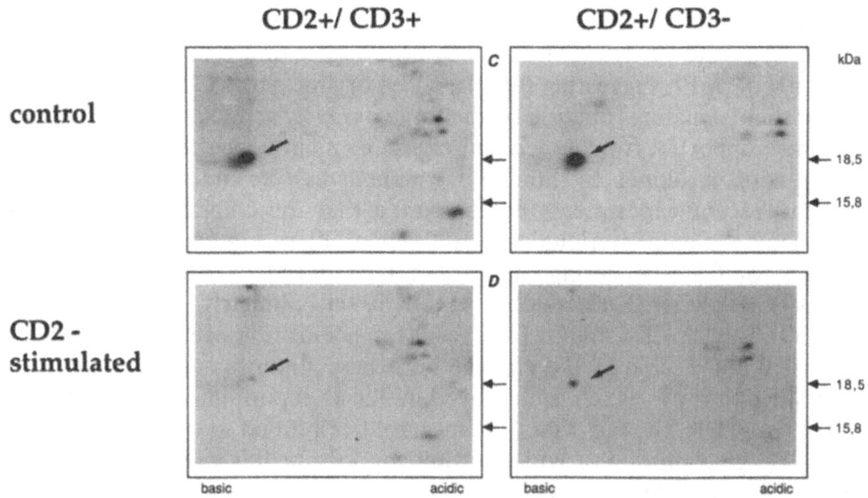

Fig. 5. Dephosphorylation of pp19 occurs in CD3/TCR negative lymphocytes. Dephosphorylation of the cytosolic pp19 molecule represents an accessory signal-dependent cellular response. This reaction, which is accompanied by pp19 translocation into the nucleus, is observed upon CD2 triggering in TC3/CD3 positive T cells as well as TCR/CD3 negative human lymphocytes

undergoes its characteristic changes following CD2 triggering by monoclonal antibodies, whether or not a T cell receptor complex is present on the cell surface (Fig. 5). Although the molecular nature of those proteins undergoing alterations by tyrosine kinases and a serine phosphatase remains to be elucidated, one can clearly conclude from these experiments that CD2 subserves a T cell receptor independent signaling function. Importantly, these latter events may be crucially involved in the functional consequences of accessory receptor dependent signaling processes.

Dephosphorylation of pp19: A Common Second Signal Inducible by Several Accessory Receptors

Given the multitude of accessory receptors expressed in the membrane of immunocompetent cells, one could expert some degree of redundancy to exist at this level. This means that for the production of particular crucial signals required to activate T lymphocytes several receptors might share common intracellular signaling pathways. To address this question, pp19 dephosporylation which was identified as a T cell receptor independent event inducible through CD2 was employed as a read-out system.

As recently demonstrated, coaggregation of CD3-TCR with either CD4 or CD8 produces a functional response which is distinct from T cell receptor triggering alone (Samstag et al. 1988).

Importantly, when compared with activation by CD2, cross-linking of TCR-CD3 with CD4 and/or CD8 was also capable of promoting dephosphorylation of pp19, suggesting that the accessory receptors CD4 and CD8 may exert their signaling function by the same pathway as CD2. Such a notion is further supported from functional experiments in which responsiveness to exogenous cytokines by human T lymphocytes was investigated. In this regard, recent experiments demonstrated that the comitogenic effects of interleukin-1 and interleukin-6 on T cell proliferation represent a consequence of CD2 triggering but cannot be induced by activation through CD3/TCR alone (Endler-Jobst et al. 1991). Similarly, cross-linking of CD3/TCR with CD4 and/or CD8 results in acquisition of responsiveness to interleukin-6 (Table 1). Taken together, these findings suggest a common signaling pathway which is employed by the Ig superfamily members CD2, CD4 and CD8. The fact that ζ chains have been found to coprecipitate with the CD4 glycoprotein provides further support for this view (Burgess et al. 1991). Recent results in which such experiments were extended to additional accessory receptors indicate that intracellular adhesion molecule (CD54), another member of the Ig superfamily, may also be linked to the pathway inducing interleukin-6 responsiveness (van Seventer et al. 1991). Finally, molecular associations of the TCR-CD3 with CD2, CD4, or CD8 and CD5 have most recently been detected in experimental animal studies as well (Beyers 1992).

Table 1. Stimuli able to induce responsiveness to interleukin-6 also result in dephosphorylation of pp19

Monoclonal antibody stimulation	Interleukin-6 (U/ml)	[^{3}H]Thymidine uptake		
		Donor 1	Donor 2	Donor 3
CD2	0	65 480	12 467	1209
CD2	10	47 440	25 740	2599
CD2	100	31 516	28 440	6791
CD2	1000	23 340	43 610	9745
CD3	0	288	78	ND
CD3	1000	134	138	ND
CD3 × CD4 × CD8	0	56 003	16 571	ND
CD3 × CD4 × CD8	1000	13 126	51 930	ND

Whether these two processes are directly linked with each other is unkown at present. Interestingly, in vitro responses obtained with T lymphocytes from the three different donors vary considerably depending on the extent of spontaneous DNA synthesis to stimulation with CD2 monoclonal antibodies alone. Nevertheless the various samples behaved strictly analogously suggesting further a functional linkage between the CD2 and the CD4/CD8 dependent accessory pathways. Results are expressed as cpm [^{3}H]thymidine uptake (means of triplicate cultures). The reason for downregulation of proliferation by interleukin-6 (donor 1) is unknown but might be related to the production of suppressive molecules such as transforming growth factor-β.

How Does the T Cell Receptor Exert Control over Accessory Receptors?

Since T cell responses are antigen specific and therefore must be controlled by the T cell receptor, the presence of a number of potential signaling molecules in the CD2 molecular complex cannot be sufficient to constitute a functional signaling unit. Otherwise, the interaction of CD2 with its natural ligand, CD58 (LFA-3) which is abundandtly present throughout the organism (Autschbach et al. 1991), would result in permanent polyclonal lymphocyte activation. Preliminary experimental evidence now suggests a mechanism by which the T cell receptor exerts control over accessory receptors, at least with regard to the induction of clonal T cell proliferation. Thus, the data delineated above (Fig. 3) demonstrated that T cell receptor modulation results in uncoupling of the ζ and ε chains from the CD2 molecular complex while leaving additional signaling molecules unaffected. As shown before (Meuer et al. 1984 c; Schraven et al. 1992 b), in this transient functional state T cell proliferation is no longer inducible by CD2 (Fig. 6).

TCR/CD3 modulation can be induced not only by monoclonal CD3 or Ti antibodies but also by the phorbol myristate acetate ester (PMA). Interestingly, under the latter conditions, triggering of T cells by CD2 to undergo DNA synthesis is still possible, if not enhanced, despite uncoupling of ζ and ε from CD2 (Liang et al. 1991). What are the differences in the signaling machinery in CD3 monoclonal antibody versus PMA-modulated T cells? A comparison of the state of CD2-associated signaling molecules may yield initial informations on this apparant paradox (Fig. 6). As shown, at variance with CD3 monoclonal antibody modulated T lymphocytes, PMA-treated T cells acquire a conformation of $p56^{lck}$ and pp29-32 which is characteristic for the activated state (i.e., transiently $p56^{lck}$ moves to $p60^{lck}$ and pp29-32 becomes pp30-31). This finding can be interpreted such that acquisition of the activated state by $p56^{lck}$ and pp29-32 represent a requirement for CD2 to exert its signaling function with regard to T cell proliferation. The induction of an intermediate activation state in these signaling molecules may be linked to a pathway involving the ζ and ε chains.

The fact that T cells can be experimentally triggered by CD2 by combinations of monoclonal antibodies in vitro could then be interpreted by induction of molecular changes in the signaling apparatures of CD2, which under physiologic conditions occurs only by TCR/CD3 dependent signals (Fig. 6). Such a concept would no longer require a physiologically occurring second ligand to explain the triggering mode induced by CD2 in vitro. The existence of such a second CD2 ligand is, in addition, unlikely since multiple mitogenic combinations of CD2 monoclonal antibodies have now been identified. With regard to their epitope specificity, these monoclonal antibody combinations are clearly distinct from each other and their mitogenic effects rather empirical (own observations).

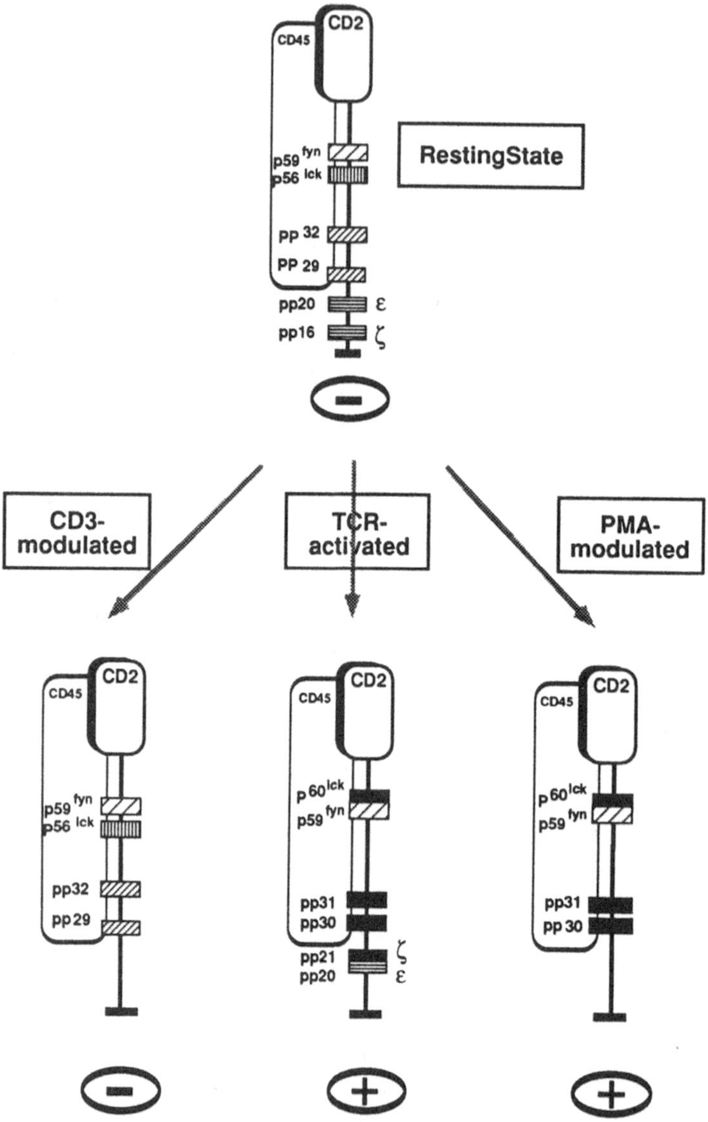

Fig. 6. Transient changes of the CD2 molecular signaling apparatus – a prerequisite for signal transduction? A number of potential signaling molecules have been identified which are linked with CD2 in untransformed resting human T lymphocytes. Since accessory molecules under physiologic conditions should not mediate clonal T cell expansion independently, the mere presence of these molecules cannot constitute a functional signaling receptor. Given that the T cell receptor complex must exert control over accessory receptors, characteristic changes in the CD2 molecular complex must be performed to allow for accessory receptor signaling. TCR activation produces transient modifications of $p56^{lck}$ and pp29-32. Under these conditions CD2 can fulfill its signaling function. Analogously, incubation of T lymphocytes with PMA induces molecular weight changes of $p56^{lck}$ and pp29-32. Again, in this functional state activation by CD2 to undergo proliferation is possible. In contrast, incubation of T cells with a nonmitogenic yet modulatory antibody

Conclusions

The important consequences of accessory receptor triggering in the immune response makes these molecules the first targets for future strategies of immunotherapy. Given that the respective ligands for T cell accessory receptors are not equally distributed throughout the organism, one can expect to define on their basis novel approaches for local immune intervention. A number of strategic consequences with regard to immunotherapy result from the observations delineated above.

1. Due to the redundancy that appears to exist at the level of accessory receptors on the cell surface, approaches to immunosuppression which are based on blocking one particular accessory receptor with monoclonal antibodies or recombinant receptor variants may not be very efficient in vivo. Thus, crucial signals required for T cell activation could still be transmitted by another, uninfluenced surface receptor due to the various options that enable the T lymphocyte to process a central signal for clonal expansion and cytokine production.
2. Elucidation of the intracellular pathways that are utilized by the various types of accessory receptors in human T cells represents a prerequisite for rational immunomodulation. Thus, to obviate a particular signaling pathway one would have to interfere simultaneously with several accessory receptors at the cell surface level. This would require the introduction of more than one blocking reagent. Alternatively, the identification of common intracellular signaling determinants could provide appropriate targets for immune intervention by low molecular weight organic compounds interfering with enzymatic processes that occur during lymphocyte activation.
3. With regard to immunostimulation, triggering of one receptor by an appropriate reagent may be sufficient to produce a critical signal which is absent in particular states of immunodeficiencies.

Clinical immune intervention at the level of accessory receptors provides potential options for novel and efficient ways of treatment. However, much has yet to be learned regarding molecular functions of these molecules. A tremendous degree of complexity will have to be analyzed in the future. This complexity exists in many ways since accessory receptors do not function independently but associate physically and functionally on the cell surface – likely controlled by a given local microenvironment.

---

directed at the T cell antigen receptor which leads to uncoupling of the ζ and ε chains from the CD2 complex and leaves $p56^{lck}$ and pp29-32 in their "resting state" leads to unresponsiveness with regard to cell proliferation induced by CD2 dependent stimuli. It seems tempting to speculate that the ζ and ε chains provide a connection between accessory receptors and the T cell receptor, which perhaps is responsible for inducing the characteristic changes in the CD2 associated signaling molecules $p56^{lck}$ and pp29-32, which might be a prerequisite for transmission of secondary signals

Another as yet poorly understood phenomenon is their tremendous variability in cell surface density. With regard to in vitro experiments, cell surface expression of accessory molecules is in general upregulated during cell activation although some exceptions to this rule also exist. Initial investigations on their expression in vivo have demonstrated a tremendous enhancement during inflammatory processes (Autschbach et al. 1991) whereas on malignant cells downregulation to almost undetectable levels has been observed (Schirren et al. 1992). Soluble mediators of the immune response appear to be potent regulators of expression of accessory receptors.

So far, most receptor structures have been investigated independently of each other. Therefore, our present knowledge on their functions remains a very limited view. Nevertheless, given the substantial progress that has been made in this area during a very short period of time, it seems justified to expect in the near future that novel strategies for immune intervention in chronic inflammatory disorders, autoimmune disease, transplant rejection, tumor immunology, and immunodeficiency disorders can be defined.

References

Albert-Wolf M, Meuer SC, Wallich R (1991) Dual function of recombinant human CD58: inhibition of T cell adhesion and activation via the CD2 pathway. Intern Immunol 3: 1353–1347

Altevogt P, Schreck J, Schraven B, Meuer SC, Schirrmacher V, Mitsch A (1990) Association of CD2 and T200 (CD45) in mouse T lymphocytes. Intern Immunol 2: 353–360

Altmann A, Coggeshall KM, Mustelin T (1990) Molecular events mediating T cell activation. Adv Immunol 48: 227–241

Autschbach F, Meuer SC, Moebius U, Manns M, Hess G, Meyer zum Büschenfelde K-H, Thoenes W, Dienes H-P (1991) Hepatocellular expression of lymphocyte function-associated antigen 3 in chronic hepatitis. Hepatology 14: 223–230

Beyers AD, Spruyt LL, Williams AF (1992) Molecular associations between the T-lymphocyte antigen receptor complex and the surface antigens CD2, CD4, or CD8 and CD5. Proc Natl Acad Sci 89: 2945–2949

Bierer BE, Burakoff SJ (1988) T cell adhesion molecules. Faseb 2: 2584–2590

Brown MH, Cantrell DA, Brattsand MJ, Crumpton MJ, Gullberg M (1989) The CD2 antigen associates with the T cell antigen receptor CD3 complex on the surface of human T-lymphocytes. Nature 339: 551–553

Burgess KE, Odysseos AD, Zalvan C, Druler BJ, Anderson P, Schlossman SF, Rudd CE (1991) Biochemical identification of a direct physical interaction between the CD4:$p56^{lck}$ and Ti/TcR/CD3 complexes. Eur J Immunol 21: 1663–1668

Endler Jobst B, Schraven B, Hutmacher B, Meuer SC (1991) Human T cell responses to IL-1 and IL-6 are dependent on signals mediated through CD2. J Immunol 146: 1736–1742

Gückel B, Berek C, Lutz M, Altevogt P, Schirrmacher V, Kyewski BA (1991) Anti-CD2 antibodies induce T cell unresponsiveness in vivo. J Exp Med 174: 957–967

Hemler ME (1990) VLA proteins in the integrin family: structures, functions, and their role on leukocytes. Annu Rev Immunol 8: 365–400

Hughes CC, Savage CO, Pober JS (1990) Endothelial cells augment T cell interleukin-2 production by a contact-dependent mechanism involving CD2/LFA-3 interaction. J Exp Med 171: 1453–1467

Jenkins MK (1992) The role of cell division in the induction of clonal anergy. Immunol Today 13: 69–73
Liang Q, Schurmann G, Betzler M, Meuer SC (1991) Downregulating of protein kinase C activation in human lamina propria T lymphocytes: influence of intestinal mucosa on T cell reactivity. Eur J Immunol 21: 2385–2389
Meuer SC (1992) Accessory receptors: regulators of the local immune response. In: Wegner C (ed) Handbook of immunopharmacology. Academic, New York (in press)
Meuer SC, Meyer zum Büschenfelde KH (1986) T cell receptor triggering induces responsiveness to interleukin 1 and interleukin 2 but does not lead to T cell proliferation. J Immunol 136: 4106–4112
Meuer SC, Hodgdon JC, Hussey RE, Protentis JP, Schlossman SF, Reinherz EL (1983) Antigen-like effects of monoclonal antibodies directed at receptors on human T cell clones. J Exp Med 158: 988–993
Meuer SC, Acuto O, Hercend T, Schlossman SF, Reinherz EL (1984a) The human T-cell receptor. Annu Rev Immunol 2: 23–50
Meuer SC, Hussey RE, Cantrell DA, Hodgdon JC, Schlossman SF, Smith KA, Reinherz EL (1984b) Triggering of the Ti-T3 antigen receptor complex results in clonal T cell proliferation via an interleukin 2 dependent autocrine pathway. Proc Natl Acad Sci USA 81: 1509–1513
Meuer SC, Hussey RE, Fabbi M, Fox D, Acuto O, Fitzgerald KA, Hodgdon JC, Protentis JP, Schlossman SF, Reinherz EL (1984c). An alternative pathway of T-cell activation: a functional role for the 50 kd T11 sheep erythrocyte receptor protein. Cell 36: 897–906
Moingeon P, Chang HC, Sayre PH, Clayton LK, Alcover A, Gardner P, Reinherz EL (1989) The structural biology of CD2. Immunol Rev 111: 111–144
Mueller DL, Jenkins MK, Schwartz RH (1989) Clonal expansion versus functional clonal inactivation: a costimulatory signalling pathway determines the outcome of T cell antigen receptor occupancy. Annu Rev Immunol 7: 445–480
Reinherz EL, Meuer S, Fitzgerald KA, Hussey RE, Levine H, Schlossman SF (1982) Antigen recognition by human T lymphocytes is linked to surface expression of the T3 molecular complex. Cell 30: 735–743
Samstag Y, Emmrich F, Staehelin T (1988) Activation of human T lymphocytes: differential effects of CD3- and CD8-mediated signals (published erratum appears). Proc Natl Acad Sci USA 85: 9689–9693
Samstag Y, Bader A, Meuer SC (1991) A serine phosphatase is involved in CD2-mediated activation of human T lymphocytes and natural killer cells. J Immunol 147: 788–794
Schirren A, Völpel H, Meuer SC (1992) Adhesion molecules on freshly recovered T leukemias promote tumor-directed lympholysis. Blood 79: 138–143
Schraven B, Roux M, Hutmacher B, Meuer SC (1989) Triggering of the alternative pathway of human T cell activation involves members of the T200 family of glycoproteins. Eur J Immunol 19: 397–403
Schraven B, Samstag Y, Altevogt P, Meuer SC (1990) Association of CD2 and CD45 on human T lymphocytes. Nature 345: 71–74
Schraven B, Kirchgessner H, Gaber B, Samstag Y, Meuer S (1991) A functional complex is formed in human T lymphocytes between the protein tyrosine phosphatase CD45, the protein tyrosine kinase $p56^{lck}$ and pp32, a possible common substrate. Eur J Immunol 21: 2469–2477
Schraven B, Schirren A, Kirchgessner H, Gaber B, Meuer SC (1992) Four CD45/$p56^{lck}$ associated phosphorproteins (pp29-32) undergo changes in human T cell activation. Eur J Immunol 22: 1857–1863
Schraven B, Wild M, Kirchgessner H, Siebert B, Wallich R, Samstag Y, Meuer SC (1993) Physiologic T cell unresponsiveness is associated with uncoupling of the CD3ζ and CD3ε-chains from the CD2 molecular complex. Eur J Immunol 23: 119–123
Schwartz RA (1990) A cell culture model for T lymphocyte clonal anergy. Science 248: 1349–1356
Springer TA (1990) Adhesion receptors of the immune system. Nature 346: 425–434

Telfer JC, Rudd CE (1991) A 32-kD GTP-binding protein associated with the CD4-p56^{lck} and CD8-p56^{lck} receptor complexes. Science 254: 439–441
Van Seventer GA, Newman W, Shimizu Y, Nutman TB, Tanaka Y, Horgan KJ, Gopal TV, Ennis E, O'Sullivan D, Grey H, Shaw S (1991) Analysis of T cell stimulation by superantigen plus major histocompatibility complex class II molecules or by CD3 monoclonal anibody: costimulation by purified adhesion ligands VCAM-1, ICAM-1, but not ELAM-1. J Exp Med 174: 901–913
Waldman H (1989) Manipulation of T cell responses with monoclonal antibodies. Annu Rev Immunol 7: 407–444

Induction of Selective Immunosuppression by Administration of MHC Class II Binding Peptides

L. Adorini

Introduction

Antigen processing and presentation entail a complex set of events leading to the activation of specific T cells by a binary ligand formed by antigenic peptides bound to major histocompatibility complex (MHC) encoded molecules [1, 2]. Over the past few years considerable progress has been made in understanding antigen processing and presentation [3–6]. The essential steps involve intracellular antigen proteolysis in antigen-presenting cells (APC), association of peptides to MHC molecules, and expression on the APC surface of the peptide-MHC complexes. Peptides bound to class I or class II MHC molecules on the surface of APC serve as ligands for the α/β T cell receptors (TCR) of $CD8^+$ or $CD4^+$ cells, respectively.

The recent progress in understanding antigen presentation to T cells has fostered a new generation of immunosuppressive agents potentially useful in the prevention and/or treatment of autoimmune diseases. A number of suitable attack points for selective immunointervention aiming at inhibition of inappropriate T cell activation have been identified: selective immunosuppression of T cell responses can be obtained by interfering with MHC, TCR, CD4/CD8, and other accessory molecules [7]. All these molecules could be targeted in different ways, but two approaches are most commonly used. The first relies on administration of monoclonal antibodies specific for molecules involved in antigen recognition and/or T cell activation [8]. The second type of approach utilizes synthetic peptides designed passively to block MHC class II restricted activation of T cells [9] or actively to induce regulatory T cells able to suppress the activity of $CD4^+$ pathogenic T cells [10].

Thus, the antigen-presenting function of MHC class II molecules could be inhibited by anti-MHC antibodies, or by blocking the MHC binding site with a competitor ligand. Similarly, the T cell receptor could be targeted by specific antibodies against TCR variable regions or by antagonists binding to the TCR but inducing anergy rather than cell activation. Moreover, the interaction between CD4 and MHC class II could be inhibited by antibodies directed against either structures or by compounds preventing their interaction. All these immunointervention strategies have been used successfully to prevent and/or treat experimental autoimmune diseases [11]. Based on these results considerable expectations have been raised for exploiting the same strategies to inhibit the activation of autoreactive T cells involved in human autoimmune diseases. Some of these expectations have already been fulfilled, for example, treatment of established human autoimmune diseases by anti-CD4 monoclonal antibody therapy is certainly promising, at least for some clinical indications (see Reithmüller et al., this volume).

The final goal of selective immunosuppression in autoimmune diseases and in control of allograft rejection is to reestablish or to establish tolerance at the T cell level. The cycling of remission and relapses typical of most autoimmune diseases may be viewed as an effort of the immune system to restore a balanced regulation. Selective immunosuppressive strategies should aim at facilitating this effort. Monoclonal antibodies anti-CD4 or anti-CD8 could be instrumental in this respect since, at least in experimental models, it has been shown that they may favor induction of tolerance to antigens coadministered with them [8]. Since autoantigens are already available within the individuals affected by autoimmune diseases, it can be predicted that anti-CD4 treatment should induce long-lasting tolerance to any autoantigen and eventually should reprogram the immune system to discriminate appropriately between self and nonself. The numerous clinical trials being performed to test this hypothesis in established human autoimmune diseases should soon provide an answer and indicate the feasibility of this approach.

Selective immunosuppression can also be induced by administration of synthetic peptides. This represents a particularly attractive mode of selective immunointervention since peptides can be appropriately designed, and in general they should be devoid of nonspecific toxic effects. Weak points of peptide-based therapies are their relatively short half-life in vivo and the need for parentheral administration, but these unfavorable characteristics could be compensated at least in part by appropriate delivery systems [12]. As presented in Fig. 1, selective immunosuppression by peptides can be distinguished in three major categories:

a) passive treatments aimed at inhibiting T cell activation by blocking the MHC binding site to any antigenic peptide, including autoantigens;
b) treatments aimed at functionally incapacitating the autoreactive T cells, either by administration of autoantigenic peptides in tolerogenic form, or by TCR antagonists able to induce selective T cell anergy;
c) vaccinationlike treatments aimed at inducing or enhancing regulatory T cells able to control the activity of pathogenic, autoreactive T cell.

At present, only the MHC blockade approach can be developed for clinical testing since information on the autoantigens involved in human autoimmune diseases is still fragmentary and not fully verified. It is hoped that the active research in this area may soon permit the identification of reliable autoantigen candidates. To this end, the possibility to separate and sequence fentomolar amounts of peptides eluted from the MHC binding site, by using a combination of microcapillary HPLC, electrospray ionization, and tandem mass spectrometry [13], may represent a real breakthrough. An obvious application of this technology would be to identify the peptides bound to the class II molecules expressed by APC infiltrating the autoimmune lesion.

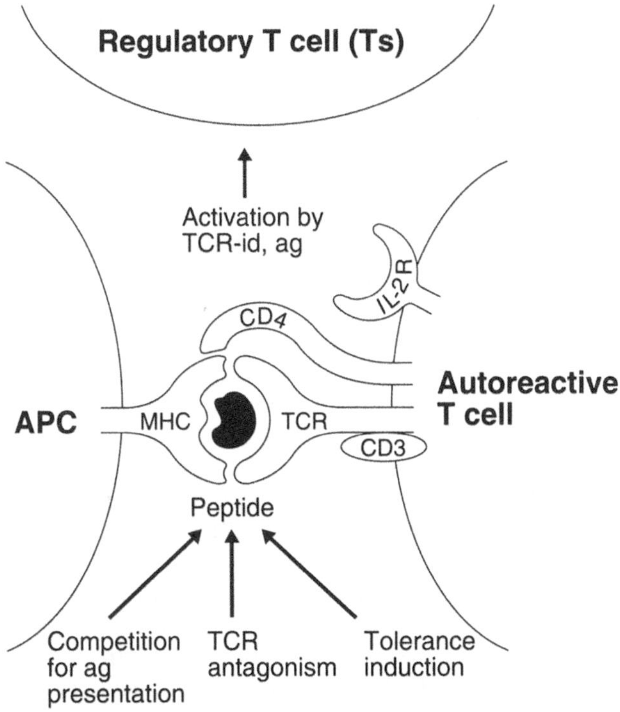

Fig. 1. Immunosuppression by MHC class II-binding synthetic peptides. Possible attack points for selective immunointervention potentially applicable to the treatment of autoimmune diseases are indicated

Induction or enhancement of immunoregulatory T cells is also being attempted, in multiple sclerosis patients, by injection of synthetic peptides derived from TCR specific for myelin basic protein [14]. However, the issue of restricted TCR usage by T cells from multiple sclerosis patients is far from resolved [15–18], suggesting that this approach may prove to be more problematic than previously anticipated.

Immunosuppression by MHC Class II Binding Peptides

Immunosuppression by MHC class II binding peptides has been tested in a variety of experimental systems, examining their effect on T cell activation in vivo either in responses to conventional antigens [19, 20] or in autoimmune disease models [21–23].

These experimental systems can be divided in two groups, based on the presence of structural homology between the peptides used to inhibit and to induce T cell responses. Accordingly, inhibition of T cell activation by injection of class II binding peptides may reflect different immunosuppressive mechanisms.

In situations in which the inhibitor peptide is structurally closely related to the antigenic peptide, antigen-specific rather than MHC-specific mechanisms may be involved in the inhibition of T cell activation by administration of class II binding peptides. These include induction of T cell tolerance [24], induction of suppressor T cells [10], or production by T cells of different lymphokines [25], such as interleukin-10, inhibiting Th1-type T cell clones. In addition, it is possible that homology between antigen and inhibitor could result in antagonism at the T cell receptor level [26], as also suggested by prevention of experimental allergic encephalomyelitis (EAE) upon administration of an analogue of the encephalitogenic peptide [27].

In mice of H-2^u haplotype the acetylated N-terminal peptide (amino acid residues 1–9) of myelin basic protein is able to induce encephalitogenic T cells [28]. Using this experimental model, several authors have demonstrated that injection of encephalitogenic peptides together with nonpathogenic analogues can prevent the clinical development of EAE. Disease prevention has been related to competition for binding of encephalitogenic peptides to I-A^u molecules [21, 22], with the consequent failure to activate encephalitogenic T cells. The evidence for this mechanism was based on the observation that peptides able to prevent EAE induction bind to I-A^u better than encephalitogenic peptides, both in assays using purified class II molecules [21] and in competition for antigen presentation in vitro [22]. However, since inhibitor and encephalitogenic peptides were highly homologous, induction of T cell tolerance or of suppressor T cells as well as antagonism at the TCR level by the competitor peptide could also account for disease prevention [26, 27, 29].

If inhibitory and antigenic peptides are non homologous, but the inhibitory peptide is immunogenic, inhibition of the T cell response to antigen could result from MHC blockade or from clonal dominance induced by the inhibitory peptide. This situation is exemplified by the study of Lamont et al. [23], using a peptide derived from the murine proteolipid protein (PLP 139–151) to induce EAE in H-2^s mice. Coadministration of this encephalitogenic peptide together with an unrelated peptide binding to I-A^s prevents EAE induction [23]. Since in this case encephalitogenic and competitor peptides do not share sequence homology, induction of T cell anergy or suppression by the competitor peptide does not appear to be the mechanism of disease prevention, and indeed this is most likely accounted for by MHC blockade. However, the inhibitory peptides used were themselves immunogenic, leaving open the possibility for a mechanism of clonal dominance in preventing induction of encephalitogenic T cells.

Collectively, these results indicate that several mechanisms, in addition to MHC blockade, may be responsible for in vivo inhibition of T cell activation by administration of MHC class II binding peptides. Our previous experiments have utilized a nonimmunogenic class II binding peptide unrelated to the antigen, strongly suggesting MHC blockade as the cause for inhibition of T cell activation [19, 20]. Data reviewed in the following section now provide direct evidence for this mechanism.

Evidence for MHC Blockade In Vivo

To directly demonstrate MHC blockade, we first established an experimental model to detect complexes of naturally processed antigenic peptides generated in vivo and expressed by MHC class II molecules on the surface of APC. This was accomplished by immunizing mice with hen egg-white lysozyme (HEL) in CFA and assessing ex vivo the expression of antigenic complexes in APC draining the injection site by their ability to activate HEL peptide-specific, class II-restricted T cell hybridomas. The basic experimental design relied on the hypothesis that lymph node cells from HEL-primed mice include APC expressing on the cell surface detectable complexes of naturally processed HEL peptides bound to class II MHC molecules. To test this hypothesis C3H and DBA/2 mice were immunized with HEL-CFA, and eight days later draining lymph node cells were irradiated and incubated in the absence of added antigen with the T cell hybridoma 3A9, recognizing the HEL peptide 46-61 together with I-A^k molecules, or with the T cell hybridoma 1H11.3, recognizing the HEL peptide 108–116 together with I-E^d molecules. The results show that lymph node cells from HEL-primed mice contain APC-expressing complexes of HEL peptides and class II MHC molecules recognized by the appropriate T cell hybridomas [30].

Having established that detectable antigenic complexes are formed in vivo between class II MHC molecules and peptides derived from HEL processing, we examined the effect of administering a peptide competitor unrelated to the antigenic peptide on the formation of antigenic complexes. Results demonstrate that injection of a peptide binding to a defined MHC class II molecule selectively inhibits the in vivo formation of antigenic complexes by peptides binding to the blocked class II molecule [30]. Importantly, in vivo MHC class II blockade is equally effective in inhibiting antigen presentation to T cell hybridomas and to bulk T cells, indicating the relevance of this immunosuppressive mechanism.

MHC Blockade as a Possible Treatment for Autoimmune Diseases

Since MHC blockade occurs in vivo, this could represent a promising approach to prevent and possibly also to treat HLA-associated autoimmune diseases. Selective MHC blockade can be induced by administering peptide competitors either in depot [19, 20] or in soluble form [31]. Moreover, exogenous competitors can inhibit in vitro equally well presentation of exogenous or endogenous antigens, the latter being likely the most relevant in the induction of autoreactive T cells leading to HLA-associated autoimmune diseases [32].

However, several points need still to be addressed to evaluate the practical feasibility of this form of immunointervention. For example, thus far MHC blockade has been evaluated only by its effect on T cell activation. It is not known whether in vivo competition for antigen presentation can also prevent induction of T cell mediated antibody responses.

We have examined the effect of MHC class II blockade on the antibody response to T cell-dependent antigens and found that administration of MHC binding peptides profoundly inhibits the antibody response to antigens presented by the blocked MHC molecule. As for T cell responses, inhibition of antibody production is selective for the MHC class II molecules to which the competitor peptide binds, and its extent depends on the molar ratio between antigenic and competitor peptides (Guéry et al., manuscript in preparation).

Inhibition of antibody responses by MHC blockade may have practical implications, since in some autoimmune diseases, for example, in myasthenia gravis, pathogenic effects are mediated primarily by autoantibodies rather than by autoreactive T cells.

In conclusion, MHC class II binding peptides administered in vivo can be effective and selective inhibitors of T cell activation. We have demonstrated that injection of a class II binding peptide can induce MHC blockade in vivo, resulting in inhibition of T cell activation and of T cell dependent antibody responses. MHC blockade modulates T cell activation by interfering with the binding of antigenic peptides to class II molecules, and this represents a promising approach to induce selective immunosuppression in HLA-associated autoimmune diseases [33, 34].

The direct demonstration of MHC blockade in vivo obviously does not exclude the possible involvement of other peptide-mediated immunoregulatory mechanisms in experimental autoimmune models, particularly when antigen homologues are used as inhibitors of T cell responses. However, since a detailed characterization of human autoantigens is not yet available, clinical development of antigen-specific immunosuppressive strategies is not possible at present. Conversely, MHC blockade is already a validated approach to prevent experimental autoimmune diseases, although it remains to be seen whether MHC blockers can also modify the course of human autoimmune diseases. Since HLA class II blockers are currently being developed for clinical testing by several groups, the answer should be forthcoming.

References

1. Bjorkman PJ, Saper MA, Samraoui B, Bennet WS, Strominger JL, Wiley DC (1987) Structure of the human class I histocompatibility antigen, HLA-A2. Nature 329: 506
2. Brown JH, Jardetzky T, Saper MA, Samraoui B, Bjorkman P, Wiley DC (1988) A hypothetical model of the foreign antigen binding site of class II histocompability molecules. Nature 332: 845
3. Moller G (ed) (1988) Antigen processing. Immunol Rev 106: 1–157
4. Adorini L (1990) The presentation of antigen by MHC class II molecules. Year Immunol 6: 21
5. Brodsky FM, Guagliardi L (1991) The biology of antigen processing and presentation. Annu Rev Immunol 9: 707

6. Unanue ER, Braciale TJ (ed) (1992) Antigen recognition. Curr Opin Immunol 4: 57–92
7. Adorini L, Barnaba V, Bona C, Celada F, Lanzavecchia A, Sercarz E, Suciu-Foca N, Wekerle H (1990) New perspectives on immunointervention in autoimmune diseases. Immunol Today 11: 383
8. Waldmann H, Cobbold SP, Qin S, Bejamin RJ, Wise M (1989) Tolerance induction in the adult using monoclonal antibodies to CD4, CD8, and CD11a (LFA-1). CSH Symp Quant Biol 54: 885
9. Adorini L, Nagy ZA (1990) Peptide competition for antigen presentation. Immunol Today 11: 21
10. Janeway C (1989) Immunotherapy by peptides. Nature 341: 482
11. Wraith DC, McDevitt HO, Steinman L, Acha-Orbea H (1989) T cell recognition as the target for immunointervention in autoimmune disease. Cell 57: 709
12. Illum L, Davis SS (1991) Drug delivery. Curr Opin Biotech 2: 254
13. Hunt DF, Henderson RA, Shabanowitz J, Sakaguchi K, Michel H, Sevilir N, Cox AL, Appella E, Engelhard VH (1992) Characterization of peptides bound to the class I MHC molecule HLA-A2.1 by mass spectrometry. Science 255: 1261
14. Kotzin BL, Karuturi S, Chou YK, Lafferty J, Forrester JM, Better M, Nedwin GE, Offner H, Vandenbark AA (1991) Preferential T cell receptor-chain variable gene use in myelin basic protein-reactive T cell clones from patients with multiple sclerosis. Proc Natl Acad Sci USA 88: 9161
15. Oskenberg JR, Stuart S, Begovich AB, Bell RB, Erlich HA, Steinman L, Bernard CCA (1990) Limited heterogeneity of rearranged T cell receptor V transcripts in brains of multiple sclerosis patients. Nature 345: 344
16. Wucherpfennig, KW, Ota K, Endo N, Seidman JG, Rosenzweig A, Weiner HL, Hafler DA (1990) Shared human T cell receptor V usage to immunodominant regions of myelin basic protein. Science 248: 1016
17. Ben-Nun A, Liblau RS, Cohen L, Lehmann D, Tournier-Lasserve E, Rosenzweig A, Jingwu Z, Raus JCM, Bach M-A (1991) Restricted T cell receptor V gene usage by myelin basic protein-specific T cell clones in multiple sclerosis: predominant genes vary in individuals. Proc Natl Acad Sci USA 88: 2466
18. Giegerich G, Pette M, Meinl E, Epplen JT, Wekerle H, Hinkkanen A (1992) Diversity of T cell receptor and chain genes expressed by human T cells specific for similar myelin basic protein peptide/major histocompatibility complexes. Eur J Immunol 22: 753
19. Adorini L, Muller S, Cardinaux F, Lehmann PV, Falcioni F, Nagy ZA (1988) In vivo competition between self peptides and foreign antigens in T cell activation. Nature 334: 623
20. Adorini L, Appella E, Doria G, Nagy ZA (1988) Mechanisms influencing the immunodominance of T cell determinants. J Exp Med 168: 2091
21. Wraith DC, Smilek DE, Mitchell DJ, Steinman L, McDevitt HO (1989) Antigen recognition in autoimmune encephalomyelitis and the potential for peptide-mediated immunotherapy. Cell 59: 247
22. Sakai K, Zamvil SS, Mitchell DJ, Hodgkinson S, Rothbard JB, Steinman L (1989) Prevention of experimental encephalomyelitis with peptides that block interaction of T cells with major histocompatiblity complex protein. Proc Natl Acad Sci USA 86: 9470
23. Lamont AG, Sette A, Fujinami R, Colon SM, Miles C, Grey HM (1990) Inhibition of experimental autoimmune encephalomyelitis induction in SJL/J mice by using a peptide with high affinity for I-A^s molecules. J Immunol 145: 1687
24. Koshland DE Jr (ed) (1990) Tolerance in the immune system. Science 248: 1335
25. Evavold BD, Allen PM (1991) Separation of IL-4 production from T cell proliferation by an altered T cell receptor ligand. Science 252: 1308
26. De Magistris MT, Alexander J, Coggeshall M, Altman A, Gaeta FCA, Grey HM, Sette A (1992) Antigen analog – major histocompatibility complexes act as antagonists of the T cell receptor. Cell 68: 625

27. Smilek DE, Wright DC, Hodgkinson S, Dwivedy S, Steinman L, McDevitt HO (1991) A single amino acid change in a myelin basic protein peptide confers the capacity to prevent rather than induce experimental autoimmune encephalomyelitis. Proc Natl Acad Sci USA 88: 9633
28. Zamvil SS, Mitchell DJ, Lee NE, Moore AC, Kitamura K, Steinman L, Rothbard JB (1986) T cell epitope of the autoantigen myelin basic protein that induces encephalomyelitis. Nature 324: 258
29. Smilek DE, Lock BL, McDevitt HO (1990) Antigenic recognition and peptide-mediated immunotherapy in autoimmune disease. Immunol Rev 118: 37
30. Guéry JC, Sette A, Leighton J, Dragomir A, Adorini L (1992) Selective immunosuppression by administration of major histocompatibility complex (MHC) class II binding peptides. I. Evidence for in vivo MHC blockade preventing T cell activation. J Exp Med 175: 1345
31. Muller S, Adorini L, Juretic A, Nagy ZA (1990) Selective in vivo inhibition of T cell activation by class II MHC-binding peptides adminstered in soluble form. J Immunol 145: 4006
32. Adorini L, Moreno J, Momburg F, Hammerling GJ, Guéry J-C, Valli A, Fuch S (1991) Exogenous peptides compete for the presentation of endogenous antigens to major histocompatibility class II-restricted T cells. J Exp Med 174: 945
33. Adorini L (ed) (1990) The molecular basis of antigen presentation to T lymphocytes: novel possibilities for immunointervention. Int Rev Immunol 6: 1–88
34. Gefter ML (ed) (1991) Major histocompatibility complex and peptides in immunotherapy. Sem Immunol 3: 193–255

Interferon-Gamma Therapy of Rheumatoid Arthritis

E.-M. Lemmel

Introduction of a new therapeutic regimen into clinical use should be supported by knowledge of the mechanisms of the pathophysiological conditions to be treated or by an explanation of the pharmacotherapeutic intervention to be offered. In the case of interferon-gamma and its introduction into the therapeutic regimens of rheumatoid arthritis in about 1983, both of these standards of classical pharmacotherapy were missing. Very little was known about the pathophysiology of rheumatoid arthritis, and interferon was known rather as an activator of inflammatory and immunological reactions (for review see [1, 9, 10, 16, 21, 23]). Thus it was rather alarming to rheumatologists when the first anecdotal reports from tumor centers raised the attention of the popular news media: patients suffering from tumors and treated with interferon-gamma claimed improvement of concomitant "rheumatic problems" when exposed to interferon-gamma (O. Klein, K. Wilms, personal communications).

Rheumatologists of several centers in the Federal Republic of Germany (FRG) then collaborated to conduct supervised trials with interferon-gamma in rheumatoid arthritis for the evalution of safety and later for dose finding and efficacy, initially to protect their patients from "hazardous" therapy with interferon-gamma. However, there were two surprises to most of the participants. No activation of the disease under interferon-gamma was observed, and some well-documented cases of rheumatoid arthritis in these early open trials showed an improvement under treatment with interferon-gamma [17].

The following years brought more convincing evidence of the efficacy and safety of interferon-gamma in the treatment of rheumatoid arthritis, mostly in multicenter efforts in the FRG. After additional open trials for safety ([26]; H.-R. Müller-Faßbender, personal communication) it was decided to document in several stages the possible effects in an open short-term study [11]. Consequently, a double-blind, placebo-controlled, short-term (4-week) study was designed [12] to determine whether the claimed positive effects were statistically significant or due merely to chance. If this study resulted in a positive finding, the further goal of this German Interferon Study Group was to conduct a double-blind, placebo-controlled, long-term (3-month) study [8, 14].

M. M. Eibl, C. Huber, H. H. Decker, U. Wahn (Eds.)
Symposium in Immunology I
Symposium in Immunology II

Open Short-Term Study

In an open, nonrandomized clinical trial conducted at multiple centers in the FRG 49 patients with classical rheumatoid arthritis were treated with recombinant interferon-gamma for 20 days. The study was carried out in two substudies. In the first the total daily dose of interferon-gamma was 50 μg and in the second 100 μg. Of the 49 cases, 40 were evaluable for statistical analysis; 24 of these patients (60%) responded to therapy, according to the criteria of succesful outcome laid down in the study protocol and were classified as responders. In responders, the clinical parameters investigated improved with both dosages. The lower dose differed from the higher one in having a markedly lower incidence of side effects such as fever, chills, and nausea, all of temporary duration and none severe in extent.

The results of this study led to the conclusion that a randomized double-blind, placebo-controlled clinical trial should be performed. In addition, after extensive discussion of the results of this study and of earlier open dose-finding evalutions it was concluded that a better effect in suppressing disease activity could be achieved if interferon-gamma were dosed low and at a later stage of treatment further decreased by extending the intervals between injections. In retrospect, this decision was of major importance for the evalution of efficacy of interferon-gamma in the treatment of rheumatoid arthritis [13].

Placebo-Controlled, Double-Blind Short-Term Study

A multicenter, placebo-controlled, double-blind study was conducted in the FRG in 1986, including 91 patients with classical rheumatoid arthritis. Treatment was given for 28 days with interferon-gamma or placebo, with 50 μg/day administered for the first 20 days, followed by 50 μg every other day for the next 8 days, administered subcutaneously. Of these patients 79 were evaluable, 40 of whom had received interferon-gamma. Inclusion criteria were classical rheumatoid arthritis not sufficiently treated with nonsteroidal anti-inflammatory drugs. Patients were allowed to be on disease-modifying drugs, providing they had been receiving treatment long enough to be stabilized (20% of the patients were receiving such drugs).

The criterion for classification as a responder was improvement in Richy or Lansbury Index by at least 30% at day 28. Of the 40 patients in the interferon-gamma group 23 (58%) were responders whereas only 11 of the 39 placebo-treated patients (28%) were responders. These results were significant in favor of the interferon-gamma group (Table 1). The side effects documented in this trial were distributed equally in the two treatment arms. These were basically the normal side effects of interferon, including nausea, fatigue, headache, and increase in body temperature, which were all temporary and of mild extent. Only one patient discontinued treatment in the interferon-gamma group due to an adverse experience – a local skin reaction

Table 1. Results of the short-term (28-day) study of nonsteroidal anti-inflammatory drugs (NSAID) and interferon-gamma (IFN-γ): n=79 (from [12])

	Responders (n=34)	Nonresponders (n=45)
NSAID + IFN-γ (n=40)	23	17
NSAID + placebo (n=39)	11	28

$X^2 = 6.91$; $\alpha = 0.01$

with erythema and induration at the injection site, which, again, was of short duration.

In general, this trial also indicated that interferon-gamma is safe in rheumatoid arthritis and showed its superiority over placebo with statistical significance.

Double-Blind, Placebo-Controlled Long-Term Study [8]

This controlled clinical trial was part of a multicenter clinical and theoretical scientific project to further evaluate the mechanisms of actions of interferon-gamma in clinical conditions such as rheumatoid arthritis and a number of experimental conditions. The study was sponsored by the German Federal Minister of Science and Technology, directed by a standing commission of the president of the Max-Planck-Gesellschaft, and coordinated by the Max-Planck-Institut für Biochemie, Munich. Overall, 249 patients with classical rheumatoid arthritis were enrolled by 16 participating hospitals. In addition to nonsteroidal anti-inflammatory drugs, patients were randomly given either interferon-gamma or placebo. In the interferon-gamma group 107 patients and in the control group 116 patients were evaluated.

The response rate after 3 months of treatment (30% or more improvement in joint indices) was significantly higher in the interferon group, with an error probability of 1% (Table 2). Compared with the control group, the interferon-gamma group benefited in all standard outcome measurements. There were more drop-outs in the placebo group than in the interferon-gamma group. In the interferon-gamma group it was possible to reduce the quantity of corticosteroids administered (allowed dosage of prednisolone 7.5 mg less;

Table 2. Results of the long-term (3-month) study of nonsteroidal anti-inflammatory drugs (NSAID) and interferon-gamma (IFN-γ): n=223 (from [8, 14])

	Responders (n=93)	Nonresponders (n=130)
NSAID + IFN-γ (n=107)	53	54
NSAID + placebo (n=116)	40	76

$X^2 = 5.19$; $\alpha = 0.01$

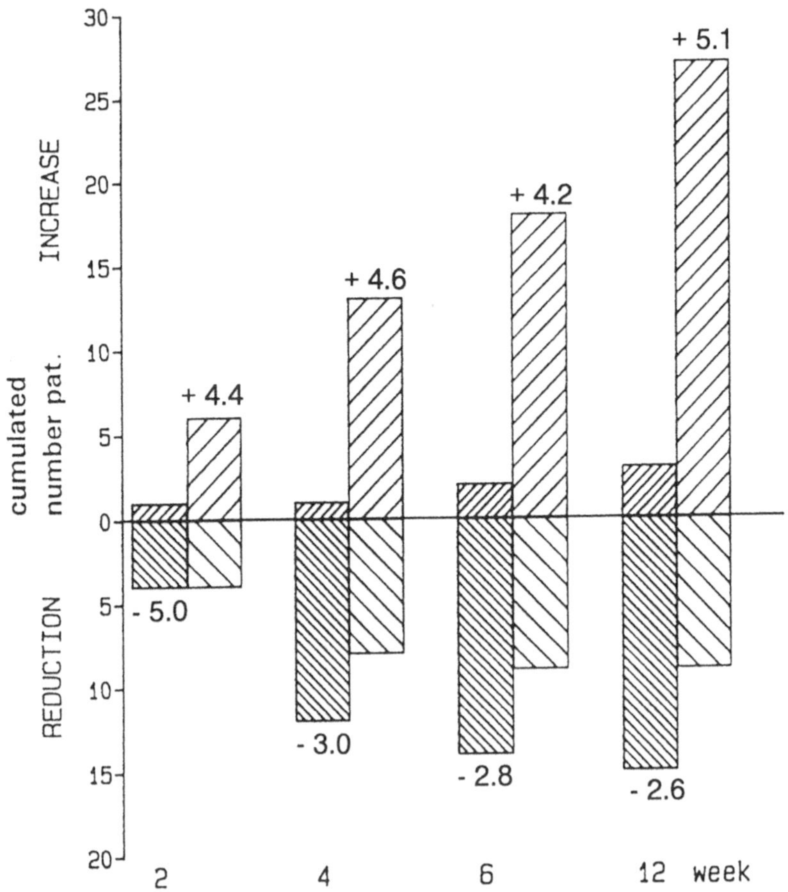

Fig. 1. Change in corticosteroid dose over the 3-month trial comparing the group under nonsteroidal anti-inflammatory drug (NSAID) plus interferon-gamma (*darker columns*) with the group under NSAID plus placebo (*lighter columns*). Cumulative number of patients with increased or decreased dose compared with baseline. *Numbers at the bars*, mean increase/reduction in weekly steroid dosage. (From [8])

Fig. 1). Side effects were of clinically unimportant nature; they were similar in both treatment groups. Influenza-like symptoms including increased temperature were more frequent in the interferon-gamma group.

In summary, the three multicenter studies conducted in the FRG resulted in evidence for a therapeutic efficacy of interferon-gamma, surpassing the response rate in the placebo groups to a statistically significant degree. In addition, long-term observations for more than 1 year including 120 patients [20, 22] and those from a field study including 476 patients [19] demonstrate the possibility of maintaining patients with rheumatoid arthritis on therapy with interferon-gamma for an extended period without the necessity of introducing more aggressive therapeutic regimens.

International Studies

Between 1985 and 1986 a single-blind dose-finding study was conducted by Wolfe et al. in Witchita, Kansas [25]. This study compared the safety and efficacy of 10 μg interferon-gamma with 100 μg interferon-gamma given subcutaneously fives times per week for 4 weeks. Thirty patients completed the 4-week treatment period. Patients in the 100-μg group experienced more improvement in all efficacy parameters than those in the 10-μg group. However, because of the small number of patients in each group, these differences were not statistically significant.

In 1985/1986 Veys et al. [24] conducted a dose-finding single-center, double-blind, placebo-controlled trial over a treatment period of 24 weeks. There were two treatment groups of equal size (13 each). One group was treated with 100 μg interferon-gamma for 5 days/week for the first week followed by two doses per week for the next 23 weeks. The control group was treated with placebo by the same schedule. In each group 11 patients completed the 24-week treatment. Although there was a tendency to superiority in several clinical disease parameters, the differences between groups did not reach statistical significance, very likely because of the small numbers of patients in the trial.

Between 1986 and 1988 Machold and coworkers [15] conducted a double-blind, placebo-controlled cross-over study in Vienna, enrolling 33 patients. Although the study design of this trial was different to those of all other studies discussed here (every patient serving as his own control, comparing efficacy and safety of interferon-gamma versus placebo in consecutive phases of the study), these researchers reached the conclusion that interferon-gamma was superior to placebo to a statistically significant extent in several of the standard measurements of clinical disease activity.

The most challenging comparison to our own clinical trials was the study by Cannon and coworkers, conducted between 1986 and 1989 [5, 6]. This was a multicenter, double-blind, placebo-controlled 12-week trial of interferon-gamma in 105 patients with classical rheumatoid arthritis. There were two treatment groups of equal size, one injected subcutaneously with 100 μg interferon-gamma for 5 days per week for 12 weeks and the other a control group treated with placebo by the same schedule. The patients were allowed to be on treatment with nonsteroidal anti-inflammatory drugs or corticosteroids (equivalent to 10 mg prednisone per day or less) for 1 month or more, and/or treatment with a stable dose of disease-modifying drugs for 3 months or more. Forty-one patients in each group completed the 12-week trial.

The analysis of the results in the course of this trial are of great interest. In their summary Cannon et al. stated that after 12 weeks of treatment, "although the improvement with rHu gamma-IFN was greater than that with placebo, the differences were generally not statistically significant." If one, however, looks at the group differences after 4 and 8 weeks of treatment, the difference in the treatment groups strongly favored the interferon group in several important clinical parameters (joint tenderness, joint swelling, morning stiffness). It is interesting to evaluate why these differences in treatment arms were increased or continued to the end of the trial after 12 weeks of treatment, as was the case in our own study with very similar design. It is felt that the overall result of the Cannon study supports our own data as well as our underlying hypothesis for the dosing schedule. It must be stressed that in the Cannon study 100 μg interferon-gamma was given five times per week for 12 weeks. No decrease in dosage or increase in dosing intervals was included in the schedule. Thus, it is suggested that the optimum efficacy of interferon, 100 μg subcutaneously per day, is reached after 4–6 weeks of treatment. If at this time the dose is not decreased, the down-regulatory effect of interferon on the disease activity may be counter balanced by the activating potential of interferon-gamma on a more inactivated immune-inflammatory system.

Cannon and coworkers [7] have published long-term observations of patients under treatment with interferon-gamma for 3 years (in individual cases for more than 5 years) demonstrating that in a considerable percentage of patients initially responding to interferon-gamma this type of treatment is able to control the disease for prolonged periods without the neccessity of changing to more aggressive therapeutic regimens.

Discussion of the Clinical Findings

The clinical data summarized in this review are mainly those from clinical studies, the earlier ones conducted as open trials and the majority under double-blind, mostly placebo-controlled conditions. The overall experience with interferon-gamma in rheumatoid arthritis has been extended largely by individual protocols of open-treated patients.

The treatment has generally been very well tolerated; side effects are mainly those of the influenza-like syndrome, of temperary duration and clinically mild in nature (headache, nausea, mild increase in body temperature, chills). In a sizable proportion of patients the disease was not sufficiently controlled by interferon-gamma, and they thus had to be withdrawn from the trial. However, there has been no evidence so far of that which one could consider a true activation of immunoinflammatory activity of the disease due to interferon-gamma administration. Activation of the disease had been the original concern when interferon-gamma was introduced into the treatment of rheumatoid arthritis in 1983, since at that time the basic biological mechanism of interferon-gamma was considered to be the activation of macrophages and the enhancement of the immune response.

Since these seemingly "paradoxical" results in patients, in which the immune and inflammatory system is known to be hyperactive, many experimental datasets have emerged, concluding that the biological activity of interferon-gamma on the immune and inflammatory systems depends very much on the activity state of both of these systems: activation in resting state, down-regulation in an activated situation. Even in the early years of the FRG trials with interferon-gamma for the treatment of rheumatoid arthritis this concept of a "double-faced mediator" in inflammatory [2–4, 18] was the basic concept for the dosing regimen. Compared to dose in tumor conditions, the initial dose in rheumatoid arthritis was low (50–100 μg daily five times per week subcutaneously) and was still reduced and extended in injection intervals during the continued therapy. It is suggested that this adjusted dosing controls dysregulated hyperactive immune and inflammatory systems, which then can be maintained in a down-regulated state of activity by decreased continued administration of interferon-gamma.

According to the data discussed above it can now be concluded that interferon-gamma indeed provides some inhibitory therapeutic potential in several clinical and serological measurements of disease activity in rheumatoid arthritis. The therapeutical power of interferon-gamma may not be considered as overwhelming, however. The observed side effects are rather minor. It should also be born in mind that, mainly for safety reasons, most of the clinical studies included patients at later stages of the disease and with negative response to conventional therapies. It seems reasonable to assume that the early disease would respond better to immunological regulators, although this still needs to be confirmed clinically. In addition, there are no data so far as to the effect of interferon-gamma administration on progression of the natural course of the disease.

In conclusion, it can be stated that the main value of the data collected in the treatment of rheumatoid arthritis with interferon-gamma is the knowledge that the administration of a natural partner of the regulatory network of mediators of the immune and inflammatory systems can be used therapeutically with benefit to the overall clinical condition. In regard to the treatment of rheumatoid arthritis this experience opens a completely new approach for therapeutic intervention. Better knowledge of the regulatory systems, better tools for the evaluation of individual susceptibility for immunoregulatory intervention, and possibly the determination of a more specific regulatory partner can increase the therapeutic power of the immunoregulatory therapeutic approach without necessarily increasing its unwanted effects.

References

1. Billiau A (1987) Interferons and inflammation. J Interferon Res 7: 559–567
2. Browning J (1987) Interferons and rheumatoid arthritis: insight into interferon biology? Immunol Today 8: 372–373
3. Brzoska J, Obert HJ (1987) Interferon gamma: ein janusköpfiger Mediator bei Entzündungen. Arzneimittelforsch/Drug Res 37 (II): 1410–1416
4. Brzoska J, Obert HJ (1990) Immunomodulating effects of interferons: conclusions for therapy. In: Gross G, Jablonska S, Pfister H, Stegner HE (eds) Genital papillomavirus

infections: modern diagnosis and treatment. Springer, Berlin Heidelberg New York, pp 379–391
5. Cannon GW, Schindler JD, Emkey RD, Denes A, Cohen SA, Wolfe F, Saway A, Jaffer AM, Weaver AL, Cogen L (1987) Double-blind trial of recombinant interferon-gamma versus placebo in rheumatoid arthritis. Arthritis Rheum 30 [Suppl]: 18
6. Cannon GW, Pincus SH, Emkey RD, Denes A, Cohen SA, Wolfe F, Saway PA, Jaffer AM, Weaver AL, Cogen L, Schindler JD (1989) Double-blind trial of recombinant gamma-interferon versus placebo in the treatment of rheumatoid arthritis. Arthritis Rheum 32: 964–973
7. Cannon GW, Emkey RD, Denes A, Cohen SA, Saway PA, Wolfe F, Jaffer AM, Weaver AL, Cogen L, Gulinello J, Kennedy SM, Schindler JD (1990) Prospective two-year followup of recombinant interferon-gamma in rheumatoid arthritis. J Rheumatol 17 [Suppl 3]: 304–310
8. German Lymphokine Study Group (1992) Double-blind controlled phase III multicenter clinical trial with interferon gamma in rheumatoid arthritis. Rheumatol Int (in press)
9. Heremans H, Dijkmans R, Sobis H, Vandekerckhove F, Billiau A (1987) Regulations by interferons of the local inflammatory response to bacterial lipopolysaccharide. J Immunol 138: 4175–4179
10. Heremans H, Billiau A (1989) The potential role of interferons and interferon antagonists in inflammatory disease. Drugs 38: 957–972
11. Lemmel EM, Franke M, Gaus W, Hartl PW, Hofschneider PH, Miehlke K, Machalke K, Obert HJ (1987) Results of a phase-II clinical trial on treatment of rheumatoid arthritis with recombinant interferon-gamma. Rheumatol Int 7: 127–132
12. Lemmel EM, Brackertz D, Franke M, Gaus W, Hartl PW, Machalke K, Mielke H, Obert HJ, Peter HH, Sieper J, Sprekeler R, Stierle H (1988 a) Results of a multicenter placebocontrolled double-blind randomized phase III clinical study of treatment of rheumatoid arthritis with recombinant interferon-gamma. Rheumatol Int 8: 87–93
13. Lemmel EM, Ober HJ, Hofschneider PH (1988 b) Low dose gamma interferon treatment of rheumatoid arthritis. Lancet I: 598
14. Lemel E-M, Gaus W, Hofschneider PH (1991) Multicenter double blind trial of interferon gamma versus placebo in the treatment of rheumatoid arthritis. Arthritis Rheum 34: 1621–1622
15. Machold KP, Graninger W, Flener R, Smolen JS (1988) Recombinant human gamma-interferon in the treatment of rheumatoid arthritis – a double-blind placebo-controlled cross-over study. Clin Res 36: 534 A
16. National Institutes of Health (1980) Interferon nomenclatures. Nature 286: 110
17. Obert HJ, Hofschneider PH (1985) Interferon bei chronischer Polyarthritis. Positive Wirkung in der klinischen Prüfung. Dtsch Med Wochenschr 110: 1766–1769
18. Obert HJ, Brzoska J (1986) Interferon-gamma in der Therapie der chronischen Polyarthritis. Arzneimittelforsch/Drug Res 36 (II): 1557–1560
19. Obert HJ, Brzoska JF (1989) Behandlung der chronischen Polyarthritis mit Interferon-gamma. Ergebnisse einer Therapiestudie der Phase II bei 476 Patienten. Rheuma 9: 286–292
20. Obert HJ, Brzoska JF (1989) Interferon-gamma in der Therapie der chronischen Polyarthritis. Die Langzeitbehandlung in der Praxis. Arzneimittelforsch/Drug Res 39 (II): 819–822
21. Schindler JD, Faller DV (1990) Gamma interferon: mechanism of action and use in rheumatoid arthritis. In: Furst DE, Weinblatt ME (eds) Immunomodulators in the rheumatic diseases. Decker, New York
22. Sprekeler R, Lemmel EM, Obert HJ (1990) Correlation of clinical and serological findings in patients with rheumatoid arthritis treated for one year with interferon-gamma. Z Rheumatol 49: 1–7
23. Trinchieri G, Perussia B (1985) Immune interferon: a pleiotropic lymphokine with multiple effects. Immunol Today 6: 131–136

24. Veys EM, Mielants H, Verbruggen G, Grosclaude JP, Luyten F, Meier W, Fiers W, Galazka AR (1987) Recombinant interferon gamma in rheumatoid arthritis. A double-blind study comparing Immuneron (recombinant interferon gamma) with placebo. Clin Exp Rheumatol 5 [Suppl 2]: 53
25. Wolfe F, Cathey MA, Hawley DJ, Balser JP, Schindler JD (1986) Clinical trial with r-IFN-gamma in rheumatoid arthritis. In: Pincus SH, Pisetsky DS, Rosenwasser LJ (eds) Biologically based immunomodulators in the therapy of rheumatic diseases. Elsevier, New York, pp 379–395
26. Zilly A, Obert HJ (1986) Therapie der chronischen Polyarthritis. Ergebnisse einer Pilot-Studie mit Lymphokinen. MMW 128: 87–89

Subject Index

GPSR Compliance

The European Union's (EU) General Product Safety Regulation (GPSR) is a set of rules that requires consumer products to be safe and our obligations to ensure this.

If you have any concerns about our products, you can contact us on ProductSafety@springernature.com

In case Publisher is established outside the EU, the EU authorized representative is:

Springer Nature Customer Service Center GmbH
Europaplatz 3
69115 Heidelberg, Germany

Batch number: 10704711

Printed by Printforce, the Netherlands